# Suicide in Children and Adolescents

In an epoch when rates of death and illness among the young have steadily decreased in the face of medical progress, it is a tragic irony that persistently high rates of youth suicide and suicide attempts remain among the leading causes of death and morbidity in this otherwise vigorous age group. This worrisome trans-national pattern poses both an urgent clinical and theoretical challenge.

How can these deaths be prevented? Can they be anticipated? Are there perceptible patterns of risk and vulnerability? What role do families, gender, culture, and biology play? What are the treatments for and outcomes of suicide attempters?

To address these questions, experts from around the world in all areas of psychiatry, including epidemiology, neurobiology, genetics and psychotherapy, have brought together their current findings in *Suicide in Children and Adolescents*.

**Robert A. King** is Professor of Child Psychiatry and Psychiatry at the Yale Child Study Center at Yale University.

**Alan Apter** is Director of the Feinberg Department of Child and Adolescent Psychiatry at the Schneider Children's Medical Center of Israel, and Professor of Psychiatry at the Sackler School of Medicine, University of Tel-Aviv.

# Cambridge Child and Adolescent Psychiatry

Child and adolescent psychiatry is an important and growing area of clinical psychiatry. The last decade has seen a rapid expansion of scientific knowledge in this field and has provided a new understanding of the underlying pathology of mental disorders in these age groups. This series is aimed at practitioners and researchers both in child and adolescent mental health services and developmental and clinical neuroscience. Focusing on psychopathology, it highlights those topics where the growth of knowledge has had the greatest impact on clinical practice and on the treatment and understanding of mental illness. Individual volumes benefit both from the international expertise of their contributors and a coherence generated through a uniform sytle and structure for the series. Each volume provides firstly an historical overview and a clear decriptive account of the psychopathology of a specific disorder or group of related disorders. These features then form the basis for a thorough critical review of the etiology, natural history, management, prevention and impact on later adult adjustment. Whilst each volume is therefore complete in its own right, volumes also relate to each other to create a flexible and collectable series that should appeal to students as well as experienced scientists and practitioners.

## Editorial board

**Series editor** Professor Ian M. Goodyer *University of Cambridge*

### Associate editors

Professor Donald J. Cohen
*Yale Child Study Center*

Professor Dr Helmut Remschmidt
*Klinikum der Philipps-Universität, Marburg, Germany*

Dr Robert N. Goodman
*Institute of Psychiatry, London*

Professor Dr Herman van Engeland
*Academisch Ziekenhuis Utrecht*

Professor Barry Nurcombe
*The University of Queensland*

Dr Fred R. Volkmar
*Yale Child Study Center*

## Already published in this series:

*Hyperactivity and Attention Disorders of Childhood* second edition edited by Seija Sandberg
0521789613 PB

*Outcomes in Neurodevelopmental and Genetic Disorders* edited by Patricia Howlin
0521797217 PB

*Practical Child and Adolescent Psychopharmacology* edited by Stan Kutcher
0521655420 PB

*Specific Learning Disabilities and Difficulties in Children and Adolescents: Psychological Assessment and Evaluation* edited by Alan and Nadeen Kaufman
0521658403 PB

*Psychotherapy with Children and Adolescents* edited by Helmut Remschmidt
0521775582 PB

*The Depressed Child and Adolescent* second edition edited by Ian M. Goodyer
0521794269 PB

*Schizophrenia in Children and Adolescents* edited by Helmut Remschmidt
0521794285 PB

*Anxiety Disorders in Children and Adolescents: Research, Assessment and Intervention* edited by Wendy Silverman and Philip Treffers
0521789664 PB

*Conduct Disorders in Childhood and Adolescence* edited by Jonathan Hill and Barbara Maughan
0521786398 PB

*Autism and Pervasive Developmental Disorders* edited by Fred R. Volkmar
0521553865 HB

*Cognitive Behaviour Therapy for Children and Families* edited by Philip Graham
0521572525 HB    0521576261 PB

# Suicide in Children and Adolescents

Edited by

## Robert A. King
*Yale Child Study Center, Yale University*

and

## Alan Apter
*Schneider Children's Medical Center of Israel and
University of Tel-Aviv Medical School*

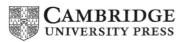
**CAMBRIDGE**
UNIVERSITY PRESS

PUBLISHED BY THE PRESS SYNDICATE OF THE UNIVERSITY OF CAMBRIDGE
The Pitt Building, Trumpington Street, Cambridge, United Kingdom

CAMBRIDGE UNIVERSITY PRESS
The Edinburgh Building, Cambridge CB2 2RU, UK
40 West 20th Street, New York, NY 10011-4211, USA
477 Williamstown Road, Port Melbourne, VIC 3207, Australia
Ruiz de Alarcón 13, 28014 Madrid, Spain
Dock House, The Waterfront, Cape Town 8001, South Africa

http://www.cambridge.org

First published 2003

Printed in the United Kingdom at the University Press, Cambridge

*Typefaces* Dante 11/14 pt and Dax     *System* LaTeX $2_\varepsilon$   [TB]

*A catalogue record for this book is available from the British Library*

ISBN 0 521 62226 3 paperback

Every effort has been made in preparing this book to provide accurate and up-to-date information that is in accord with accepted standards and practice at the time of publication. Nevertheless, the authors, editors and publisher can make no warranties that the information contained herein is totally free from error, not least because clinical standards are constantly changing through research and regulation. The authors, editors and publisher therefore disclaim all liability for direct or consequential damages resulting from the use of material contained in this book. Readers are strongly advised to pay careful attention to information provided by the manufacturer of any drugs or equipment that they plan to use.

This volume is dedicated to the memory of our friends and teachers
Donald J. Cohen, M.D. and Joseph D. Noshpitz, M.D.

*M'dor l'dor*
*From one generation to the next*

# Contents

# Contributors

**Robert A. King, M.D.**
Professor of Child Psychiatry and Psychiatry
Yale Child Study Center
230 South Frontage Road
POB 207900
New Haven, CN 06511 USA
tel: +1-203-785-5880
fax: +1-203-737-5104
e-mail: robert.king@yale.edu

**Alan Apter, M.D.**
Professor of Psychiatry
Sackler School of Medicine
University of Tel-Aviv Medical School
Chairman, Dept. of Child and Adolescent
    Psychiatry
Schneider Children's Medical Center of Israel
14 Kaplan St.
Petah Tikva, Israel 49202
e-mail: eapter@clalit.org.il

**Alan L. Berman, Ph.D.**
Executive Director
American Association of Suicidology
4201 Connecticut Ave., N.W.
Washington, DC, 20008 USA
tel: +1-202-237-2280
fax: +1-202-237-2282
e-mail: berman@suicidology.org

**Julie Boergers, Ph.D.**
Clinical Assistant Professor
Brown Medical School
Rhode Island Hospital
593 Eddy Street
Providence, RI 02903 USA
tel: +1-401-444-4515
fax: +1-401-444-7018
e-mail: Julie Boergers@brown.edu

**David A. Brent, M.D.**
Academic Chief, Child and Adolescent
    Psychiatry
Western Psychiatric Institute and Clinic
Professor of Psychiatry, Pediatrics
    and Epidemiology
University of Pittsburgh School of
    Medicine
3811 O'Hara Street, Suite 112
Pittsburgh, PA 15213 USA
tel: +1-412-624-5172
fax: +1-412-624-7997
e-mail: brentda@msx.upmc.edu

**Derek Chambers M.A.**
Research & Resource Officer
National Suicide Review Group
Western Health Board
Office 10 Orantown Centre
Oranmore, Galway, Ireland
tel: +353-91-787056
e-mail: derek.chambers@whb.ie

**Cornelia L. Gallo, M.D.**
Assistant Clinical Professor of Child
    Psychiatry

Yale Child Study Center
230 South Frontage Road
POB 207900
New Haven, CN 06511 USA

**Madelyn S. Gould, Ph.D., M.P.H.**
Professor
Psychiatry and Public Health (Epidemiology)
Columbia University
New York State Psychiatric Institute
1051 Riverside Drive Unit 72
New York, NY 10032 USA
tel: +1-212-543-5329
fax: +1-212-543-5966
e-mail: gouldm@child.cpmc.columbia.edu

**Ted Greenberg, M.P.H.**
Research Scientist
Columbia University
New York State Psychiatric Institute
722 West 168th Street
New York, NY 10032 USA
tel: +1-212-543-5931
e-mail: greenbet@child.cpmc.columbia.edu

**Richard Harrington, M.B.B.S.**
University Department of Child Psychiatry
Royal Manchester Children's Hospital
Pendlebury, Manchester, UK
tel: +44-161-727-2401
e-mail: r.c.harrington@man.ac.uk

**Michael J. Kelleher, M.D., M.Phil.,**
    **F.R.C.P.I., F.R.C. Psych. (*deceased*)**
National Suicide Research Foundation
Perrott Avenue
College Road
Cork
Ireland

**J. John Mann, M.D.**
Dept. of Neuroscience / Psychiatry
NY State Psychiatric Institute
Columbia Presbyterian Medical Center
722 W. 168th St., Box 28

New York, NY 10032 (011-61-3) 9527-2867 USA
tel: +1-212-543-5000 / 5571
fax: +1-212-543-6017 or (212) 781-0503
e-mail: jjm@columbia.edu

**Israel Orbach, Ph.D.**
Professor, Department of Psychology
Bar-llan University
Ramat-Gan, Israel 52900
tel: +972-353-18174
fax: +972-353-50267
e-mail: orbachi@mail.biu.ac.il

**Cynthia R. Pfeffer, M.D.**
Professor of Psychiatry, Director of the
    Childhood Bereavement Program
Weill Medical College of Cornell University
New York Presbyterian Hospital
21 Bloomingdale Road, White Plains
NY 10605 USA
e-mail: cpfeffer@med.cornell.edu

**Vladislav V. Ruchkin, M.D., Ph.D.**
Assistant Professor
Institute of Psychiatry
Northern State Medical University,
    Arkhangelsk, Russia currently also:
Hewlett Research Fellow in the Program on
    International Child and Adolescent Mental
    Health
Yale Child Study Center
230 South Frontage Road
POB 207900
New Haven, CN 06511 USA
tel: +1-203-785-2545
e-mail: vladislav.ruchkin@yale.edu

**Younus Saleem**
University Department of Child Psychiatry
Royal Manchester Children's Hospital
Pendlebury, Manchester UK
tel: +44+161-727-2401

**Mary E. Schwab-Stone, M.D.**
Associate Professor of Child Psychiatry and
    Psychology

Yale Child Study Center
230 South Frontage Road
POB 207900
New Haven, CN 06511 USA
tel: +1-203-785-2545
e-mail: mary.schwab-stone@yale.edu

**David Shaffer, M.B., B.S.,**
**F.R.C.P., F.R.C. Psych**
Irving Philips Professor of Psychiatry
Columbia University
Director of Child Psychiatry
New York State Psychiatric Institute
1051 Riverside Drive
New York, NY 10032 USA
tel: +1-212-543-5947
fax: +1-212-543-5966
e-mail: shafferd@child.cpmc.columbia.edu

**Anthony Spirito, Ph.D.**
Director, Clinical Psychology Training
    Program
Potter Building
Box G-BH

Brown University
Providence, RI 02906 USA
tel: +1-401-444-1833
fax: +1-401-444-1888
e-mail: Anthony_Spirito@brown.edu

**Danuta Wasserman, M.D., Ph.D.**
Professor of Psychiatry and Suicidology and
    Chairmen of the Department of Public
    Health Sciences at the Karolinska Institute
Head of the Swedish National Centre for
    Suicide Research and Prevention of Mental
    Illness, at the National Institute for
    Psychosocial Medicine
Director of the WHO Collaborating
    Centre for Suicide research and
    promotion of mental health
Karolinska Institute
Box 230
171 77 Stockholm, Sweden
tel: +46-8-7287026
fax: +46-8-30-64-39
e-mail: danuta.wasserman@ipm.ki.se

# Preface

In an epoch when rates of death and illness among the young have steadily decreased in the face of medical progress, the persistently high rates of youth suicide and suicide attempts in the West remain a tragic irony and a challenge to both our clinical practice and theoretical understanding. The purpose of this monograph is to present the current state of scientific and clinical knowledge regarding suicidal behavior in children and adolescents.

Clinical epidemiology now makes it possible to examine rates of completed suicide, as well as rates of suicidal ideation and attempts of varying degrees of severity in defined community populations of adolescents and children. Beyond prevalence rates, these studies provide important data on the demographic and psychosocial correlates of suicidal behavior, uncontaminated by the selection biases inherent in clinical samples. Despite the innate limitations posed by the unavailability of the key informant, modern postmortem psychological autopsy techniques also now give us systematic information concerning psychopathology and other risk factors in young suicides.

Although no single factor explains youth suicide, progress has been made in beginning to tease apart the tangle of intersecting domains of vulnerabilities that are associated with suicidal behavior in the young. Suicide is the most dramatic of the spectrum of self-destructive and health-endangering behaviors that unfortunately characterize adolescence. One of the editors' goals is to examine youth suicidal behavior in the context of this spectrum. The perspective of developmental psychopathology emphasizes the interaction of risk and protective factors over the life span and we discuss the importance of this perspective for understanding the shared and distinctive factors that confer resilience or vulnerability to suicidal and other risk behaviors. Separate chapters describe our current understanding of predisposing genetic, neurobiological, cultural, and psychodynamic factors. A chapter on the case study method underlines the challenge of understanding how these various factors intersect in the life story of any given individual.

This volume also addresses the clinical challenges posed by youthful suicidal behavior. Despite the clear need for effective interventions to prevent these avoidable forms of mortality and morbidity, the wide prevalence of risk factors for suicide in adolescents (depression, impulsivity, affective lability, substance use), as well as the frequency of suicidal ideation make it difficult to target preventive programs effectively and efficiently. Although suicidal ideation and attempts in the young are dismayingly common, completed suicide is statistically rare, making outcome studies of community suicide prevention programs difficult.

Careful evaluation of suicidal children and adolescents is a crucial prerequisite for effective treatment and a chapter is devoted to the special assessment issues posed by such youngsters. Systematic treatment studies dealing with suicidal behavior in children and adolescents are only recently beginning to be available. The adaptation of cognitive behavioral treatment and related approaches to suicidal youngsters is described, as well as the special issues involved in treating this age group. Adolescent suicide attempters are notoriously difficult to engage effectively in treatment. A review of follow-up studies of adolescent attempters suggests that many such youngsters remain at risk for repeat attempts, as well as a host of other difficulties. In light of these worrisome findings, methods of improving treatment adherence and other elements of after-care are discussed, as well as cross-national patterns of after-care.

Finally, all too often, treatment is not sought or fails, resulting in a completed suicide, with devastating consequences for surviving family members. These consequences may be particularly ominous for children. The suicide of a family member appears to place young close relatives at increased risk for subsequent suicide, most likely for experiential as well as genetic reasons. A final chapter therefore discusses methods of postvention to help children and families cope with the suicide death of a family member.

# 1

# The epidemiology of youth suicide

Madelyn S. Gould, David Shaffer, and Ted Greenberg

## Introduction

This chapter reviews three major sources of data that are used to derive the epidemiology of completed suicide in children and adolescents – official mortality statistics, the psychological autopsy literature, and general population epidemiologic surveys of nonlethal suicidal behavior. A presentation of the rates and patterns of completed and attempted suicide will be followed by a discussion of the risk factors for youth suicide. This information on the epidemiology of youth completed and attempted suicide can be applied to planning of services, the drawing of causal inferences or the identification of developmental phenomena.

## Suicide rates and patterns

### Completed suicide

**Leading causes of adolescent and young adult death in the U.S.**

Unintentional injuries, suicide and homicide are consistently the leading causes of death among youth aged 10–24 in the U.S. (Table 1.1). Suicide was the fourth leading cause of death among 10- to 14-year-olds, and the third leading cause of death among 15- to 19-year-olds and among 20- to 24-year-olds in 1999. The rankings vary by gender and ethnicity: suicide accounts for more deaths among males and whites. Age, gender, and ethnic differences in incidence will be discussed further below.

**Age**

The incidence of suicide varies markedly by age. In 1999, 192 boys and 50 girls aged between 10 and 14 committed suicide in the U.S., accounting for 5.8% (242/4121) of all deaths occurring in this age group. The age-specific mortality rate from suicide was 1.2 per 100 000. Although 10- to 14-year-olds represented

**Table 1.1.** Leading causes of death by age in the U.S., 1999*

| Causes of death | Total | | Whites | | | | African-Americans | | | |
| | Rank[a] | Rate[b] | Males | | Females | | Males | | Females | |
| | | | Rank[a] | Rate[b] | Rank[a] | Rate[b] | Rank[a] | Rate[b] | Rank[a] | Rate[b] |
|---|---|---|---|---|---|---|---|---|---|---|
| 10–14 years | | | | | | | | | | |
| Accidents | 1 | 8.3 | 1 | 10.4 | 1 | 5.8 | 1 | 13.6 | 1 | 6.4 |
| Suicide | 4 | 1.2 | 3 | 2.1 | 6 | 0.6 | 7 | 1.4 | 7 | – |
| Homicide | 3 | 1.3 | 4 | 1.2 | 4 | 0.8 | 2 | 3.5 | 4 | 1.6 |
| 15–19 years | | | | | | | | | | |
| Accidents | 1 | 33.9 | 1 | 53.5 | 1 | 23.6 | 2 | 37.1 | 1 | 13.4 |
| Suicide | 3 | 8.2 | 2 | 13.9 | 3 | 2.9 | 3 | 10.0 | 5 | 1.6 |
| Homicide | 2 | 10.6 | 3 | 8.7 | 4 | 2.4 | 1 | 63.2 | 2 | 10.2 |
| 20–24 years | | | | | | | | | | |
| Accidents | 1 | 38.7 | 1 | 60.6 | 1 | 17.9 | 2 | 54.5 | 1 | 16.0 |
| Suicide | 3 | 12.7 | 2 | 22.1 | 4 | 3.5 | 3 | 19.4 | 6 | 2.3 |
| Homicide | 2 | 16.1 | 3 | 12.5 | 3 | 3.7 | 1 | 110.6 | 2 | 12.8 |

* Unless otherwise noted, mortality statistics from 1999 are presented.

[a] Ranking within the 10 leading causes of death.

[b] Per 100 000.

*Sources:* CDC National Center for Injury Prevention and Control, Office of Statistics and Programming. CDC Wonder Mortality Data Request Screen. Available at http://wonder.cdc.gov/mortsql.ghtml (accessed 10 April 2002).

7.2% of the U.S. population, the 242 child suicides represented only 0.8% (242/29 199) of all suicides. Only two children under the age of 10 committed suicide in 1999. Among 15- to 19-year-olds, 1347 boys and 268 girls committed suicide, yielding a suicide mortality rate of 8.2 per 100 000. This is nearly seven times as common as in the younger age group. The percentage of all suicides represented by 15- to 19-year-olds (5.5%) is nearly equal to the percentage of 15- to 19-year-olds in the total population (7.2%). Among 20- to 24-year-olds, 1979 males and 307 females between the ages of 20 and 24 committed suicide, yielding an overall mortality rate of 12.7 per 100 000. This age group represents 6.6% of the total population; the suicides in this age group represent 7.2% of all suicides.

Figure 1.1 presents variations in incidence by specific age, gender, and ethnic group in the U.S. in 1998. Suicide is uncommon in childhood and early adolescence. Within the 10- to 14-year-old group, most suicides are aged between 12 and 14. Suicide incidence increases markedly in the late teens and continues to rise until the early twenties, reaching a level that is maintained throughout

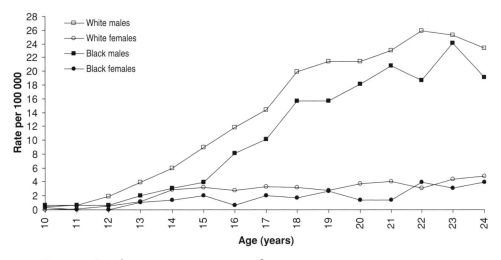

Figure 1.1  Suicide rates, ages 10–24 years, as of 1998.
*Source:* Populations Branch, Populations Division, U.S. Bureau of the Census, U.S. population estimates by ages, sex, race, and Hispanic origin: 1990–1998.
*Source:* National Center for Health Statistics, Vital Statistics of the United States, Volume II; *Mortality,* 1998.

adulthood, until the beginning of the sixth decade when the rates increase markedly among men.

The age difference in completed suicide rates is a universal phenomenon, as can be seen by the ratio of late adolescent/young adult (15–24 years) to child/young adolescent (5–14 years) suicides in countries with data published by the World Health Organization (2001) (Table 1.2). The similar age pattern in the international data suggests that cultural factors are unlikely to explain the rarity of suicide before puberty (Shaffer and Hicks, 1994). Shaffer et al. (1996) suggest that the most likely reason underlying the age of onset of suicide appears to be the age of onset of depression or exposure to drugs and alcohol. These two significant risk factors for suicide in adults (e.g., Barraclough et al., 1974; Robins et al., 1959) and in adolescents (to be discussed later in the chapter) are rare in very young children and become prevalent only in later adolescence.

### Gender

In the U.S., nearly six times more 15- to 19-year-old boys than girls commit suicide. The ratio of boys to girls steadily increases from prepuberty to young adulthood (see Figure 1.1). The same pattern of sex differences does not exist in all countries (see Table 1.2). Among 15- to 24-year-olds, in North America, Western Europe, Australia, and New Zealand, suicide is more common in males

**Table 1.2.** Youth suicide rates* by age, sex, and country

| Country | Year | 5–14 years | | | 15–24 years | | | 15–24: 5–14 Ratio | |
|---|---|---|---|---|---|---|---|---|---|
| | | Males | Females | M:F | Males | Females | M:F | Males | Females |
| Australia | 1997 | 0.5 | 0.5 | 1.0 | 30.0 | 6.6 | 4.5 | 60.0 | 13.2 |
| Austria | 1999 | 0.4 | 0.2 | 2.0 | 20.3 | 5.3 | 3.8 | 50.8 | 26.5 |
| Canada | 1997 | 1.9 | 0.6 | 3.2 | 22.4 | 4.5 | 5.0 | 11.8 | 7.5 |
| Chile | 1994 | 0.1 | 0.3 | 0.3 | 10.9 | 1.5 | 7.3 | 109.0 | 5.0 |
| China (urban) | 1998 | 0.3 | 0.4 | 0.8 | 3.4 | 4.4 | 0.8 | 11.3 | 11.0 |
| China (rural) | 1998 | 0.9 | 1.0 | 0.9 | 8.4 | 15.2 | 0.6 | 9.3 | 15.2 |
| Finland | 1998 | 0.9 | 0.6 | 1.5 | 29.5 | 7.9 | 3.7 | 32.8 | 13.2 |
| France | 1997 | 0.3 | 0.3 | 1.0 | 13.4 | 4.3 | 3.1 | 44.7 | 14.3 |
| Germany | 1998 | 0.7 | 0.4 | 1.8 | 12.7 | 3.5 | 3.6 | 18.1 | 8.8 |
| Hungary | 1999 | 1.8 | 0.2 | 9.0 | 19.1 | 3.9 | 4.9 | 10.6 | 19.5 |
| Ireland | 1996 | 1.3 | – | – | 25.4 | 4.5 | 5.6 | 19.5 | – |
| Israel | 1997 | 0.4 | – | – | 12.6 | 1.6 | 7.9 | 31.5 | – |
| Italy | 1997 | 0.2 | 0.2 | 1.0 | 8.5 | 1.8 | 4.7 | 42.5 | 9.0 |
| Japan | 1997 | 0.5 | 0.3 | 1.7 | 11.3 | 5.5 | 2.1 | 22.6 | 18.3 |
| Mexico | 1995 | 0.5 | 0.3 | 1.7 | 7.6 | 2.0 | 3.8 | 15.2 | 6.7 |
| Netherlands | 1997 | 1.1 | – | – | 11.3 | 4.4 | 2.6 | 10.3 | – |
| New Zealand | 1998 | 3.0 | 1.4 | 2.1 | 38.1 | 13.3 | 2.9 | 12.7 | 9.5 |
| Norway | 1997 | 1.0 | – | – | 20.2 | 4.7 | 4.3 | 20.2 | – |
| Poland | 1996 | 1.6 | 0.4 | 4.0 | 17.2 | 2.9 | 5.9 | 10.8 | 7.3 |
| Republic of Korea | 1997 | 0.9 | 1.1 | 0.8 | 12.5 | 8.0 | 1.6 | 13.9 | 7.3 |
| Russian Federation | 1998 | 3.0 | 0.7 | 4.3 | 51.9 | 8.6 | 6.0 | 17.3 | 12.3 |
| Scotland | 1997 | – | – | – | 19.5 | 5.3 | 3.7 | – | – |
| Singapore | 1998 | 1.2 | – | – | 13.4 | 10.9 | 1.2 | 11.2 | – |
| Sweden | 1996 | 0.2 | 0.4 | 0.5 | 12.0 | 4.6 | 2.6 | 60.0 | 11.5 |
| Switzerland | 1998 | 0.9 | – | – | 24.8 | 5.6 | 4.4 | 27.6 | – |
| U.K. of Great Britain and Ireland | 1998 | 0.1 | 0.1 | 1.0 | 10.4 | 2.9 | 3.6 | 104.0 | 29.0 |
| United States | 1998 | 1.2 | 0.4 | 3.0 | 18.5 | 3.3 | 5.6 | 15.4 | 8.3 |

* per 100 000.

*Source:* World Health Organization. Suicide rates and absolute numbers of suicide by country (2001). Available at http://www.who.int/mental_health/Topic_Suicide/suicide1.html.

than in females. However, in some countries in Asia (e.g., Singapore), sex rates are equal and, in some (e.g., China), the majority of suicides are committed by females.

Both psychopathologic factors and sex-related method preferences are considered to contribute to the pattern of sex differences (Shaffer and Hicks, 1994). Suicide is often associated with aggressive behavior and alcohol abuse (see discussion below) and both are more common in males. The role of gender-related method preference is more complex. Methods of suicide favored by women, such as overdoses, tend to be less lethal than the methods favored by men, such as hanging (Moscicki, 1995). However, an overdose may have quite different implications for lethality in different societies. Where treatment resources are not readily available or when the chosen ingestant is untreatable, overdoses are more likely to be lethal than in countries with well-developed treatment facilities (Shaffer and Hicks, 1994). Thus, in the U.S. in 1999 only 11% of completed suicides resulted from an ingestion (see section below on Methods); whereas in some South Asian and South Pacific countries, the majority of suicides are due to ingestions of herbicides such as paraquat, for which no effective treatment is available (Haynes, 1987; Shaffer and Hicks, 1994). A further discussion of method preference by age, gender, and ethnicity in the U.S. is given below.

**Ethnicity**
Until 1979, the ethnic breakdown in the annual age-specific mortality statistics in the U.S. published by the National Center for Health Statistics (NCHS) was limited to whites and nonwhites. The "nonwhites" category comprised a heterogeneous group individuals, including African-Americans and other minority groups. In 1979, the ethnic breakdown was expanded to white, black, and "other." The NCHS began to routinely code Hispanic origin in vital statistics data in about 1984. Since the vital statistics data are taken from State death certificates, the NCHS has to rely on States to provide the necessary information. In 1979, only 15 States had a Hispanic origin item on the death certificate. In 1984, there were 22 States, in 1989 there were 47 States, and beginning with 1997 data all States and the District of Columbia were included in Hispanic origin tabulations. While the availability of data on suicide rates for Latino youth is still limited (Canino and Roberts, 2001), Latino youth do not appear to be overrepresented among completed suicides in the U.S. (Demetriades et al., 1998; Gould et al., 1996; Smith et al., 1985).

The *number* of deaths for Native Americans has been tabulated as far back as at least 1900, but *rates* were not available because of concerns regarding the quality of Native American *population estimates*. The Division of Vital Statistics publishes crude death rates, not cause- or age-specific rates, for Native Americans in the *"Report of Final Mortality Statistics"* (called *"Advance Report of Final Mortality Statistics"* before 1995) in the *Monthly Vital Statistics Report*. The first report was in 1992, but death rates were provided retrospectively back to 1980. Cause-specific rates, such as suicide rates, are available in special reports, such as the recent special surveillance summary from the Centers for Disease Control and Prevention (CDC), derived from data from the Indian Health Service (IHS) and the NCHS (Wallace et al., 1996). Regarding violent deaths among Native Americans residing in Indian Health Service Areas, Native American males had the highest suicide rates in the U.S. during the period 1979–1992. Native American males and females aged 15–24 years had suicide rates of 62.0 per 100 000 and 10.0 per 100 000, respectively (Wallace et al., 1996).

Youth suicide has generally been more common in whites than African-Americans in the U.S. (see Table 1.1). The historically lower suicide rate among African-Americans has been hypothesized to be due to differences in religiosity, dissimilar degrees of social integration, and differences in "outwardly" rather than "inwardly" directed aggression (Shaffer et al., 1994). However, the difference in the suicide rates between whites and African-Americans has been decreasing during the past 15 years. There was a marked increase in the suicide rate among African-American males between 1986 and 1994, a period in which the rates for white males and for African-American males started to converge. This was followed by declining rates since the mid 1990s among all ethnic groups. The postulated reasons for this secular change will be discussed in the "Secular trends" section.

### Geography

In the U.S., youth suicide rates, uncorrected for ethnicity, are highest among the Western States and Alaska and lowest in the Northeastern States (see Table 1.3). The reasons underlying this pattern are unclear. It may reflect different ethnic mixes or the varying availability of firearms (Shaffer, 1988). There is no apparent differential pattern by age or gender. The ratio of white to African-American rates is greatest in the South, consistent with earlier reports (Shaffer et al., 1994).

### Methods

Firearms are the most common method and hanging the second most prevalent method of suicide in the U.S., regardless of age or ethnicity (see Table 1.4). These two methods were the only ones used by 10- to 14-year-olds or by African-American youths in 1999. There is some variability of method by gender. Ingestions are the second most prevalent method of suicide for females overall, accounting for 30% of all female suicides, while only 6.7% of all male suicides are due to this method. Among 15- to 19-year-olds, ingestions account for 15.7 % of female suicides in contrast to 2% of male suicides and, among 20- to 24-year-olds,

Table 1.3. Regional suicide rates[a] by age, gender, and ethnicity in the U.S., 1998

| Region | Age | | Gender | | | Ethnicity | | |
|---|---|---|---|---|---|---|---|---|
| | 15–19 | 20–24 | Males[b] | Females[b] | M:F[b] | White[b] | Af.–Am.[b] | W:A[b] |
| Northeast | 6.7 | 11.7 | 15.0 | 2.9 | 5.2 | 9.5 | 8.5 | 1.1 |
| Connecticut | * | * | 14.8 | * | – | 6.8 | * | – |
| Maine | * | * | – | * | – | 13.1 | * | – |
| Massachusetts | 7.1 | 11.0 | 15.4 | * | – | 9.5 | * | – |
| New Hampshire | 5.6 | 9.7 | 12.8 | 2.2 | 5.8 | 8.7 | 5.4 | 1.6 |
| New Jersey | * | * | 35.0 | * | – | 21.7 | * | – |
| New York | 3.9 | 9.2 | 11.3 | * | – | 5.7 | * | – |
| Pennsylvania | 7.6 | 15.2 | 17.9 | 4.1 | 4.3 | 11.0 | 12.2 | 0.9 |
| Rhode Island | * | * | * | * | – | * | * | – |
| Vermont | * | * | * | * | – | * | * | – |
| Midwest | 8.9 | 13.7 | 18.7 | 3.3 | 5.7 | 11.1 | 10.8 | 1.0 |
| Illinois | 7.6 | 11.3 | 15.1 | 3.3 | 4.6 | 9.8 | 8.9 | 1.1 |
| Indiana | 8.1 | 16.8 | 20.9 | * | – | 11.4 | * | – |
| Iowa | 9.7 | 12.9 | 19.0 | * | – | 11.2 | * | – |
| Kansas | 15.7 | * | 26.5 | * | – | 15.3 | * | – |
| Michigan | 7.9 | 11.4 | 17.0 | * | – | 9.9 | * | – |
| Minnesota | 8.9 | 20.5 | 22.8 | * | – | 12.5 | * | – |
| Missouri | 11.2 | 16.7 | 21.6 | 5.6 | 3.9 | 14.6 | * | – |
| Nebraska | * | * | 21.5 | * | – | 12.2 | * | – |
| North Dakota | * | * | * | * | – | * | * | – |
| Ohio | 8.3 | 9.7 | 15.7 | * | – | 8.8 | * | – |
| South Dakota | * | * | 39.4 | * | – | * | * | – |
| Wisconsin | 5.9 | 16.3 | 17.4 | * | – | 10.9 | * | – |
| South | 9.5 | 13.5 | 19.2 | 3.3 | 5.9 | 12.8 | 7.8 | 1.6 |
| Alabama | 8.1 | 14.2 | 19.7 | * | – | 12.8 | * | – |
| Arkansas | 13.4 | 15.5 | 23.6 | * | – | 15.8 | * | – |
| Delaware | * | * | * | * | – | * | * | – |
| District of Columbia | * | * | * | * | – | * | * | – |
| Florida | 9.5 | 13.4 | 17.7 | 4.7 | 3.8 | 12.7 | 7.5 | 1.7 |
| Georgia | 8.2 | 11.9 | 16.9 | * | – | 12.5 | * | – |
| Kentucky | 9.0 | 11.6 | 18.4 | * | – | 10.6 | * | – |
| Louisiana | 10.0 | 13.9 | 20.5 | * | – | 12.7 | * | 1.2 |
| Maryland | * | 13.59 | 15.06 | * | – | 10.3 | 11.0 | 0.9 |
| Mississippi | 9.1 | 18.5 | 25.1 | * | – | 19.7 | * | – |
| North Carolina | 6.8 | 11.3 | 15.3 | * | – | 9.3 | 8.2 | 1.1 |
| Oklahoma | 15.4 | 18.8 | 28.8 | * | – | 18.0 | * | – |

(cont.)

**Table 1.3.** (*cont.*)

| Region | Age | | Gender | | | Ethnicity | | |
|---|---|---|---|---|---|---|---|---|
| | 15–19 | 20–24 | Males[b] | Females[b] | M:F[b] | White[b] | Af.–Am.[b] | W:A[b] |
| South Carolina | 8.5 | 14.5 | 20.6 | * | – | 12.7 | * | – |
| Tennessee | 12.7 | 10.0 | 19.1 | * | – | 12.9 | * | – |
| Texas | 9.5 | 13.9 | 19.6 | 3.1 | 6.4 | 12.7 | 6.9 | 1.8 |
| Virginia | 10.5 | 13.1 | 19.3 | * | – | 13.2 | * | – |
| West Virginia | * | 16.6 | 22.6 | * | – | 14.8 | * | – |
| West | 9.4 | 14.6 | 19.6 | 3.5 | 5.7 | 12.2 | 9.6 | 1.3 |
| Arizona | 15.1 | 19.2 | 28.8 | * | – | 16.3 | * | – |
| California | 6.4 | 11.0 | 13.9 | 2.9 | 4.8 | 9.2 | 8.2 | 1.1 |
| Colorado | 13.7 | 20.1 | 28.3 | * | – | 16.8 | * | – |
| Idaho | * | * | 27.5 | * | – | 14.1 | * | – |
| Montana | * | * | * | * | – | * | * | – |
| Nevada | 18.9 | 24.0 | 34.3 | * | – | 21.2 | * | – |
| New Mexico | * | 25.4 | 30.1 | * | – | 16.8 | * | – |
| Oregon | * | 21.1 | 22.5 | * | – | 13.3 | * | – |
| Utah | 14.4 | 19.4 | 30.9 | * | – | 17.0 | * | – |
| Washington | 9.7 | 14.8 | 20.8 | * | – | 11.6 | * | – |
| Wyoming | * | * | * | * | – | * | * | – |
| Alaska | * | 55.2 | 68.2 | * | – | * | * | – |
| Hawaii | * | * | * | * | – | * | * | – |

* Figure does not meet standards of reliability or precision set by the National Center for Health Statistics (rates based on fewer than 20 deaths).

[a] Per 100 000.

[b] Af.–Am., African-American; W:A, White to African-American.

*Sources:* CDC National Center for Injury Prevention and Control, Office of Statistics and Programming. CDC Wonder Mortality Data Request Screen. Available at http://wonder.cdc.gov/mortsql.ghtml (accessed 10 April 2002).

this method accounts for 18.9% of female suicides compared to 3.2% of male suicides.

### Secular trends

Over the past three decades, there has been little change in the suicide rate among 10- to 14-year-olds (Figure 1.2); however, there have been dramatic changes among 15- to 19-year-olds (Figure 1.3). From the 1960s until 1988 there was a threefold increase in suicides among males aged 15–19 years. The rates then started to plateau until the mid 1990s, when the rates started to steadily

**Table 1.4.** Rates* of suicide methods by age, gender, and ethnicity in the U.S., 1999

| Method | 10–14 years | | | | | 15–19 years | | | | | 20–24 years | | | | | All ages | | | | |
|---|---|---|---|---|---|---|---|---|---|---|---|---|---|---|---|---|---|---|---|---|
| | T | M | F | W | AA | T | M | F | W | AA | T | M | F | W | AA | T | M | F | W | AA |
| Ingestions $x_{60}$–$x_{65}$, $x_{68}$, $x_{69}$ | – | – | – | – | – | 0.4 | 0.3 | 0.4 | 0.4 | 0.1** | 0.7 | 0.7 | 0.7 | 0.8 | 0.3 | 1.2 | 1.2 | 1.2 | 1.4 | 0.4 |
| Carbon monoxide and other poisoning by gases $x_{66}$, $x_{67}$ | – | – | – | – | – | 0.2 | 0.3 | 0.1** | 0.2 | – | 0.6 | 0.9 | 0.1** | 0.7 | – | 0.6 | 0.9 | 0.3 | 0.7 | 0.1 |
| Hanging $x_{70}$ | 0.6 | 1.0 | 0.2 | 0.6 | 0.7 | 2.2 | 3.4 | 0.9 | 2.2 | 1.3 | 3.0 | 5.0 | 0.9 | 3.1 | 1.8 | 2.0 | 3.4 | 0.7 | 2.1 | 1.1 |
| Firearms $x_{72}$, $x_{73}$, $x_{74}$ | 0.5 | 0.8 | 0.2 | 0.6 | – | 4.9 | 8.5 | 1.1 | 5.2 | 3.9 | 7.4 | 13.2 | 1.4 | 7.5 | 7.9 | 6.1 | 10.9 | 1.5 | 6.7 | 3.2 |
| Other (includes drowning, jumping, cutting, explosives and other) $x_{71}$, $x_{75}$, $x_{79}$, $x_{81}$–$x_{84}$, $x_{87.0}$ | – | – | – | – | – | 0.3 | 0.5 | 0.1** | 0.3 | 0.4** | 0.6 | 1.0 | 0.2 | 0.6 | 0.6** | 0.6 | 0.9 | 0.3 | 0.6 | 0.5 |

* Per 100 000.

** Fewer than 20 cases.

*Source:* CDC National Center for Injury Prevention and Control, Office of Statistics and Programming. CDC Wonder Mortality Data Request Screen. Available at http://wonder.cdc.gov/mortsql.ghtml (accessed, 10 April 2002).

Abbreviations: AA, African-American; F, female; M, male; T, total; W, White. $x_{66}$, $x_{67}$, etc. are ICD 10 mortality codes.

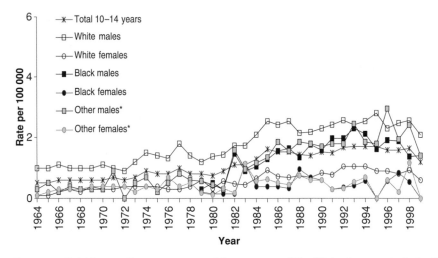

Figure 1.2  Suicide rates for 10- to 14-year-olds, 1964–1999. *The "Other" groups include all non-whites.

*Source:* National Center for Health Statistics, Vital Statistics of the United States, Volume II; Mortality, 1964–1998.

*Source:* CDC National Center for Injury Prevention and Control, Office of Statistics and Programming. CDC Wonder Mortality Data Request Screen. Available at http://wonder.cdc.gov/mortsql.ghtml (Accessed 10 April 2002).

decline among all gender/ethnic groups. Suicide rates among 20- to 24-year-olds remained relatively steady from 1980 until the mid 1990s at a level that was a twofold increase compared to 1964 rates (Figure 1.4). Since the mid 1990s, the declining rate noted among 15- to 19-year-olds has also occurred among 20- to 24-year-olds.

A considerable number of causal explanations, involving diagnostic, social or familial factors, have been posited for the dramatic secular trends in youth suicidal behavior (Berman and Jobes, 1995; Diekstra et al., 1995). The reasons proposed for the increase include changes in the prevalence of substance abuse (Shaffer et al., 1996) and increased availability of firearms (Boyd, 1983; Boyd and Moscicki, 1986; Brent et al., 1987, 1991). There was evidence that the rate of suicide by firearms rose faster than the suicide rate by other methods (Boyd, 1983; Boyd and Moscicki, 1986; Brent et al., 1987), and that guns were twice as likely to be found in the homes of suicide victims as in the homes of attempters or psychiatric controls (Brent et al., 1991).

Similar factors have been proposed for the recent declines in teenage suicide rates. The restriction of the availability of lethal methods (e.g., firearms) at first seems a possible explanation (Brent et al., 1999) because the decrease in youth

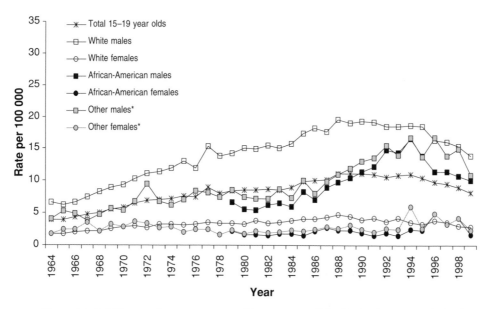

Figure 1.3  Suicide rates for 15- to 19-year-olds, 1964–1999. *The "Other" groups include all non-whites.

*Source:* National Center for Health Statistics, Vital Statistics of the United States, Volume II; *Mortality, 1964–1998.*

*Source:* CDC National Center for Injury Prevention and Control, Office of Statistics and Programming. CDC Wonder Mortality Data Request Screen. Available at http://wonder.cdc.gov/mortsql.ghtml (Accessed 10 April 2002).

suicide rates largely reflects a decrease in firearm suicides (Figure 1.5). However, there are a number of reasons to question this explanation: (1) it is unclear if access to firearms has been reduced: the proportion of suicides by firearms, a plausible proxy for method availability (Cutright and Fernquist, 2000), has not changed between 1988 and 1999; (2) there has been a decline ranging from 20% to 30% in the youth suicide rates in England, Finland, Germany, and Sweden where firearms account for very few suicides (WHO, 2001); (3) a systematic examination of the proportion of suicides committed by firearms over a long period of time has shown that the proportion is only weakly related to overall changes in the rate (Cutright and Fernquist, 2000). The decline in youth suicide also does not seem to be due to a decrease in substance use: repeat benchmark studies that use similar measures and sampling methods such as the Youth Risk Behavior Survey (CDC 1995, 1996, 1998, 2000) give no indication of a decline in alcohol or cocaine use during this time. Better treatment of depression is a more likely factor underlying the decrease in suicide rates, supported by the parallel

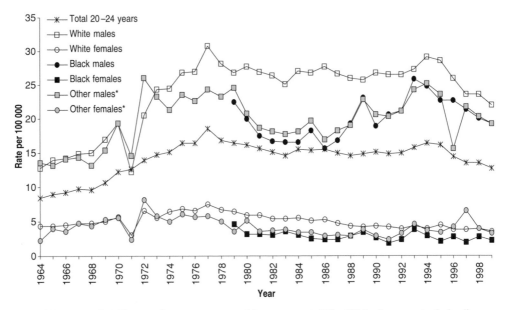

Figure 1.4  Suicide rates for 20- to 24-year-olds, 1964–1999. *The "Other" groups include all non-whites.

*Source:* National Center for Health Statistics, Vital Statistics of the United States, Volume II; *Mortality*, 1964–1998.

*Source:* CDC National Center for Injury Prevention and Control, Office of Statistics and Programming. CDC Wonder Mortality Data Request Screen. Available at http://wonder.cdc.gov/mortsql.ghtml (Accessed 10 April 2002).

increase in the number of prescriptions for antidepressants for youth during the same time period (Lonnqvist, 2000; Shaffer and Craft, 1999). The delay in the onset of the suicide decline in African-American suicides is compatible with a treatment effect because of their greater difficulty in accessing treatment resources (Goodwin et al., 2001). Other findings suggesting that more treatment may be a factor in the recent decline are that in Sweden the proportion of suicides who have received antidepressant treatment is lower than the rest of the depressed population (Isacsson, 2000).

## Nonlethal suicidal behavior

There is no surveillance system for nonlethal suicidal behavior in the U.S., with the exception of Oregon, which has mandated the reporting of all attempted suicides among persons younger than 18 years who are treated at a hospital or a hospital emergency department (Andrus et al., 1991). Nevertheless, the surge of general population studies of suicide attempters and ideators in the past decade

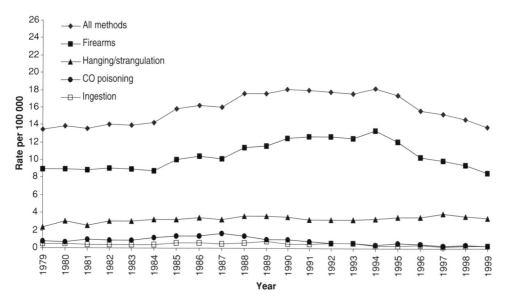

Figure 1.5  Method of suicide for white males aged 15–19 years, 1979–1999.
*Source:* CDC National Center for Injury Prevention and Control, Office of Statistics and Programming. CDC Wonder Mortality Data Request Screen. Available at http://wonder.cdc.gov/mortsql.ghtml (Accessed 10 April 2002).

has yielded reliable estimates of the rates of suicidal behavior (e.g., Andrews and Lewinsohn, 1992; CDC, 2000; Fergusson and Lynskey, 1995; Garrison et al., 1993; Gould et al., 1998; Joffe et al., 1988; Kandel et al., 1991; Kashani et al., 1989; Roberts and Chen, 1995; Swanson et al., 1992; Velez and Cohen, 1988; Windle et al., 1992). Of these studies, the largest and the most representative is the Youth Risk Behavior Survey (YRBS) (CDC, 2000), conducted by the CDC. The following estimates of suicidal ideation and attempts are from this YRBS national school-based survey of students in grades 9–12, primarily 14–18 years of age. These estimates are consistent with those cited in the epidemiologic literature (e.g., Fergusson and Lynskey, 1995; Garrison et al., 1993; Gould et al., 1998; Lewinsohn et al., 1996; Velez and Cohen, 1988). The YRBS indicated that 19.3% of high school students had "seriously considered attempting suicide" during the past year. Nearly 15% of students made a specific plan to attempt suicide, 8.3% reported any suicide attempt during the past year, and 2.6% of students made a medically serious suicide attempt that required medical attention.

### Age
The developmental trends for completed and attempted suicide vary somewhat. Suicide attempts, like completed suicides, are relatively rare among prepubertal

children, and they increase in frequency through adolescence. Suicide attempts reach a peak between 16 and 18 years of age, after which there is a marked decline in frequency as adolescents enter early adulthood (Kessler et al., 1999; Lewinsohn et al., 2001). This significant drop in frequency is evident only for young women (Lewinsohn et al., 2001). As noted earlier, the incidence of completed suicide increases until it reaches a level in early adulthood that is maintained for a few more decades.

### Gender

A gender paradox in suicide exists in the U.S. in that completed suicide is more common among males, yet suicidal ideation and attempts are more common among females (CDC, 2000; Garrison et al., 1993; Gould et al., 1998; Lewinsohn et al., 1996). The YRBS indicated that female students were significantly more likely to have seriously considered attempting suicide (24.9%), made a specific plan (18.3%), and attempted suicide (10.9%) than male students (13.7%, 10.9%, and 5.7% respectively). A possible explanation for the elevated rates of suicide attempts among teenage girls is their elevated rates of depression (Lewinsohn et al., 1996, 2001). The YRBS, however, found no significant difference by gender in the prevalence of *medically serious* attempts requiring medical attention (3.1% females, 2.1% males). Methods of suicidal behavior favored by women, such as overdoses, tend to be less lethal than the methods favored by men, such as hanging (Moscicki, 1995). These gender-related method preferences have been postulated to explain the different gender ratio in completed versus attempted suicides in the U.S.

### Race/Ethnicity

There is evidence from a few epidemiologic studies that Latino youth living in the U.S. have higher rates of suicidal ideation and attempts than other youth groups (CDC, 2000; Roberts and Chen, 1995; Roberts et al., 1997); however, as noted earlier, Latinos do not appear to be overrepresented among *completed* suicides. The YRBS reported that Latino students (19.9%) were significantly more likely than African-American students (15.3%) to have seriously considered suicide. Making a specific plan was significantly more prevalent among Latino students (17.7%) than either white (12.4%) or African-American students (11.7%). Latino students (12.8%) were more likely to have made any suicide attempt than white (6.7%) or African-American (7.3%) students; however, there was no preponderance of medically serious attempts among Latinos (3.0%), as compared to whites (1.9%) or African-Americans (2.9%). Grunbaum et al. (1998) and Walter et al. (1995) did not find a higher prevalence of suicidal ideation or attempts among

Latinos. These equivocal findings highlight the need for further research in this area.

## Risk factors

The remainder of the chapter will focus on the main risk factors for youth suicide evaluated by the psychological autopsy studies (Appleby et al., 1999; Brent et al., 1988a, 1993a, 1996, 1999; Groholt et al., 1998; Ho et al., 1995; Houston et al., 2001; Lesage et al., 1994; Marttunen et al., 1991; Rich et al., 1986; Runeson, 1989; Shaffer et al., 1996; Shafii et al., 1985) that employed direct interviews of family and/or peer informants (Table 1.5), and the general population epidemiologic surveys of nonlethal suicidal behavior (Andrews and Lewinsohn, 1992; CDC, 1995, 1998; Fergusson and Lynskey, 1995; Garrison et al., 1993; Gould et al., 1998; Joffe et al., 1988; Kaltiala-Heino et al., 1999; Kandel et al., 1991; Kashani et al., 1989; Reinherz et al., 1995; Roberts and Chen, 1995; Swanson et al., 1992; Velez and Cohen, 1988; Windle et al., 1992) (Table 1.6). The current presentation of risk factors is based on a comprehensive, but not exhaustive, review of the most relevant English-language publications through 2001.

### Psychopathology

Psychological autopsy studies have determined that the majority of those who completed suicide had significant psychiatric problems, including previous suicidal behavior, depressive disorder, substance abuse, and conduct disorder. Generally, at least 90% of youth suicides have had at least one major psychiatric disorder. Depressive disorders are consistently the most prevalent disorders: 61% in the New York study (Shaffer et al., 1996), 64% in the Finnish national study (Marttunen et al., 1991), and 49% in the Pittsburgh study (Brent et al., 1993a). Female victims are more likely than males to have had an affective disorder. Substance abuse has been found to be a significant risk factor, with the exception of the Israeli study of male military conscripts (Apter et al., 1993). Substance abuse is more prevalent in older adolescent male suicide victims (Marttunen et al., 1991; Shaffer et al., 1996). A high prevalence of comorbidity between affective and substance abuse disorders has been found consistently. Discrepant results have been reported for bipolar disorder, with the Pittsburgh study reporting relatively high rates (Brent et al., 1988a, 1993a), while other studies report no or few bipolar cases (Marttunen et al., 1991; Runeson, 1989; Shaffer et al., 1994) (see Brent 1995, for a review of the psychiatric risk factors for youth suicide). Despite the generally high risk of suicide among people with schizophrenia, schizophrenia accounts for very few of all youth suicides (Brent et al., 1993a;

**Table 1.5.** Psychological autopsy studies of youth completed suicide

| Study | Number of suicides | Location | Age range (years) | Controls | Informants |
|---|---|---|---|---|---|
| Appleby et al. (1999) | 84 total 5 < 20 | Greater Manchester | 13–34 | 64 age- and gender-matched controls obtained through the general practices of the matched cases | Family member or close contact Available records |
| Apter et al. (1993) | 43 | Israeli military service | 18–21 | – | Preinduction medical exam and psychopathologic interview with victim |
| Brent et al. (1988a) | 27 | 3 counties that include and surround Pittsburgh, Pennsylvania | <20 | 56 suicidal inpatients (ages 13–19) | Parents or parental figure; peers or siblings Available records |
| Brent et al. (1993a) | 67 | 28 counties of western Pennsylvania (including Pittsburgh) | <20 | 67 age-, sex-, SES-, and county of residence-matched community controls | Parents or parental figure; siblings; friends; community controls Available records |
| Brent et al. (1996) | 58 total 37 new cases | See Brent et al. (1993a) | <20 | 58 controls from original sample | Primary caretaking parent, siblings, relatives, professional contacts |
| Brent et al. (1999) | 140 total 9 new cases | See Brent et al. (1993a) | <20 | 131 age-, sex, SES-, and county of residence-matched community controls | Parents or parental figure; siblings; friends; community controls Available records |
| Groholt et al. (1998) | 129 | Norway (nationwide) | 8–19 | 889 sex- and age-matched controls | Family, friends, health authorities Available records |
| Ho et al. (1995) | 239 total 139 < 20 | Hong Kong | 10–24 | No controls | Parents; relatives; friends; classmates; doctors Available records |

| Study | Sample size | Location | Age range | Controls | Sources of information |
|---|---|---|---|---|---|
| Houston et al. (2001) | 27 total 9 < 20 | 4 counties in the UK that include Northamptonshire, Berkshire, Buckinghamshire, and Oxfordshire | 15–24 | 22 deliberate self harm patients matched for age | Relatives; friends Available records |
| Lesage et al. (1994) | 75 total ?:<20 | Greater Montreal and Quebec City | 18–35 | Age-, marital-, occupation matched community controls | Parents; siblings; spouse; friends or other relatives Available records |
| Marttunen et al. (1991) | 53 | Finland (nationwide) | 13–19 | – | Parents; health professionals Available records |
| Rich et al. (1986) | 133 under age 30 14 < 20 | San Diego County, California | <30 vs ≥30 (subset <20) | – | Family members; spouses; acquaintances; employers; other witnesses; physicians, and other professionals Available records |
| Runeson (1989) | 58 total 9 < 20 | Gothenburg, Sweden | 15–29 | – | Parents; siblings; others; spouses; relatives; friends; employers; professionals Available records |
| Shaffer et al. (1996) | 120 | New York City and 28 surrounding counties in New York State, New Jersey, and Connecticut | <20 | 147 age-, sex-, and ethnic-matched community controls; 101 similarly matched hospitalized suicide attempters | Parents or other adult member of household; sibling or friend; school teacher; community control; attempter control Available records |
| Shafii et al. (1985) | 20 | Louisville and surrounding Jefferson County, Kentucky | 12–19 | 17 friends as matched-pair controls (closely matched for age, sex, education, SES, and religious background) | All members of family; friends; other relatives; significant others |

Abbreviations: SES, Socioeconomic status.

**Table 1.6. Epidemiologic studies of youth suicidal ideation/aftermath**

| Study | N | Age or grade | Location | Assessment |
|---|---|---|---|---|
| Andrews and Lewinsohn (1992) | 1 710 | 14–18 years old | U.S.–Oregon | School-based survey |
| CDC (2000) | 15 349 | Grades 9–12 | U.S.–Nationwide | School-based survey |
| Fergusson and Lynskey (1995) | 954 | Birth to 16 years old | New Zealand | Household survey |
| Garrison et al. (1991) | 1 542 | 12–14 years old | U.S.–South Carolina | School-based survey |
| | | | | Stage 2–home interview |
| Garrison et al. (1993) | 3 764 | 9th–12th grades | U.S.–South Carolina | School-based survey |
| Gould et al. (1998) | 1 285 | 9–17 years old | U.S.–CT, GA, NY, PR | Household survey |
| Joffe et al. (1988) | 1 256 | 12–16 years old | Canada–Ontario | Household survey |
| Kaltiala-Heino et al. (1999) | 16 410 | 14–16 years old | Finland | School-based survey |
| Kandel et al. (1991) | 593 | 9th and 11th grades | U.S.–Northeast | School-based survey |
| Kashani et al. (1989) | 210 | 8, 12, and 17 years old | U.S.–Missouri | Household survey |
| Reinherz et al. (1995) | 400 | Primarily 9th and 12th grades | U.S.–Northeast | School-based survey |
| Roberts and Chen (1995) | 2 614 | 6th–8th grades | U.S.–New Mexico | School-based survey |
| Swanson et al. (1992) | 4 157 | 12–17 years old | U.S.–Texas and New Mexico | School-based survey |
| Velez and Cohen (1988) | 752 | 9–18 years old | U.S.–New York | Household survey |
| Windle et al. (1992) | 11 400 | 8th and 10th grades | U.S.–20 states | School-based survey |

Shaffer et al., 1996). Between one-quarter and one-third of youth suicide victims have made a prior suicide attempt (Brent, 1995; Brent et al., 1993a; Shaffer et al., 1996). Prior suicidal behavior confers a particularly high risk for boys (i.e., a 30-fold increase); for girls, the risk is also elevated (i.e., approximately threefold), but it is not as potent a risk factor as major depression (Shaffer et al., 1996).

The psychiatric problems of suicide *attempters* are quite similar to those of adolescents who *complete* suicide, and the gender-specific diagnostic profiles of suicide attempters parallel those of suicide victims (e.g., Andrews and Lewinsohn, 1992; Beautrais et al., 1996; Gould et al., 1998). However, despite the overlap between suicidal *attempts* and *ideation* (Andrews and Lewinsohn, 1992; Reinherz et al., 1995) and the significant prediction of future attempts from ideation (Lewinsohn et al., 1994; Reinherz et al., 1995), the diagnostic profiles of attempters and ideators are somewhat distinct (Gould et al., 1998). In particular, substance abuse/dependence is more strongly associated with suicide attempts than with suicidal ideation (Garrison et al., 1993; Gould et al., 1998; Kandel, 1988).

## Cognitive factors

Hopelessness has been shown to be associated with completed suicide in youth (Shaffer et al., 1996). However, the vast majority of the victims who expressed hopelessness before their death had met criteria for a mood disorder; thus, it is unclear whether hopelessness per se or depression accounts for the association. Within clinical (Rotheram-Borus and Trautman, 1988) and nonclinical samples of youth (Cole, 1988; Lewinsohn et al., 1994; Reifman and Windle, 1995), hopelessness has not consistently proven to be an independent predictor of suicidality, once depression is taken into account. Other dysfunctional cognitive styles have been reported to differentiate suicidal from nonsuicidal youth (Asarnow et al., 1987; Rotheram-Borus et al., 1990). Poor interpersonal problem-solving ability has been found to be associated with suicidality within clinical samples of adolescents (Asarnow et al., 1987; Rotheram-Borus et al., 1990). Rotheram-Borus and colleagues (1990) reported that female attempters from minority groups generated fewer alternatives to solving stressful problems than both a consecutive series of nonsuicidal adolescent outpatients and community controls. Depression did not account for these cognitive differences.

## Stressful life events

The psychological autopsy research generally supports the association of life stressors, such as interpersonal losses (e.g., breaking up with a girlfriend or boyfriend) and legal or disciplinary problems, with suicide (Brent et al., 1993b;

Gould et al., 1996; Marttunen et al., 1993; Rich et al., 1988; Runeson, 1990). The prevalence of specific stressors has been reported to vary depending on the psychiatric disorder of the suicide victim (Brent et al., 1993b; Gould et al., 1996; Marttunen et al., 1994; Rich et al., 1988; Runeson, 1990). Interpersonal losses are consistently reported to be more common among suicide victims with substance abuse disorders (Brent et al., 1993b; Gould et al., 1996; Marttunen et al., 1994; Rich et al., 1988). Legal or disciplinary crises were more common in victims with disruptive disorders (Brent et al., 1993b; Gould et al., 1996) or substance abuse disorders (Brent et al., 1993b). Despite these associations, specific stressors, such as legal and disciplinary problems, are still associated with an increased risk of suicide, even after adjusting for psychopathology (Brent et al., 1993b; Gould et al., 1996).

Similar stressful life events have been reported to be risk factors for suicide attempts among adolescents (Lewinsohn et al., 1996; Beautrais et al., 1997). Beautrais and her colleagues (1997) reported that interpersonal losses and conflicts and legal problems remained significant risk factors for serious suicide attempts after controlling for antecedent social, family, and personality factors.

## Family factors
### Family history
A family history of suicidal behavior greatly increases the risk of completed suicide, as reported in several studies (Brent et al., 1988a, 1994; Gould et al., 1996; Shaffer, 1974; Shafii et al., 1985). The reasons for this familial aggregation are not yet known. It may reflect a genetic factor, rather than a general index of family chaos and psychopathology, since a family history has been shown to increase suicide risk even when studies have controlled for poor parent–child relationships and parental psychopathology (Brent, 1996; Gould et al., 1996). Furthermore, familial aggregation seems more likely to be due to genetic factors than imitation, based on Schulsinger's (1980) adoption study that reported a greater concordance of suicidal behavior with biologic relatives than adoptive relatives.

Studies have also found high rates of parental psychopathology, particularly depression and substance abuse, to be associated with completed suicide in adolescence (Brent et al., 1988a, 1994; Gould et al., 1996), as well as with suicidal ideation and attempts (e.g., Fergusson and Lynskey, 1995; Joffe et al., 1988; Kashani et al., 1989). Brent and his colleagues (1994) reported that a family history of depression and substance abuse significantly increased the risk of completed suicide, even after controlling for the victim's psychopathology. They concluded that familial psychopathology adds to suicide risk by mechanisms other than merely increasing the liability for similar psychopathology in an adolescent. In contrast, Gould and her colleagues (1996) found that the impact of parental psychopathology no longer contributed to the youth's suicide risk after the study controlled for the youth's psychopathology. To date, it is unclear precisely how familial psychopathology increases the risk for suicide.

### Parental divorce

Two large-scale studies with general population controls (Brent et al., 1993a, 1994; Gould et al., 1996) have found that suicide victims are more likely to come from nonintact families of origin, although the overall impact of separation/divorce on suicide risk is small. In the New York Study (Gould et al., 1996), the association between separation/divorce and suicide decreased when accounting for parental psychopathology. This is consistent with the reported association of divorce and parental depression (Weissman et al., 1992). Brent et al. (1994) also showed a trend towards higher rates of mental disorder in the parents of both suicide victims and community controls in nonintact families of origin, and reported that a nonintact family of origin was not associated with increased suicide risk after controlling for family history of psychopathology (Brent et al., 1994). Overall, the impact of divorce on suicide risk is quite small in the psychological autopsy studies.

### Parent–child relationships

The New York and Pittsburgh studies, which are the two large controlled studies that have been conducted to date, both report problematic parent–child relationships. The New York Study (Gould et al., 1996) reported that suicide victims had significantly less frequent and less satisfying communication with their mothers and fathers. There was no evidence of more negative interactions between victims and their parents, nor was there a greater history of severe physical punishment. The Pittsburgh study (Brent et al., 1994) reported that suicide victims were more likely to be exposed to parent–child discord and physical abuse. The reason for the discrepancies regarding parent–child conflict and physical abuse in the New York and Pittsburgh studies is unclear since the studies used a similar methodology with demographically matched community controls and comparable informants. Family aggression has been noted to be prevalent in suicidal children identified in the general community (Beautrais et al., 1996), as well as in suicidal children seen in clinical settings (see Spirito et al., 1989, for a review).

## Contagion

Research has indicated that "outbreaks" or clusters of completed suicides in the U.S. occur primarily among teenagers and young adults, with only sporadic and minimal effects beyond 24 years of age (Gould et al., 1990a, 1990b). Similar age-specific patterns have been reported for clusters of *attempted* suicides (Gould et al., 1994). Estimates of the percentage of teenage suicides that occur in clusters average between 1% and 2%, with considerable variation by State and year, yielding estimates from less than 1% to 13% (Gould et al., 1990a). These estimates only reflect mortality data and, thus, do not include clusters of attempted suicides (Gould et al., 1994). While most of the research on clustering of youth suicide has reported significant clustering (Brent et al., 1989; Gould et al., 1990a, 1990b, 1994), one study has found no clustering of adolescent suicides within a particular locale for a specified time frame (Gibbons et al., 1990). Given the relative rarity of suicide clusters, the examination of one location does not yield enough statistical power to clearly detect clustering.

There is considerable evidence that suicide stories in the mass media, including newspaper articles (Barraclough et al., 1977; Blumenthal and Bergner, 1973; Etzersdorfer et al., 1992; Ganzeboom and de Hann, 1982; Ishii, 1991; Jonas, 1992; Motto, 1970; Phillips, 1974, 1979, 1980; Stack, 1989, 1990; Wasserman, 1984), television news reports (Bollen and Phillips, 1982; Phillips and Carstensen, 1986), and fictional dramatizations (Gould and Shaffer, 1986; Gould et al., 1988; Holding, 1974, 1975; Schmidtke and Hafner, 1988), are followed by a significant increase in the number of suicides (see Gould, 2001; Schmidtke and Schaller, 2000; Stack, 2000 for reviews). These studies generally employ an "ecological" analysis of death certificate data, in which comparisons are made between the number of suicides in geographic areas with and without a media exposure, or in the same locale before and after an exposure. The magnitude of the increase appears to be proportional to the amount of publicity given to the story (Bollen and Phillips, 1981; Motto, 1970; Phillips, 1974, 1979; Wasserman, 1984). The impact of suicide stories on subsequent completed suicides has been reported to be greatest for teenagers (Phillips and Carstensen, 1986). Despite this ample body of literature supportive of the hypothesis that suicides dramatized in the media encourage imitation, a few studies did not report an association between media reports and subsequent suicides (Berman, 1988; Phillips and Paight, 1987) or found only an association among adolescent, not adult, suicides (Kessler et al., 1989). Interactive factors that may moderate the impact of media stories include characteristics of the stories, individual reader/viewer attributes, and the social context of the stories (Gould, 2001).

Recently, alternative research strategies have been introduced to study suicide contagion. In contrast to the ecological designs that utilize death certificate data to study differential community suicide rates, the newer paradigms include experimental designs that examine youths' reactions to media dramatizations or written vignettes about suicide (e.g., Biblarz et al., 1991; Gibson and Range, 1991), content-analytic studies that assess the impact of specific display and content characteristics of media stories (Fekete and Schmidtke, 1995), and case–control psychologic autopsies of suicide clusters (Davidson et al., 1989; Gould et al., 1995). An ongoing psychological autopsy study funded by the National Institute of Mental Health, examining 53 suicide clusters that occurred in the U.S. between 1988 and 1996, should soon be able to identify the factors that initiate a suicide "outbreak" (Gould, 1999).

## Socioenvironmental factors

### Socioeconomic status

Little information is available in the psychological autopsy literature on the association of socioeconomic status (SES) and suicide. Psychological autopsy studies either matched the cases and controls on this factor (e.g., Brent et al., 1993a) or did not report it. There are two studies with available information: Brent and his colleagues (1988a) reported no difference between suicide victims and suicidal inpatients in SES, and Gould et al. (1996) reported a differential ethnic effect in a comparison between suicide victims and community controls. Only African-American, but neither white nor Latino suicide victims, had a significantly higher SES than their general population counterparts. Specifically, there was an overrepresentation of the middle class and an underrepresentation of the poorest strata among the African-American suicides.

Higher rates of sociodemographic disadvantage have been found among youth making serious suicide attempts compared to community controls (Beautrais et al., 1996). Specifically an increased risk of suicide attempts was found among youth who lacked formal educational qualifications, had low annual incomes, and had changed residence within the previous six months.

### School and work problems

Significant suicide risks are posed by difficulties in school, not working, not being in school, and not going to college (Gould et al., 1996). Youngsters who are "drifting," affiliated with neither a school nor a work institution, appear to be at substantial risk for completing suicide. Shaffer (1974) noted that many suicides among children under the age of 15 took place after a period of absence from school and that a similar phenomenon had been reported for children who had attempted suicide (Teicher and Jacobs, 1966), suggesting that social isolation associated with absence from school may facilitate suicidal behavior.

Individuals who have made suicide attempts also appear more likely to have difficulties in school. Beautrais et al. (1996) reported that serious suicide attempters were more likely to have "no formal educational qualification," which is roughly equivalent to dropping out of high school, or not going to college. Lewis et al. (1988) found that suicide attempters in a community-based sample had significantly lower school achievement than nonattempters. However, the relationship between attempted suicide and low school achievement was explained by the effects of depression.

## Sexual orientation

The New York Study (Shaffer et al., 1995) is the only psychological autopsy study of youth suicide, to date, to examine the association of sexual orientation and suicide. Homosexuality was defined as having had homosexual experiences or having declared a homosexual orientation. Three suicide victims and no controls met these criteria. This difference was not statistically significant. All three suicide victims demonstrated evidence of significant psychiatric disorder before death, and in no instance did the suicide directly follow an episode of stigmatization. Given the opportunities for underreporting by informants, the psychological autopsy paradigm is somewhat limited in its capacity to assess the role of sexual orientation.

Recent epidemiologic studies suggest a significant association between sexual orientation and nonlethal suicidal behavior. In a survey of Minnesota high school students, Remafedi et al. (1998) reported a significantly higher rate of suicide attempts among gay/bisexual males compared to heterosexual males. Utilizing the YRBS in Massachusetts, Faulkner and Cranston (1998) and Garofalo and colleagues (1998) also found higher rates of suicide attempts among homosexual and bisexual adolescents. In a 21-year longitudinal study of a birth cohort of 1265 children born in Christchurch New Zealand, gay, lesbian, and bisexual youth were at increased risks of suicidal ideation and suicide attempts (Fergusson et al., 1999).

## Biological risk factors

There is evidence that abnormalities in the serotonergic system are associated with suicide, as well as with impulsivity and aggression (e.g., Blumenthal, 1990; Mann and Stoff, 1997). Low levels of serotonin among suicide attempters have been found to be predictive of future completed suicide (Asberg et al., 1986). This dysregulation in the serotonergic system appears to occur in a range of psychiatric disorders. The examination of biologic factors associated with suicide has largely been limited to studies of adults (see Mann and Stoff (1997), for a comprehensive review of these studies). The few studies examining children and adolescents suggest a similar association between serotonin abnormalities and suicidal behavior. Pfeffer et al. (1998) reported that whole blood tryptophan levels were significantly lower in prepubertal children with a recent history of a suicide attempt. Greenhill et al. (1995) found a relationship between serotonin measures and medically serious attempts within a small sample of adolescent suicide attempter inpatients with major depressive disorder. Further research is needed to determine whether serotonin-related measures could be predictive of youth suicidal behavior.

## Analysis of research

This section will evaluate the sources of data and research used to yield our current knowledge of the risk factors for suicidal behavior in youth. We review three major sources of information – official mortality statistics, psychological autopsy studies, and epidemiologic surveys of suicide attempters.

### Official mortality statistics

There is a continuing concern and debate regarding the validity of suicide mortality data (Jobes et al., 1987; Mohler and Earls, 2001; Monk, 1987; O'Carroll, 1989; O'Donnell and Farmer, 1995; Phillips and Ruth, 1993; Sainsbury, 1983). The problem of underreporting or biased reporting of suicides in official mortality statistics has been the focus of many investigations (see Jobes et al., 1987; O'Carroll, 1989; for reviews). Efforts to develop operational criteria for the determination of suicide by coroners or medical examiners have attempted to address these problems (Rosenberg et al., 1988). There is still some suggestion that underreporting or misclassification of death verdicts may vary as a function of the method of death (O'Carroll, 1989; Phillips and Ruth, 1993), the race/ethnicity of the victim (Mohler and Earls, 2001; Phillips and Ruth, 1993), and the victim's age (Mohler and Earls, 2001). However, Mohler and Earls (2001) found that, despite misclassification, recent official mortality data reflect the true direction of trends in youth suicide: the increase in suicide rates for male adolescents between 1979 and 1994 was supported after correcting for misclassification.

Barraclough (1973) suggested that the combination of the cause of death labeled "injury undetermined whether accidentally or purposefully inflicted" with suicide is likely to provide the most accurate representation of the "true" suicide rate, and that the comparison of these two categories can provide a current estimate of the magnitude of possible underreporting. Table 1.7 presents the rates of these two categories for populations of different ages, gender and ethnicity. Using this procedure, the suicide rate per 100 000 for 10- to 14-year-olds in 1999 would be increased from 1.2 to 1.4; in 15- to 19-year-olds from

**Table 1.7.** Rates* of suicide and undetermined deaths by age in the U.S., 1999

|  | 1999 | | |
|---|---|---|---|
|  | Suicide | Undetermined | Total |
| **10–14** |  |  |  |
| Total | 1.2 | 0.2 | 1.4 |
| Males | 1.9 | 0.3 | 2.2 |
| Females | 0.5 | – | 0.5 |
| Whites | 1.3 | 0.2 | 1.5 |
| African-Americans | 0.9 | – | 0.9 |
| **15–19** |  |  |  |
| Total | 8.2 | 0.8 | 9.0 |
| Males | 13.3 | 1.3 | 14.6 |
| Females | 2.8 | 0.3 | 3.1 |
| Whites | 8.6 | 0.8 | 9.4 |
| African-Americans | 5.9 | 0.8 | 6.7 |
| **20–24** |  |  |  |
| Total | 12.7 | 1.5 | 14.2 |
| Males | 21.6 | 2.3 | 23.9 |
| Females | 3.5 | 0.7 | 4.2 |
| Whites | 13.1 | 1.5 | 14.6 |
| African-Americans | 10.8 | 1.7 | 12.5 |

* Per 100 000.

*Source:* CDC National Center for Injury Prevention and Control, Office of Statistics and Programming. CDC Wonder Mortality Data Request Screen. Available at http://wonder.cdc.gov/mortsql.ghtml (accessed 10 April 2002).

8.2 to 9.0; in the population age 20- to 24-year-olds, from 12.7 to 14.2. Thus, the magnitude of potential underreporting appears to be minimal. There is little variation in the pattern of underreporting deaths by gender or ethnicity in 1999. In summary, although possible sources of bias may remain, suicide mortality data is considered a fairly robust source of information (Monk, 1987; Moscicki, 1995; O'Carroll, 1989; Sainsbury, 1983; Shaffer and Hicks, 1994).

## Psychological autopsy studies

The psychological autopsy method has been an important research strategy for the identification of psychiatric and psychosocial risk factors for suicide. It is a procedure to reconstruct the social and psychological circumstances of a suicide victim by interviewing surviving informants and abstracting information from records collected during the victim's life. Within the past decade, there have been several psychological autopsy studies of youth suicide that have employed direct interviews of family and/or peer informants within an epidemiologic sampling frame of consecutively determined suicides in a predefined geographical area (Apter et al., 1993; Brent et al., 1988a, 1993a; Marttunen et al., 1991; Rich et al., 1986; Runeson, 1989; Shaffer et al., 1996; Shafii et al., 1985). Other postmortem investigations that employed review of records rather than informant interviews (e.g., Hawton et al., 1999) are not included in the review. Of the psychological autopsy studies, five had more than 50 cases of adolescent suicide (Brent et al., 1993a, 1996, 1999; Groholt et al., 1998; Ho et al., 1995; Marttunen et al., 1991; Shaffer et al., 1996); eight were controlled (Appleby et al., 1999; Brent et al., 1988a, 1993a, 1996, 1999; Groholt et al., 1998; Houston et al., 2001; Lesage et al., 1994; Shaffer et al., 1996; Shafii et al., 1985); five were performed in the U.S. (Brent et al., 1988a, 1993a, 1996, 1999; Rich et al., 1986; Shaffer et al., 1996; Shafii et al., 1985); five in England and Europe (Appleby et al., 1999; Groholt et al., 1998; Houston et al., 2001; Marttunen et al., 1991; Runeson, 1989); one in Israel (Apter et al., 1993); one in Hong Kong (Ho et al., 1995); and one in Canada (Lesage et al., 1994).

Few reports describe the reliability and validity of the psychological autopsy method (Beskow et al., 1990, Brent et al., 1988b; Velting et al., 1998). Brent et al. (1988b) found that neither the informants' affective symptomatology nor the time interval between the death and the interview affected the reports about the victims. Velting et al. (1998) reported that the unavailability of the victim's perspective leads to an underestimation of the prevalence of psychopathology in general, and major depression and alcohol abuse in particular. The employment of multiple informants, including peers, attempts to address this limitation by providing a broader base of information than can be provided by the parent (or other adult) alone.

Overall, the consistency in the results across different psychological autopsy studies of youth suicide, reported earlier in the chapter, reinforces our confidence in the validity of the methodology.

## Epidemiological surveys of nonlethal suicidal behavior

Epidemiologic population-based surveys provide a means to estimate the prevalence and identify the risk factors of suicidal behavior. Clinical samples of suicide attempters can provide information regarding the course of suicidal behavior in a referred population, and, obviously, they are also an important source for treatment trials of suicidal behavior. However, a major limitation of research on clinical samples is that it does not include the vast majority of suicide attempters in the community. Among all attempters, only about one-third have received any mental health services (Velez and Cohen, 1988) and as few as 12% of attempters receive medical treatment following their attempt (Smith and Crawford, 1986). Furthermore, due to higher referral rates of individuals with multiple problems (Berkson, 1946), these problems can appear to be associated in referred samples, even though they may not be associated in population-based samples (Fleiss, 1981).

There have been several epidemiologic population-based surveys of youth suicide. These vary with regard to the sampling frame (household vs. school); generalizability (local communities vs. national); assessments (time frame, severity criteria, mode, comprehensiveness, anonymity); and informant (multiple vs. self-report only). The differential impact of these methodological features will be discussed below.

### Sampling frame

There have been fewer household-based surveys (five to date: Fergusson and Lynskey, 1995; Gould et al., 1998; Joffe et al., 1988; Kashani et al., 1989; Velez and Cohen, 1988) than school-based surveys (at least 30 to date: e.g., Andrews and Lewinsohn, 1992; CDC, 1995; Garrison et al., 1993; Kandel et al., 1991; Roberts and Chen, 1995; Swanson et al., 1992; Windle et al., 1992). Household surveys are generally more expensive and less efficient than school-based surveys, a probable explanation for the preponderance of the latter. The vast majority of students attend schools, thus school-based surveys offer the unique opportunity to access large populations of youths in centralized locations. Nevertheless, household samples can capture youngsters not in school (e.g., dropouts), and lend themselves to longer, comprehensive assessments using multiple informants. All of the houshold-based surveys have employed interviews with youth and parents, whereas the school-based surveys, with few exceptions (Andrews and Lewinsohn, 1992; Garrison et al., 1991; Reinherz et al., 1995), have employed self-report questionnaires. The estimates of suicide attempts derived from the household surveys (3%) are at the lower bound of the estimates from the school-based surveys (3% to 8%). Methodological features in some of the school-based surveys, such as the use of *anonymous* questionnaires, may account for the higher estimates (see below).

### Generalizability

The only nationally representative surveys of youth in the U.S. are the school-based surveys conducted by the CDC, utilizing the YRBS (CDC, 2000). However, there have been several other large-scale studies, not limited to one community (e.g., Andrews and Lewinsohn, 1992; Garrison et al., 1991; Gould et al., 1998; Swanson et al., 1992; Windle et al., 1992). With rare exception (Smith and Crawford, 1986; Windle et al., 1992), the school-based studies have only included public schools, with commensurate limitations to their generalizability. Also, school-based surveys have not included individuals who have dropped out of school, a subgroup who are at higher suicidal risk (Gould et al., 1996).

## Assessments

The *time frame* of the assessments, per se, does not appear to affect prevalence estimates. It is unclear why estimates derived from studies employing lifetime estimates do not exceed those from studies using a time frame of "the past year," unless the participants are essentially ignoring the time frame.

The employment of a *severity criterion on* substantially reduces estimates of attempts and ideation. Estimates of attempts resulting in injuries or medical attention (CDC, 1995, 1998; Garrison et al., 1993) are 75% less than estimates of *any* attempt. Similarly, actually having a plan is less prevalent than "serious" ideation, which is more rare than any ideation.

The *mode* of the assessments (interview vs. questionnaire) is confounded with the sampling frame (household vs. school-based) and informants (multiple vs. self-report only), as described previously; therefore, it is unclear why estimates from studies employing interviews tend to yield lower estimates than studies using self-administered questionnaires. There is some research to suggest that individuals admit more sensitive behaviors and feelings on a paper-and-pencil questionnaire than to a person administering an interview (Cain, 1989; Sudman and Bradburn, 1974; Turner et al., 1992).

The *comprehensiveness* of the assessment, with regard to correlates and risk factors of suicidal behavior, greatly varies across studies. Diagnostic information is routinely assessed during the interview protocols (Andrews and Lewinsohn, 1992; Fergusson and Lynskey, 1995; Gould et al., 1998; Joffe et al., 1988; Kashani et al., 1989; Reinherz et al., 1995; Velez and Cohen, 1988) but appears to be beyond the scope of the vast majority of school-based studies employing questionnaires. Stressful life events, symptom scales, hopelessness, and other risk behaviors are included in most studies.

The *anonymity* of the questionnaire assessment has a critical impact on prevalence estimates (Safer, 1997). The highest estimates of suicide attempts and ideation have been derived largely from studies employing anonymous assessments (Adcock et al., 1991; CDC, 2000; Dubow et al., 1989; Felts et al., 1992; Harkavy Friedman et al., 1987; Riggs et al., 1990; Smith and Crawford, 1986;

Swanson et al., 1992). If the estimates from anonymous assessments are more valid, then prevention efforts incorporating screening procedures, which by design have to identify the youngster, might be missing some vulnerable individuals.

### Informant

Although it is recognized that multiple informants provide the most comprehensive assessment of a child or adolescent, the sole employment of youths' self-reports does not appear to compromise the assessment of suicidal behavior and ideation. Self-identification of problems by adolescents is highly correlated with a clinician's determination of need for treatment (Bird et al., 1990). Moreover, adolescents have been shown to be more likely than parents and other informants to identify suicidal ideation and past suicidal behavior (Andrews et al., 1993; Velez and Cohen, 1988), as well as depressive symptoms (Bird et al., 1990; Weissman et al., 1987a, 1987b). Thus, for suicidal ideation and behavior, and their major risk factors, it is likely that the adolescents can provide the most clinically relevant assessments of their psychological distress.

## Conclusions

Differences in the suicide rate by age, sex, and broad secular trends have been identified in national and international mortality statistics. The psychological autopsy studies and general population epidemiologic surveys of nonlethal suicidal behavior have highlighted mental illness, family characteristics, and stressful life events as key risk factors for youth suicide. These epidemiologic paradigms, using official mortality statistics, psychological autopsy interviews, and general population epidemiologic surveys of nonlethal suicidal behavior have yielded portraits of high-risk individuals (such as older males who are depressed and abusing alcohol and/or drugs), in high-risk situations (such as living in homes or communities with easy access to firearms, or where other suicides have occurred) who need to be targeted for prevention and treatment efforts.

## Acknowledgements

This work was made possible by NIMH Child Research Center Grant 5P50MH43878-08 and NIMH Project Grant R01 MH47559. Portions of the chapter were adapted from Gould and Kramer (2001). Youth suicide prevention. *Suicide and Life-Threatening Behavior*, **31**(Supplement), Spring: 6–31.

## REFERENCES

Adcock, A. G., Nagy, S., and Simpson, J. A. (1991). Selected risk factors in adolescent suicide attempts. *Adolescence*, **26**, 817–828.

Andrews, J. A. and Lewinsohn, P. M. (1992). Suicidal attempts among older adolescents: prevalence and co-occurrence with psychiatric disorders. *Journal of the American Academy of Child and Adolescent Psychiatry*, **31**, 655–662.

Andrews, V. C., Garrison, C. Z., Jackson, K. L., Addy, C. L., and McKeown, R. E. (1993). Mother–adolescent agreement on the symptoms and diagnoses of adolescent depression and conduct disorders. *Journal of the American Academy of Child and Adolescent Psychiatry*, **32**, 731–738.

Andrus, J. K., Fleming, D. W., Heumann, M. A., Wassell, J. T., Hopkins, D. D., and Gordon, J. (1991). Surveillance of attempted suicide among adolescents in Oregon, 1988. *American Journal of Public Health*, **81**, 1067–1069.

Appleby, L., Cooper, J., Amos, T., and Faragher, B. (1999). Psychological autopsy study of suicides by people aged under 35. *British Journal of Psychiatry*, **175**, 168–174.

Apter, A., Bleich, A., King, R., Kron, S., Fluch, A., Kotler, M., and Cohen, D. J. (1993). Death without warning? A clinical postmortem study of suicide in 43 Israeli adolescent males. *Archives of General Psychiatry*, **50**, 138–142.

Asarnow, J., Carlson, G., and Guthrie, D. (1987). Coping strategies, self perceptions, hopelessness, and perceived family environments in depressed and suicidal children. *Journal of Consulting and Clinical Psychology*, **55**, 361–366.

Asberg, M., Nordstrom, P., and Traskman-Bendz, L. (1986). Biological factor in suicide. In Roy, A. (ed.), *Suicide* (pp. 47–71). Baltimore, MD: Williams and Wilkins.

Barraclough, B. M. (1973). Differences between national suicide rates. *British Journal of Psychiatry*, **122**, 95–96.

Barraclough, B. M., Bunch, J., Nelson, B., and Sainsbury, P. (1974). A hundred cases of suicide: clinical aspects. *British Journal of Psychiatry*, **125**, 355–373.

Barraclough, B. M., Shepherd, D., and Jennings, C. (1977). Do newspaper reports of coroners' inquests incite people to commit suicide? *British Journal of Psychiatry*, **131**, 258–532.

Beautrais, A. L., Joyce, P. R., and Mulder, R. T. (1996). Risk factors for serious suicide attempts among youths aged 13 through 24 years. *Journal of the American Academy of Child and Adolescent Psychiatry*, **35**(9), 1174–1182.

Beautrais, A. L., Joyce, P. R., and Mulder, R. T. (1997). Precipitating factors and life events in serious suicide attempts among youths aged 13 through 24 years. *Journal of the American Academy of Child and Adolescent Psychiatry*, **36**(11), 1543–1551.

Berkson, J. (1946). Limitations of the application of fourfold table analysis to hospital data. *Biometrics Bulletin*, **2**, 47–53.

Berman, A. L. (1988). Fictional depiction of suicide in television films and imitation effects. *American Journal of Psychiatry*, **145**, 982–986.

Berman, A. L. and Jobes, D. A. (1995). Suicide prevention in adolescents (age 12–18). *Suicide and Life-Threatening Behavior*, **25**(1), 143–154.

Beskow, J., Runeson, B., and Asgard, U. (1990). Psychological autopsies: methods and ethics. *Suicide and Life-Threatening Behavior*, **20**(4), 307–323.

Biblarz, A., Brown, R. M., Biblarz, D. N., Pilgrim, M., and Baldree, B. F. (1991). Media influence on attitudes toward suicide. *Suicide and Life-Threatening Behavior*, **21**, 374–384.

Bird, H. R., Yager, T., Staghezza, B., and Gould, M. S. (1990). Impairment in the epidemiological measurement of childhood psychopathology in the community. *Journal of the American Academy of Child and Adolescent Psychiatry*, **29**, 796–803.

Blumenthal, S. J. (1990). Youth suicide: risk factors assessment, and treatment of adolescent and young adult suicidal patients. *Psychiatric Clinics of North America*, **13**, 511–556.

Blumenthal, S. and Bergner, L. (1973). Suicide and newspaper: a replicated study. *American Journal of Psychiatry*, **130**, 468–471.

Bollen, K. A. and Phillips, D. P. (1981). Suicidal motor vehicle fatalities in Detroit: a replication. *American Journal of Sociology*, **87**, 404–412.

Bollen, K. A. and Phillips, D. P. (1982). Imitative suicides: a national study of the effect of television news stories. *American Sociological Review*, **47**, 802–809.

Boyd, J. H. (1983). The increasing rate of suicide by firearms. *New England Journal of Medicine*, **308**, 872–874.

Boyd, J. H. and Moscicki, E. K. (1986). Firearms and youth suicide. *American Journal of Public Health*, **76**, 1240–1242.

Brent, D. A. (1995). Risk factors for adolescent suicide and suicidal behavior: mental and substance abuse disorders, family environmental factors, and life stress. *Suicide and Life-Threatening Behavior*, **25**, 52–63.

Brent, D. A. (1996). Familial factors in suicide and suicidal behavior. *Lifesavers: The Quarterly Newsletter of the American Suicide Foundation*, **8**, 2–3.

Brent, D. A., Perper, J. A., and Allman, C. J. (1987). Alcohol, firearms, and suicide among youth: temporal trends in Allegheny County, PA, 1960–1983. *Journal of the American Medical Association*, **257**, 3369–3372.

Brent, D. A., Perper, J. A., Goldstein, C. E., Kilko, D. J., Allan, M. J., Allman, C. J., and Zelenak, J. P. (1988a). Risk factors for adolescent suicide: a comparison of adolescent suicide victims with suicidal inpatients. *Archives of General Psychiatry*, **45**, 581–588.

Brent, D. A., Perper, J. A., Kolko, D. J., and Zelenak, J. P. (1988b). The psychological autopsy: methodological considerations for the study of adolescent suicide. *Journal of the American Academy of Child and Adolescent Psychiatry*, **27**(3), 362–366.

Brent, D. A., Kerr, M. M., Goldstein, C., Boxigar, J., Wartella, M., and Allan, M. J. (1989). An outbreak of suicide and suicidal behavior in a high school. *Journal of the American Academy of Child and Adolescent Psychiatry*, **28**(6), 918–924.

Brent, D. A., Perper, J. A., Allman, C. J., Moritz, G. M., Wartella, M. E., and Zelenak, J. P. (1991). The presence and accessibility of firearms in the homes of adolescent suicides: a case–control study. *Journal of the American Medical Association*, **266**, 2989–2995.

Brent, D. A., Perper, J. A., Moritz, G., Allan, C., Friend, A., Roth, B. S., Schweers, J., Balach, L., and Baugher, M. (1993a). Psychiatric risk factors for adolescent suicide: a case control study. *Journal of the American Academy of Child and Adolescent Psychiatry*, **32**(3), 521–529.

Brent, D. A., Perper, J. A., Moritz, G., Baugher, M., Roth, C., Balach, L., and Schweers, J. (1993b). Stressful life events, psychopathology and adolescent suicide: a case control study. *Suicide and Life-Threatening Behavior*, **23**(3), 179–187.

Brent, D. A., Perper, J. A., Moritz, G. M., Baugher, M., Schweers, J., and Ross, C. (1993c). Firearms and adolescent suicide, a community case control study. *American Journal of Diseases of Children*, **147**, 1066–1071.

Brent, D. A., Perper, J. A., Moritz, G., Liotus, L., Schweers, J., Balach, L., and Roth, C. (1994). Familial risk factors for adolescent suicide: a case–control study. *Acta Psychiatrica Scandinavica*, **89**, 52–58.

Brent, D. A., Bridge, J., Johnson, B. A., and Connolly, J. (1996). Suicidal behavior runs in families: a controlled family study of adolescent suicide victims. *Archives of General Psychiatry*, **53**, 1145–1152.

Brent, D. A., Baugher, M., Bridge, J., Chen, T., and Chiappetta, L. (1999). Age- and sex-related risk factors for adolescent suicide. *Journal of the American Academy of Child and Adolescent Psychiatry*, **38**, 1497–1505.

Cain, V. S. (1989). In Fowler, F. J. (ed.), *Methodological Experiments in the National Survey of Health and Sexual Behavior* (pp. 241–258). Washington D.C: Department of Health and Human Services.

Canino, G. and Roberts, R. E. (2001). Suicidal behavior among Latino youth. *Suicide and Life-Threatening Behavior*, **31** (Supplement), 122–131.

Centers for Disease Control and Prevention (CDC) (1995). Youth Risk Behavior Surveillance – United States, 1993. *MMWR Morbidity and Mortality Weekly Report*, **44** (SS01), 1–56.

Centers for Disease Control and Prevention (CDC) (1996). Youth Risk Behavior Surveillance – United States, 1995. *MMWR Morbidity and Mortality Weekly Report*, **45** (SS04), 1–84.

Centers for Disease Control and Prevention (CDC) (1998). Youth Risk Behavior Surveillance – United States, 1997. *MMWR Morbidity and Mortality Weekly Report*, **47** (SS03), 1–89.

Centers for Disease Control and Prevention (CDC) (2000). Youth Risk Behavior Surveillance – United States, 1999. *MMWR Morbidity and Mortality Weekly Report*, **49** (SS05), 1–96.

Cole, D. A. (1988). Hopelessness, social desirability, depression, and parasuicide in two college student samples. *Journal of Consulting and Clinical Psychology*, **56**, 131–136.

Cutright, P., and Fernquist, R. M. (2000). Firearms and suicide: the American experience, 1926–1996. *Death Studies*, 24, 705–719.

Davidson, L. E., Rosenberg, M. L., Mercy, J. A., Franklin, J., and Simmons, J. T. (1989). An epidemiologic study of risk factors in two teenage suicide clusters. *Journal of the American Medical Association*, **262**, 2687–2692.

Demetriades, D., Murray, J., Myles, D., Chand, L., Sathyaragiswaran, L., Noguchi, T., Bongard, F. S., Vryer, G. H., and Gaspard, D. J. (1998). Epidemiology of major trauma and trauma deaths in Los Angeles County. *Journal of the American College of Surgery*, **187**, 373–383.

Diekstra, R. F., Kienhorst, C. W. M., and de Wilde, E. J. (1995). Suicide and suicidal behavior among adolescents. In Rutter, M. and Smith, D. (eds.), *Psychosocial Disorders in Young People, Time Trends and their Causes* (pp. 686–761). New York: John Wiley & Sons.

Dubow, E. F., Kausch, D. F., Blum, M. C., Reed, J., and Bush, E. (1989). Correlates of suicidal ideation and attempts in a community sample of junior high and high school students. *Journal of Clinical Child Psychology*, **18**, 158–166.

Etzersdorfer, E., Sonneck, G., and Nagel-Kuess, S. (1992). Newspaper reports and suicide. *New England Journal of Medicine*, **327**, 502–503.

Faulkner, A. H. and Cranston, K. (1998). Correlates of same-sex behavior in a random sample of Massachusetts high school students. *American Journal of Public Health*, **88**, 262–266.

Fekete, S. and Schmidtke, A. (1995). The impact of mass media reports on suicide and attitudes toward self-destruction: previous studies and some new data from Hungary and Germany. In Mishara, B. L. (ed.), *The Impact of Suicide* (pp. 142–155). New York: Springer.

Felts, W. M., Chenier, T., and Barnes, R. (1992). Drug use and suicide ideation and behavior among North Carolina public school students. *American Journal of Public Health*, **82**, 870–872.

Fergusson, D. M. and Lynskey, M. (1995). Childhood circumstances, adolescent adjustment, and suicide attempts in a New Zealand birth cohort. *Journal of the American Academy of Child and Adolescent Psychiatry*, **34**, 612–622.

Fergusson, D. M., Horwood, L. J., and Beautrais, A. L. (1999). Is sexual orientation related to mental health problems and suicidality in young people? *Archives of General Psychiatry*, **56**, 876–880.

Fleiss, J. L. (1981). *Statistical Methods for Rates and Proportions*. New York: John Wiley & Sons.

Ganzeboom, H. B. G. and de Haan, D. (1982). Gepubliceerde zelfmoorden en verhoging van sterfte door zelfmoord en ongelukken in Nederland 1972–1980. *Mens en Maatschappij*, **57**, 55–69.

Garofalo, R., Wolf, R., Cameron, M. S., Kessel, S., Palfrey, J., and DuRant, R. H. (1998). The association between health risk behaviors and sexual orientation among a school-based sample of adolescents. *Pediatrics*, **101**, 895–902.

Garrison, C. Z., Jackson, K. L., Addy, C. L., McKeown, R. E., and Waller, J. L. (1991). Suicidal behaviors in young adolescents. *American Journal of Epidemiology*, **133**(10), 1005–1014.

Garrison, C. Z., McKeown, R. E., Valois, R. F., and Vincent, M. L. (1993). Aggression, substance use, and suicidal behaviors in high school students. *American Journal of Public Health*, **83**, 179–184.

Gibbons, R. D., Clark, D. C., and Fawcett, J. A. (1990). A statistical method for evaluating suicide clusters and implementing cluster surveillance. *American Journal of Epidemiology*, **132**, 183–191.

Gibson, J. A. P. and Range, L. M. (1991). Are written reports of suicide and seeking help contagious? High schoolers' perceptions. *Journal of Applied Social Psychology*, **21**, 1517–1523.

Goodwin, R., Gould, M. S., Blanco, C., and Olfson, M. (2001). Prescription of psychotropic medications to youths in office-based practice. *Psychiatry Service*, **52**, 1081–1087.

Gould, M. S. (1999). *Psychological Autopsy of Cluster Suicides in Adolescents*. Grant R01 MH47559-04S2. Bethesda, MD: National Institute of Mental Health.

Gould, M. S. (2001). Suicide and the media. In Hendin, H., and Mann, J. J. (eds.) *Suicide Prevention: Clinical and Scientific Aspects. Annals of the New York Academy of Sciences*. New York City, NY: New York Academy of Sciences.

Gould, M. S. and Kramer, R. A. (2001). Youth suicide prevention. *Suicide and Life-Threatening Behavior*, **31**(Supplement), Spring: 6–31.

Gould, M. S. and Shaffer, D. (1986). The impact of suicide in television movies: evidence of imitation. *New England Journal of Medicine*, **315**, 690–694.

Gould, M. S., Shaffer, D., and Kleinman, M. (1988). The impact of suicide in television movies: Replication and commentary. *Suicide and Life-Threatening Behavior*, **18**, 90–99.

Gould, M. S., Wallenstein, S., and Kleinman, M. (1990a). Time-space clustering of teenage suicide. *American Journal of Epidemiology*, **131**, 71–78.

Gould, M. S., Wallenstein, S., Kleinman, M. H., O'Carroll, P., and Mercy, J. (1990b). Suicide clusters: an examination of age-specific effects. *American Journal of Public Health*, **80**, 211–212.

Gould, M. S., Petrie, K., Kleinman, M., and Wallenstein, S. (1994). Clustering of attempted suicide: New Zealand National Data. *International Journal of Epidemiology*, **23**(8), 1185–1189.

Gould, M. S., Forman, J., Kleinman, M., and Wallenstein, S. (1995). Psychological autopsy of cluster suicides in adolescents. Paper presented at the 42nd meeting of the American Academy of Child and Adolescent Psychiatry, New Orleans, LA, 17–22 October 1995.

Gould, M. S., Fisher, P., Parides, M., Flory, M., and Shaffer, D. (1996). Psychosocial risk factors of child and adolescent completed suicide. *Archives of General Psychiatry*, **53**, 1155–1162.

Gould, M. S., King, R., Greenwald, S., Fisher, P., Schwab-Stone, M., Kramer, R., Flisher, A. J., Goodman, S., Canino, G., and Shaffer, D. (1998). Psychopathology associated with suicidal ideation and attempts among children and adolescents. *Journal of the American Academy of Child and Adolescent Psychiatry*, **37**, 915–923.

Greenhill, L., Waslick, B., Parides, M., Fan, B., Shaffer, D., and Mann, J. J. (1995). Biological studies in suicidal adolescent inpatients. *Scientific Proceedings of the Annual Meeting of the American Academy of Child and Adolescent Psychiatry*, **11**, 124. New York City, NY: American Academy of Child and Adolescent Psychiatry.

Groholt, B., Ekeberg, O., Wichstrom, L., and Haldorsen, T. (1998). Suicide among children and younger and older adolescents in Norway: a comparative study. *Journal of the American Academy of Child and Adolescent Psychiatry*, **37**(5), 473–481.

Grunbaum, J. A., Basen-Engquist, K., and Pandey, D. (1998). Association between violent behaviors and substance use among Mexican-American and non-Hispanic White high school students. *Journal of Adolescent Health*, **23**, 153–159.

Harkavy Friedman, J. M., Asnis, G. M., Boeck, M., and DiFiore, J. (1987). Prevalence of specific suicidal behaviors in a high school sample. *American Journal of Psychiatry*, **144**, 1203–1206.

Hawton, K., Houston, K., and Shepperd, R. (1999). Suicide in young people. *British Journal of Psychiatry*, **175**, 271–276.

Haynes, R. H. (1987). Suicide and social response in Fiji: a historical survey. *British Journal of Psychiatry*, **151**, 21–26.

Ho, T. P., Hung, S. F., Lee, C. C., Chung, K. F., and Chung, S. Y. (1995). Characteristics of youth suicide in Hong Kong. *Social Psychiatry and Psychiatric Epidemiology*, **30**, 107–112.

Holding, T. A. (1974). The B.B.C. "Befrienders" series and its effects. *British Journal of Psychiatry*, **124**, 470–472.

Holding, T. A. (1975). Suicide and "The Befrienders". *British Medical Journal*, **3**, 751–753.

Houston, K., Hawton, K., and Shepperd, R. (2001). Suicide in young people aged 15–24: A psychological autopsy study. *Journal of Affective Disorders*, **63**, 159–170.

Isacsson, G. (2000). Suicide prevention – a medical breakthrough: *Acta Psychiatrica Scandinavica*, **102**, 113–117.

Ishii, K. (1991). Measuring mutual causation: effect of suicide news on suicides in Japan. *Social Science Research*, **20**, 188–195.

Jobes, D. A., Berman, A. L., and Josselson, A. R. (1987). Improving the validity and reliability of medical-legal certifications of suicide. *Suicide and Life-Threatening Behavior*, **17**(4), 310–325.

Joffe, R. T., Offord, D. R., and Boyle, M. H. (1988). Ontario Child Health Study: suicidal behavior in youth aged 12–16 years. *American Journal of Psychiatry*, **145**, 1420–1423.

Jonas, K. (1992). Modelling and suicide: a test of the Werther effect. *British Journal of Social Psychology*, **31**, 295–306.

Kaltiala-Heino, R., Rimpela, M., Marttunen, M., Rimpela, A., and Rantanen, P. (1999). Bullying, depression, and suicidal ideation in Finnish adolescents: school survey. *British Medical Journal*, **319**, 348–351.

Kandel, D. (1988). Substance use, depressive mood, and suicidal ideation in adolescence and young adulthood. In Stiffman, A. R. and Feldman, R. A. (eds.), *Advances in Adolescent Mental Health*. Greenwich, CT: JAI press.

Kandel, D. B., Raveis, V. H., and Davies, M. (1991). Suicidal ideation in adolescence: depression, substance abuse, and other risk factors. *Journal of Youth and Adolescence*, **20**, 289–309.

Kashani, J. H., Goddard, P., and Reid, J. C. (1989). Correlates of suicidal ideation in a community sample of children and adolescents. *Journal of the American Academy of Child and Adolescent Psychiatry*, **28**, 912–917.

Kessler, R. C., Downey, G., Stipp, H., and Milavsky, R. (1989). Network television news stories about suicide and short-term changes in total U.S. suicides. *Journal of Nervous and Mental Disorders*, **177** (Supplement 9), 551–555.

Kessler, R. C., Borges, G., and Walters, E. E. (1999). Prevalence of and risk factors for lifetime suicide attempts in the National Comorbidity Survey. *Archives of General Psychiatry*, **56**, 617–626.

Lesage, A. D., Boyer, R., Grunberg, F., Vanier, C., Morissette, R., Menard-Buteau, C., and Loyer, M. (1994). Suicide and mental disorders: a case–control study of youth men. *American Journal of Psychiatry*, **151**(7), 1063–1068.

Lewinsohn, P. M., Rohde, P., and Seeley, J. R. (1994). Psychosocial risk factors for future adolescent suicide attempts. *Journal of Consulting and Clinical Psychology*, **62**, 297–305.

Lewinsohn, P. M., Rohde, P., and Seeley, J. R. (1996). Adolescent suicidal ideation and attempts: prevalence, risk factors, and clinical implications. *Clinical Psychology Science and Practice*, **3**(1), 25–36.

Lewinsohn, P. M., Rohde, P., Seeley, J. R., and Baldwin, C. L. (2001). Gender differences in suicide attempts from adolescence to young adulthood. *Journal of the American Academy of Child and Adolescent Psychiatry*, **40**(4), 427–434.

Lewis, S. A., Johnson, J., Cohen, P., Garcia, M. and Velez, C. N. (1988). Attempted suicide in youth: its relationship to school achievement, educational goals and socioeconomic status. *Journal of Abnormal Child Psychology*, **16**(4), 459–471.

Lonnqvist, J. (2000). Suicide mortality in Finland declined by 21% from 1990 to 1998. *Psychiatria Fennica*, **31**, 5.

Mann, J. J. and Stoff, D. M. (1997). A synthesis of current findings regarding neurobiological correlates and treatment of suicidal behavior. *Annals New York Academy of Sciences*, **836**, 352–363.

Marttunen, M. J., Aro, H. M., Henriksson, M. M., and Lonnqvist, J. K. (1991). Mental disorders in adolescent suicide. *Archives of General Psychiatry*, **48**, 834–839.

Marttunen, M. J., Aro, H. M., and Lonnqvist, J. K. (1993). Precipitant stressors in adolescent suicide. *Journal of the American Academy of Child and Adolescent Psychiatry*, **32**(6), 1178–1183.

Marttunen, M. J., Aro, H. M., Henrikksson, M. M., and Lonnqvist, J. K. (1994). Psychosocial stressors more common in adolescent suicides with alcohol abuse compared with depressive adolescent suicides. *Journal of the American Academy of Child and Adolescent Psychiatry*, **33**(4), 490–497.

Mohler, B. and Earls, F. (2001). Trends in adolescent suicide: misclassifation bias? *American Journal of Public Health*, **91**(1), 150–153.

Monk, M. (1987). Epidemiology of suicide. *Epidemiologic Reviews*, **9**, 51–69.

Moscicki, E. K. (1995). Epidemiology of suicidal behavior. *Suicide and Life-Threatening Behavior*, **25**(1), 22–35.

Motto, J. A. (1970). Newspaper influence on suicide. *Archives of General Psychiatry*, **23**, 143–148.

O'Carroll, P. W. (1989). A consideration of the validity and reliability of suicide mortality data. *Suicide and Life-Threatening Behavior*, **19**(1), 1–16.

O'Donnell, I. and Farmer, R. (1995). The limitations of official suicide statistics. *British Journal of Psychiatry*, **166**, 458–461.

Pfeffer, C. R., McBride, A., Anderson, G. M., Kakuma, T., Fensterheim, L., and Khait, V. (1998). Peripheral serotonin measures in prepubertal psychiatric inpatients and normal children: associations with suicidal behavior and its risk factors. *Biological Psychiatry*, **44**, 568–577.

Phillips, D. (1974). The influence of suggestions on suicide; substantive and theoretical implications of the Werther effect. *American Sociological Review*, **39**, 340–354.

Phillips, D. (1979). Suicide, motor vehicle fatalities, and the mass media: evidence toward a theory of suggestion. *American Journal of Sociology*, **84**, 1150–1174.

Phillips, D. (1980). Airplane accidents, murder, and the mass media: towards a theory of imitation and suggestion. *Social Forces*, **58**, 1001–1004.

Phillips, D. and Carstensen, L. L. (1986). Clustering of teenage suicides after television news stories about suicide. *New England Journal of Medicine*, **315**, 685–689.

Phillips, D. and Paight, D. J. (1987). The impact of televised movies about suicide: a replicative study. *New England Journal of Medicine*, **317**, 809–811.

Phillips, D. P. and Ruth, T. E. (1993). Adequacy of official suicide statistics for scientific research and public policy. *Suicide and Life-Threatening Behavior*, **23**(4), 307–319.

Reifman, A. and Windle, M. (1995). Adolescent suicidal behaviors as a function of depression, hopelessness, alcohol use, and social support: a longitudinal investigation. *American Journal of Community Psychology*, **23**, 329–354.

Reinherz, H. A., Giaconia, R. M., Silverman, A. B., Friedman, A., Pakiz, B., Frost, A. K., and Cohen, E. (1995). Early psychosocial risks for adolescent suicidal ideation and attempts. *Journal of the American Academy of Child and Adolescent Psychiatry*, **34**, 599–611.

Remafedi, G., French, S., Story, M., Resnick, M. D., and Blum, R. (1998). The relationship between suicide risk and sexual orientation: results of a population-based study. *American Journal of Public Health*, **88**, 57–60.

Rich, C. L., Young, D., and Fowler, M. D. (1986). San Diego Suicide Study: I. Young vs old subjects. *Archives of General Psychiatry*, **45**, 577–582.

Rich, C. L., Fowler, R. C., Fogarty, L. A., and Young, D. (1988). San Diego Suicide Study: III. Relationships between diagnoses and stressors. *Archives of General Psychiatry*, **45**, 589–592.

Riggs, S., Alario, A. J., and McHorney, C. (1990). Health risk behaviors and attempted suicide in adolescents who report prior maltreatment. *The Journal of Pediatrics*, **116**, 815–821.

Roberts, R. E. and Chen, Y. (1995). Depressive symptoms and suicidal ideation among Mexican-origin and Anglo adolescents. *Journal of the American Academy of Child and Adolescent Psychiatry*, **34**, 81–90.

Roberts, R. E., Chen, Y., and Roberts, C. R. (1997). Ethnocultural differences in prevalence of adolescent suicidal behaviors. *Suicide and Life-Threatening Behavior*, **27**, 208–217.

Robins, E., Murphy, P. I., Wilkinson, R. H., Jr., Gassner, S., and Kayes, J. (1959). Some clinical considerations in the prevention of suicide based on a study of 134 successful suicides. *American Journal of Public Health*, **49**, 888–988.

Rosenberg, M. L., Davidson, L. E., Smith, J. C., Berman, A. L., Buzbee, H., Gantner, G., Gay, G. A., Moore-Lewis, B., Mills, D. H., Murray, D., O'Carroll, P. W., and Jobes, D. (1988). Operational criteria for the determination of suicide. *Journal of Forensic Sciences*, **33**(6), 1445–1456.

Rotheram-Borus, M. J. and Trautman, P. D. (1988). Hopelessness, depression and suicidal intent among adolescent suicide attempters. *Journal of the American Academy of Child and Adolescent Psychiatry*, **27**, 700–704.

Rotheram-Borus, M. J., Trautman, P. D., Dopkins, S. C., and Shrout, P. E. (1990). Cognitive style and pleasant activities among female adolescent suicide attempters. *Journal of Consulting and Clinical Psychology*, **58**, 554–561.

Runeson, B. (1989). Mental disorder in youth suicide: DSM-III-R Axes I and II. *Acta Psychiatrica Scandinavica*, **79**, 490–497.

Runeson, B. (1990). Psychoactive substance use disorder in youth suicide. *Alcohol and Alcoholism*, **25**, 561–568.

Safer, D. (1997). Self-reported suicide attempts by adolescents. *Annals of Clinical Psychiatry*, **9**, 263–269.

Sainsbury, P. (1983). Validity and reliability of trends in suicide statistics. *World Health Quarterly*, 339–348.

Schmidtke, A., and Hafner, A. (1988). The Werther effect after television films: new evidence for an old hypothesis. *Psychological Medicine*, **18**, 665–676.

Schmidtke, A., and Schaller, S. (2000). The role of mass media in suicide prevention. In Hawton, K., and van Heeringen, K. (eds.) *The International Handbook of Suicide and Attempted Suicide* (pp. 675–698). New York City, NY: John Wiley & Sons.

Schulsinger, F. (1980). Biological psychopathology. *Annual Review of Psychology*, **31**, 583–606.

Shaffer, D. (1974). Suicide in childhood and early adolescence. *Journal of Child Psychology and Psychiatry*, **15**, 275–291.

Shaffer, D. (1988). The epidemiology of teen suicide: an examination of risk factors. *Journal of Clinical Psychiatry*, **49**(9), 36–41.

Shaffer, D. and Craft, L. (1999). Methods of adolescent suicide prevention. *Journal of Clinical Psychiatry*, **60**, 70–74.

Shaffer, D. and Hicks, R. (1994). Suicide. In Pless, I. B. (ed.), *The Epidemiology of Childhood Disorders* (pp. 339–365). New York: Oxford University Press.

Shaffer, D., Gould, M., and Hicks, R. (1994). Worsening suicide rate in Black teenagers. *American Journal of Psychiatry*, **151**(12), 1810–1812.

Shaffer, D., Fisher, P., Hicks, R. H., Parides, M., and Gould, M. (1995). Sexual orientation in adolescents who commit suicide. *Suicide and Life-Threatening Behavior*, **25**, 64–71.

Shaffer, D., Gould, M. S., Fisher, P., Trautman, P., Moreau, D., Kleinman, M., and Flory, M. (1996). Psychiatric diagnosis in child and adolescent suicide. *Archives of General Psychiatry*, **53**, 339–348.

Shafii, M., Carrigan, S., Whittinghill, J. R., and Derrick, A. (1985). Psychological autopsy of completed suicide in children and adolescents. *American Journal of Psychiatry*, **142**, 1061–1064.

Smith, J. C., Mercy, J. A., and Warren, C. W. (1985). Comparison of suicides among Anglos and Hispanics in five Southwest states. *Suicide and Life-Threatening Behavior*, **15**, 14–26.

Smith, K. and Crawford, S. (1986). Suicidal behavior among "normal" high school students. *Suicide and Life-Threatening Behavior*, **16**, 313–325.

Spirito, A., Brown, L., Overholser, J., and Fritz, G. (1989). Attempted suicide in adolescence: a review and critique of the literature. *Clinical Psychology Review*, **9**, 335–363.

Stack, S. (1989). The effect of publicized mass murder and murder-suicides on lethal violence. *Social Psychiatry and Psychiatric Epidemiology*, **24**, 202–208.

Stack, S. A. (1990). A reanalysis of the impact of non-celebrity suicides: a research note. *Social Psychiatry and Psychiatric Epidemiology*, **25**, 269–273.

Stack, S. (2000). Media impacts on suicide: a quantitative review of 293 findings. *Social Science Quarterly*, **81**, 956–971.

Sudman, S. and Bradburn, N. M. (1974). *Response effects in surveys*. Chicago, IL: Aldine Publishing Company.

Swanson, J. W., Linskey, A. O., Quintero-Salinas, R., Pumariega, A. J., and Holzer III, C. E. (1992). A binational school survey of depressive symptoms, drug use, and suicidal ideation. *Journal of the American Academy of Child and Adolescent Psychiatry*, **31**, 669–678.

Teicher, J. D. and Jacobs, J. (1966). Adolescents who attempt suicide. *American Journal of Psychiatry*, **122**, 1248–1257.

Turner, C. F., Lessler, J. T., and Devore, J. W. (1992). In Turner, C. F., Lessler, J. J., and Gfroerer, J. C. (eds.), *Effects of Mode of Administration and Wording on Reporting of Drug Use* (pp. 177–220). Washington D.C.: Government Printing Office.

Velez, C. N. and Cohen, P. (1988). Suicidal behavior and ideation in a community sample of children: maternal and youth reports. *Journal of the American Academy of Child and Adolescent Psychiatry*, **27**, 349–356.

Velting, D. M., Rathus, J. H., and Asnis, G. M. (1998). Asking adolescents to explain discrepancies in self-reported suicidality. *Suicide and Life-Threatening Behavior*, **28**, 187–196.

Wallace, J. D., Calhoun, A. D., Powell, K. E., O'Neil, J., and James, S. P. (1996). *Homicide and Suicide among Native Americans, 1979–1992*. Atlanta, GA: Centers for Disease Control and Prevention, National Center for Injury Prevention and Control. Violence Surveillance Series, No. 2.

Walter, H. J., Vaughan, R. D., Armstrong, B., Krakoff, R. Y., Maldonado, L. M., Tiezzi, L., and McCarthy, J. F. (1995). Sexual, assaultive, and suicidal behaviors among urban minority junior high school students. *Journal of the American Academy of Child and Adolescent Psychiatry*, **34**, 73–80.

Wasserman, I. M. (1984). Imitation and suicide: a reexamination of the Werther effect. *American Sociological Review*, **49**, 427–436.

Weissman, M. M., Wickramaratne, P., Warner, V., John, K., Prusoff, B. A., Merikangas, K. R., and Gammon, G. D. (1987a). Assessing psychiatric disorders in children: discrepancies between mothers' and children's reports. *Archives of General Psychiatry*, **44**(8), 747–753.

Weissman, M. M., Gammon, G., Davis, J. K., Merikangas, K. R., Warner, V., Prusoff, B. A., and Sholomskas, D. (1987b). Children of depressed parents: increased psychopathology and early onset of major depression. *Archives of General Psychiatry*, **44**(10), 847–853.

Weissman, M. M., Fendrich, M., Warner, V., and Wickramaratne, P. (1992). Incidence of psychiatric disorder in offspring at high and low risk for depression. *Journal of the American Academy of Child and Adolescent Psychiatry*, **31**, 640–648.

Windle, M., Miller-Tutzauer, C., and Domenico, D. (1992). Alcohol use, suicidal behavior, and risky activities among adolescents. *Journal of Research on Adolescence*, **2**, 317–330.

World Health Organization. Suicide rates and absolute numbers of suicide by country (2001). Available at http://www3.who.int./whosis/whsa/ftp/download.htm [accessed 8 March 2001].

## 2

# Suicide and the "continuum of adolescent self-destructiveness": is there a connection?

Robert A. King, Vladislav V. Ruchkin, and Mary E. Schwab-Stone

## Introduction

The adolescent period in contemporary Western society is characterized by a distinctive pattern of morbidity and mortality. Suicidal behavior and completed suicide are more common in adolescence than in any other developmental epoch (save, for males, in old age). It is also notable that the leading causes of adolescent deaths (at least in the U.S.) – accidents, homicide, and suicide – are preventable ones, frequently associated with life-styles characterized by impulsivity, reckless-ness, and substance or alcohol use. (Cultural contributions to this pattern are apparent in the U.S., where the low legal age for driving and easy availability of guns contribute to the high national adolescent mortality rates from motor vehi-cle fatalities, homicide, or suicide.) In addition to high rates of suicidal attempts and ideation, adolescence in the industrialized world is also characterized by increased health-threatening behaviors, such as tobacco, alcohol, and drug use; unprotected sex; fighting; reckless driving; and, in the U.S., weapon-carrying (Centers for Disease Control and Prevention, 2002).

In attempting to integrate these striking epidemiological observations, Holinger (1979) and others have postulated a "continuum of selfdest-ructiveness" in adolescence ranging from the covert (e.g., substance use, unprotected and precocious sexual activity, reckless driving) through the overt (e.g., self-mutilation and suicide attempts). Holinger's account, however, leaves open what underlying factors might account for this proposed association. Jes-sor (1991, 1998) and others (summarized in Dryfoos, 1990) have attempted to explain the frequent association in adolescence between various forms of "problem" or risk behaviors, but these accounts have generally not consid-ered suicidal behavior as part of the constellation of "problem" behaviors or as one of the outcomes to be explained by the various vulnerability models proposed.

A clearer understanding of the possible relationship of suicidal behavior and ideation to various other health-threatening risk behaviors is critically important from the theoretical, clinical, and preventive points of view.

From a theoretical point of view, with few exceptions, most of the literature on adolescent suicidality is strangely a-developmental. Hence, it would be an important advance to be able to examine adolescent suicidal behavior from the perspectives of developmental psychopathology and the multi-factorial, transactional models that have been developed to explain other adolescent risk behaviors (Cairns et al. 1998; Cicchetti and Cohen, 1995; Jessor, 1991, 1998; Perris, 1994).

From a clinical point of view, given the very high prevalence levels of adolescent risk behaviors, as well as suicidal ideation, it is important for clinicians to understand how these forms of psychopathology may interact or amplify each other.

From a preventive point of view, a clearer understanding of the "structure of risk behaviors" (including suicidality) would permit more efficient identification of high-risk youth as well as more fundamental means of intervention. For example, although depression and suicidal ideation in teens often go undetected by parents and other adults, substance use, minor delinquencies, and other reckless behaviors are much more likely to capture adults' attention. Finally, identifying the shared vulnerability and protective factors that may underlie the hypothesized "spectrum of self-destructive behaviors" would facilitate integrating prevention programs to go beyond what Jessor has characterized as the "problem of the week" approach ("Just say 'No' to teen suicide, or drugs, or tobacco, or drunk driving, or unsafe sex, . . . ").

## Overview of chapter

This chapter will examine the nature and extent of the associations between overt suicidal thoughts and behavior and various other forms of adolescent health-impairing behavior.

We will begin by reviewing the epidemiological data linking suicidal behavior and adolescent risk behaviors, evidence compatible with the notion of a "continuum of self-destructiveness." Next we will argue that suicidality is linked to the continuum of other adolescent problem behaviors for multiple reasons.

First, suicidal behaviors and other risk behaviors share an association with psychiatric diagnoses such as mood, disruptive, substance use, and anxiety disorders.

Second, problem behaviors have a cumulative deleterious impact on adolescent development, increasing negative interactions with significant others, undermining coping skills, and increasing the likelihood of stressful life events and emotional crises.

Third, and perhaps most important, we propose that the predisposition to suicidal ideation and suicide attempts and other problem behaviors often co-occur because they share common developmental antecedents and risk factors. Among these are negative environmental influences (family, peers, neighborhood) that, in interaction with specific personality or temperamental traits, promote the development of impulsivity, increased risk-taking, and egotism, as well as thwart the development of adaptive emotional coping skills and adequate cognitive and moral development. This adverse developmental process fosters an underlying personality structure with increased levels of behavioral activation and lack of behavioral inhibition or cognitive control over one's own behavior. Such environments often also present an increased level of hassles and stressful live events which, especially when amplified by a reactive emotional style, increase the cumulative burden of negative life experiences.

## Studies supporting the notion of a "continuum of self-destructiveness"

Adolescent problem behaviors such as truancy, substance use, high-risk or early onset of sexual activity, and delinquency frequently co-occur (Donovan et al., 1988; Dryfoos, 1990; Jessor, 1991). For example, as discussed later, Donovan et al. (1988) concluded that the correlation between different types of adolescent problem behaviors could be explained by a single common factor. The extent of association between problem behaviors, however, differs with the behaviors involved, suggesting that etiological factors vary to some extent with gender, demographic group, and the specific type of problem behavior (Barone et al., 1995; Ensminger, 1990; Garnefski and Diekstra, 1997; McGee and Newcomb, 1992). Thus, in a New Zealand community sample of 15-year-olds, Fergusson et al. (1994) found a significant association between early sexual activity, alcohol abuse, cannabis use, conduct disorder, and police contacts. Youngsters who demonstrated one type of problem behavior were at increased risk for the other problem behaviors, with the odds ratios between pairs of problem behaviors ranging from 4.19 to 20.12. However, using latent class analysis, Fergusson et al. (1994) also distinguished four groups: (1) the first group, consisting of 85.4% of the population, had very low probabilities of any problem behavior; (2) the second group (5.2% of the sample) was characterized by an accelerated transition to adult hedonic behaviors, with elevated risks for early sexual activity, alcohol abuse, and cannabis use; (3) the third group (6.7% of the sample) consisted of adolescents whose problem behaviors involved antisocial and delinquent behaviors (high risk of cannabis use, conduct problems, and police contact); (4) the fourth group (2.7% of sample) consisted of multi-problem youngsters with elevated risks for all of the problem behaviors. Girls predominated in the second group, while boys predominated in the third group; similar rates of boys and girls were found in the fourth, multi-problem group).

Epidemiologic studies of self-reported risk behaviors also provide empirical support for the relationship between suicidal ideation or attempts and other potentially health-compromising risk behaviors. The Centers for Disease Control and Prevention's (2002) periodic Youth Risk Behavior Survey (YRBS) provides data on the epidemiology of risk behaviors and suicidal ideation and attempts in successive large national samples of high-school students. The potential utility of these data for studying the associations between suicidal ideation/attempts and other forms of adolescent risk behavior is only beginning to be exploited. For example, examining the CDC YRBS data for 3054 Massachusetts high-school students, Woods et al. (1997) found lifetime suicide attempts were significantly associated with physical fights in the past year, regular tobacco use, lack of seatbelt use, gun carrying, substance use before last sexual activity, and lifetime drug use. An analysis of the national cross-sectional survey data on 11 631 high-school students found significant and substantial correlations between suicide attempts and gun carrying, multiple sexual partners, condom non-use, fighting resulting in injury, driving while intoxicated, and cocaine use (Sosin et al., 1995). Orpinas et al. (1995) examined the YRBS data for 2075 Texas high-school students and found that weapon-carrying and fighting resulting in injury were associated with suicidal ideation, as well as with alcohol use, number of sexual partners, and low academic performance. Using the YRBS survey self-report data from 3764 South Carolina high-school students, Garrison et al. (1993) found aggressive behaviors, illicit drug use, drinking frequency, and cigarette use associated with suicidal ideation and attempts, with odds ratios generally increasing in magnitude with severity of reported suicidal behavior.

Similar findings emerge from other surveys of adolescent community populations. For example, in a survey of 3738 predominantly minority junior high students in an economically disadvantaged New York City school district, Walter et al. (1995) found significant associations between suicide attempts/ideation and assaultive behavior, academic difficulties, and sexual intercourse. Examining the risk of involvement in assaultive behavior, sexual intercourse, and suicide ideation/attempts for both genders, the risk of involvement in each behavior was substantially increased by involvement in the other two behaviors. Similarly, in a population study of 1699 15- to 16-year-old Australian students, Patton et al. (1997) found that antisocial behavior and substance use were associated with self-harm in girls (but not boys), while sexual activity was independently associated with deliberate self-harm in both sexes.

Whatever the pathogenic basis for the association between suicidality and other health-endangering behaviors, it may persist over time, even many years. For example, adolescent suicide attempters are at ongoing risk for injury and death from motor vehicle accidents, substance abuse, homicide, etc. (see Chapter 12). Prospective studies demonstrate a shared set of social, developmental, and psychopathological risk factors predicting completed or attempted suicide and unintentional injury or death (Fergusson and Lynskey, 1995a,b; Neeleman et al., 1998). Similarly, smoking in adolescence or young adulthood has a significant association with suicide, even years later (Clayton, 1998) (whether by virtue of a link with impulsivity, aggression, or other psychiatric comorbidity or neurobiological trait remains uncertain).

## Psychiatric diagnoses common to suicidality and problem behaviors

One likely important source of apparent association between suicidal behavior and other risk behaviors is their shared association with predisposing psychiatric conditions, such as depression, disruptive disorders, or anxiety.

As discussed at length in other chapters (Chapters 1, 3, and 4), the presence of a psychiatric disorder, such as a mood, disruptive, anxiety, or substance abuse disorder, is one of the most significant risk factors for attempted and completed suicide in children and adolescents, with over 90% of adolescent suicide completers having at least one Axis I diagnosis (Brent et al., 1993a; Gould et al., 1998; Shaffer et al., 1996).

Axis I pathology is also an important risk factor for suicide attempts and ideation. For example, data from the NIMH Methods for the Epidemiology of Child and Adolescent Mental Disorders (MECA) Study of 1285 randomly selected children and adolescents aged 9–17 years were analyzed with respect to suicidal ideation and attempts, psychiatric diagnosis, and psychosocial risk factors; as in other studies, mood, anxiety, and substance abuse/dependence disorders independently increased the risk for suicide attempts. Disruptive disorders were not independently associated with suicide attempts, but were associated with suicidal ideation, while substance abuse/dependence differentiated suicide attempters from those with suicidal ideation alone (Gould et al., 1998). Some of these diagnoses, such as substance abuse or conduct disorder, are, of course, synonymous with or highly associated with potentially life- and health-threatening behavior in their own right. Mood disorders in children and adolescents are also associated with increased disruptive diagnoses (Puig-Antich, 1982) and, in adolescents, substance abuse (e.g., Flament et al., 2001). Although depressive symptoms and major depressive disorder are significant risk factors for attempted suicide, the additional presence of a comorbid disruptive behavior disorder or substance abuse increases the risk of attempted suicide even further (Lewinsohn et al., 1996; Wagner et al., 1996).

Historically, psychiatric diagnosis has been perhaps the most systematically studied risk factor for adolescent suicide completers and attempters (Chapter 1), in part because the DSM (Diagnostic and Statistical Manual)/ICD (International Classification of Diseases) framework has provided a uniform nosology suitable for international use and in part because Axis I diagnoses rely on symptoms whose presence or absence can be determined to a considerable extent from surviving informants. However, as we shall discuss, although critically important when present, Axis I diagnoses may represent simply the tip of the pathogenic iceberg, with other important personality and psychosocial risk factors less readily apparent or well studied.

## Caveat regarding the heterogeneity of adolescent suicidal behavior

There are many developmental paths into adolescent suicidal ideation, attempts, or completion and no single explanatory account is likely to fit all cases. Although, taken as a whole, youth suicides and suicide attempts show a strong association with aggression and mood, disruptive, and substance abuse disorders (Chapter 1; Brent et al., 1993a, 1999; Clark and Horton-Deutsch, 1992; Gould et al., 1996, 1998; Shaffer et al., 1988, 1996), a small number of adolescent suicide completers (Apter et al., 1993a; Brent et al., 1993b), as well as a fair number of adolescent suicide attempters or ideators in community samples do not have any diagnosable psychopathology (Reinherz et al., 1995; Velez and Cohen, 1988).

Adolescent suicides and suicide attempters are thus not a homogeneous group and can be divided into various descriptive subgroups that differ with respect to their profile of risk and protective factors, including diagnosis, personality style, and family and environmental factors (Engstrom et al., 1996). The proportional admixture of psychiatric diagnoses and symptoms, family pathology, and other adverse environmental factors varies widely from youngster to youngster. At one extreme, for example, clinical experience suggests that there are youngsters with severe depression or psychosis who may be prone to attempt suicide to escape intolerable psychic pain, even without much additional contribution from negative family or life events, substance use, or other problem behaviors; indeed, such youngsters' families may be intact and supportive. In contrast, there are other suicidal children and adolescents who experience multiple stressors, such as physical or sexual abuse, multiple losses or disruptions of attachment; poor family communications and parent–child relationships; and other forms of social adversity (Cohen-Sandler et al., 1982; Wagner, 1997). This chronically traumatic upbringing in many cases reflects parental psychopathology, which may be mirrored – on either a genetic or experiential basis – in the child (see Chapter 4).

## Diverse patterns of diagnostic comorbidity

The heterogeneity of patterns of diagnostic comorbidity is apparent in clinical samples and community studies of attempters and completers. Such studies demonstrate that patterns of diagnostic comorbidity influence the extent to which other problem behaviors are associated with suicidality.

Apter et al. (1995), for example, distinguished two types of suicidal behavior in adolescent inpatients: the first characterized by a wish to die and common in depressive disorders, the second characterized by impulse control problems and associated with externalizing disorders. In a series of studies, Apter and colleagues (1988, 1991, 1995) found that in violent inpatients, suicidality was not correlated with depression or sadness and that, indeed, conduct-disordered adolescent inpatients, who showed little depression, had more suicidal behaviors than did their peers with major depressive disorder (Apter et al., 1988). Renaud et al. (1999) similarly found that although co-morbid substance abuse and a history of physical abuse were associated with completed suicide in adolescents with disruptive disorder, co-morbid major depressive disorder was not an additional risk factor in such adolescents. Pfeffer and colleagues (1989) divided a sample of adolescent inpatients according to the presence or absence of assaultive or suicidal behavior. Compared to controls, the suicidal-only group was distinguished by depression, drug use, and environmental stress; the assaultive-only group by aggression and violence; and the combined assaultive-suicidal group by both accidents and violence.

Community samples of nonreferred youngsters provide the clearest picture of patterns of comorbidity in the general population, uncontaminated by the referral biases that limit the findings from clinical samples. Using a strategy similar to that of Pfeffer et al. (1989) and Apter et al. (1988, 1991, 1993b, 1995) in a community sample, Vermeiren et al. (2003) divided a group of Belgian high-school adolescents into a suicidal-only group, a violence-only group, a combined suicidal-violent group, and a control group that was neither suicidal nor violent. Compared to the controls, all of the comparison groups had elevated levels of depression, somatization, sensation seeking, and covert aggression. The suicidal-only group manifested significantly more anxiety, alcohol abuse, covert aggression, and negative expectations of the future; the violence-only group showed significantly more overt aggression, sensation seeking and drug abuse; and the combined suicidal-violent group was significantly higher in somatization, covert, and overt aggression.

### Diverse patterns of personality vulnerabilities

Postmortem studies of youthful suicides find that over and above the high rates of Axis I psychiatric disorder, personality disorders and problematic personality traits also make a contribution. Even after controlling for Axis I diagnoses, Brent et al. (1994) found that traits such as irritability and aggression and Axis II diagnoses (especially DSM Cluster B (impulsive, dramatic disorders)) were significantly associated with adolescent completed suicide. Cluster C personality disorders (especially avoidant type) were also significantly associated with completed suicide, paralleling the findings of other studies that a significant number of adolescent suicides appear to have anxious, perfectionistic, rigid, isolative, or inhibited traits (Apter et al., 1993a; King and Apter, 1996; Shaffer, 1974; Shafii et al., 1985).

### Gender-related diversity in vulnerability factors

It should also be noted that risk factors and prognostic implications associated with adolescent suicidal behavior differ with gender. In their psychologic autopsy study of adolescent suicides, Shaffer et al. (1996) found that, for boys, completed suicide was associated with major depression, substance abuse, and/or antisocial behavior; in contrast, for girls, major depression and antisocial behavior, but not substance abuse, were associated with increased risk of suicide completion. In their longitudinal population study of Australian adolescents, Patton et al. (1997) found that antisocial behavior and substance use were associated with self-harm in girls, but not in boys. Furthermore, suicide attempts appear to carry graver prognostic implications for boys than for girls with respect to later psychosocial adaptation or subsequent completed suicide (Chapter 12; Farbstein et al., 2002).

## Cumulative and generalizing adverse impact on adolescent development

### The "vicious circle" effects of adolescent problem behaviors

Another source of association between adolescent suicidality and other problem behaviors is the cumulative deleterious effect of the latter on adolescent development. Viewed longitudinally, many adolescent problem behaviors increase the likelihood of negative interactions with significant adults (and thus the number

of disciplinary crises and other stressful life events), erode academic and proso-
cial involvements, and augment the probability of socialization to progressively
more deviant peer groups. Furthermore, in so far as the adolescent indulges in
alcohol and substance use, these in turn increase impulsivity and affective instability, decrease inhibition, and further undermine coping skills. Thus, as Dryfoos
(1988) noted, "One clear sense that can be derived is the impact of early initiation
of any one of the [problem] behaviors. Starting any one of the behaviors early
appears to produce more negative outcomes and to rapidly 'spread' to other
realms of behavior" p. 25, quoted in Hurrelmann (1989).

## Pathogenic processes by which problem behaviors increase vulnerability to suicidal behavior or ideation

Certain adolescents are predisposed to suicidal ideation or attempts by virtue of
specific types of psychopathology interacting with deficient or maladaptive coping styles (Brent, 1997; Shaffer and Pfeffer, 2001; Shaffer et al., 1988). Given that
only a small minority of individuals with major depression ultimately complete
suicide, it seems likely that suicidal behavior is the outcome of an accumulation of numerous additional factors and events over and above the presence of
a psychiatric disorder. Thus, whether any given vulnerable youngster actually
progresses to attempting or completing suicide depends on certain stochastic
processes; for example, the confluence of trait-dependent vulnerability factors
(e.g., impulsivity, poor coping skills, aggressiveness), additional triggering stressors inducing intense dysphoric affects, together with permissive factors (e.g.,
contagion effects, lack of social support) and the concurrent availability of lethal
means. In terms of this process, the presence of multiple problem behaviors,
when combined with poor interpersonal skills and/or impulsivity, provides a
potent recipe for brewing a suicidal crisis. Suicidal action often takes place shortly
after a stressful event (disciplinary crisis, fight with parent or romantic partner)
induces some extreme emotions, such as desperation, rage or helplessness, but
can also follow distorted emotions from a depressed mood or intoxication with
drugs or alcohol. While some of the stressful negative events that generate intense dysphoric reactions are independent of the adolescent's control, others are
at least in part the product of the adolescent's maladaptive traits or symptoms.

The ready availability of means of self-harm is an important final permissive
factor in setting the stage for suicidal behavior. For example, firearm availability
in the home is an even greater risk factor for suicide for youngsters *without* any
apparent psychiatric diagnoses than it is for those *with* known psychopathology
(Brent, 2001; Brent et al., 1993b); presumably, ready firearm availability permits
an impulsive fatal outcome to what might otherwise be a transient suicidal mood.

## Shared antecedents and risk factors for problem behaviors and adolescent suicidality

### Shared psychopathological traits: impulsivity, recklessness, and aggression

The linkage between problem behaviors and youthful suicidal ideation or behavior is not solely due to a shared association with the presence of a psychiatric disorder. Thus, in the MECA study data described above, even after adjusting for sociodemographic status and the presence of a mood, anxiety, or disruptive disorder, a statistically significant association remained between suicidal ideation or attempts and sexual activity and even occasional recent drunkenness, smoking, and physical fighting (King et al., 2001). Another likely important source of this association between suicidal and other risk behaviors lies in an underlying shared association with pathological or maladaptive personality traits.

Studies examining possible risk factors for the development of risk-taking behaviors have focused on a variety of personality factors: impulsivity (e.g., Kahn et al., 2002; Vitaro et al., 1999; Wills et al., 2001); aggressiveness (Durant et al., 1997); self-criticism (Leadbeater et al., 1999); sensation seeking; and deficits in coping (Horesh et al., 1996), social skills, and problem-solving deficits (Kazdin, 1995). These same traits also appear to set the stage for vulnerability to suicidal ideation or behavior (See Chapter 5; Asarnow et al., 1987; Blatt, 1995; Brent 1997; Rotheram-Borus et al., 1990) .

Impulsivity, in particular, is often considered to play an important role in the development of a wide range of externalizing problems, with higher levels of childhood impulsivity predicting greater antisocial involvement in adolescence (Loeber et al., 2001; Olson et al., 1999). Several studies have similarly demonstrated the linkage of impulsivity to aggressiveness (e.g., Martin et al., 1994), as well as to substance abuse and antisocial personality disorder (e.g., Hesselbrock and Hesselbrock, 1992). Impulsivity in turn has also often been demonstrated to be highly related to suicidality (Apter et al., 1990, 1991, 1993b, 1995; Horesh et al., 1997, 1999; Kingsbury et al., 1999; Koslowsky et al., 1992), and Chapters 4 and 5 examine in detail the major role that impulsivity and its presumed neurobiologic substrate(s) (such as serotonergic dysregulation) play in relation to suicidal behavior. In the Houston Case Control Study of nearly lethal suicide attempts, impulsive attempters (i.e., those who premeditated suicide for less than five minutes before acting) were characterized by significantly more physical fighting (past 12 months), compared to nonimpulsive suicides, even after adjusting for the greater preponderance of males in the impulsive group (Simon et al., 2001). (It is interesting to note that even in nonhuman male free-ranging primates, low cerebrospinal fluid 5-hydroxyindoleacetic acid (5-HIAA) concentrations are associated with excessive mortality (Higley et al., 1996).)

Other authors have specifically emphasized the role played in both adolescent suicidality and various risk behaviors by recklessness (Clark et al., 1990; Shaffer et al., 1996), sensation-seeking, high neuroticism, hostility, and low socialization (for a review see also Verona and Patrick, 2000).

These specific personality factors, in turn, have also been suggested as providing a link to other social and family factors conferring vulnerability to the development of many kinds of risk-taking behaviors, including suicidality. Some authors, for example, have suggested that abuse in childhood may constitute an environmental risk factor for the development of trait impulsivity and aggression, as well as suicide attempts in depressed adults, or, alternatively, that impulsivity and aggression may be inherited traits underlying both a parental propensity for child abuse and subsequent adult suicidal behavior in the offspring (Brodsky et al., 2001).

The important mediating role of maladaptive traits in linking adverse early experience with later suicidality is illustrated by the work of Yang and Clum (2000). Using a structural equations approach to cross-sectionally collected data, they found that recalled early negative life events (maltreatment, family instability, and poor general family environment) were associated with later suicidal ideation; however, this link was largely accounted for by their effects on impaired psychological functioning (self-esteem, external locus of control, hopelessness, and problem-solving deficits).

## Shared family/social risk factors

Dryfoos (1990) has summarized the extensive overlap in both the prevalence and risk factors for delinquency, substance use, teen pregnancy, and school failure, including the frequent commonalities of poverty; low resistance to deviant peers; insufficient bonding and communication with parents; and insufficient, harsh or inconsistent parental discipline or monitoring.

One of the most ambitious attempts to give a general account of the underlying cause(s) of various types of behavior deviance is Jessor's Problem Behavior Theory. Jessor (1991, 1998) describes several overlapping domains of risk and protective factors for adolescent risk behaviors: biology/genetics, social environment, perceived environment, and personality.

Jessor especially emphasizes the importance of a factor he terms "conventionality-unconventionality." *Unconventionality* includes such risk factors as: association with deviant peers, orientation to peer rather than parental values, and parental tolerance of deviance. *Conventionality*, in contrast, includes such protective factors as: value on academic achievement, intolerance of deviance, involvement with church and/or community organizations, and compatibility of parent and peer values. (One cannot help remark that, in many ways, Jessor's construct of conventionality-unconventionality recalls Durkheim's concept of anomie (1966), cast in the terms that are most relevant to the social world of the adolescent.)

Based on a large body of empirical data, Jessor (1987, 1991, 1998; Jessor et al., 1997) concludes that this conventionality-unconventionality factor is highly correlated with problem behaviors, such as delinquency, alcohol and drug abuse, risky driving, and precocious sexual activity, as well as more modestly correlated with health-promoting activities such as regular exercise, adequate sleep, attention to healthy diet, and seat-belt use (Donovan et al., 1993).

Although Jessor's theory, which proposes a single unitary factor underlying a range of problem behaviors, has been examined with respect to delinquency, substance use, and precocious sexual behavior, it has not been much studied with respect to adolescent suicidal behavior.

Kandel et al. (1991) examined several of Jessor's constructs in relation to suicidal ideation in a community sample of high-school students. They found that levels of suicidal ideation were associated with a lack of either closeness to parents or dependence on them for advice; feeling better understood by peers than by parents; delinquency; risk taking, and more frequent life events. Gender-specific risk factors for suicidal ideation included, for girls, lack of religious service attendance, alienation from school, and poor self-reported health, and for boys more frequent medical visits and reported days in bed for physical illness. Although the effects of lack of closeness to parents were mediated in part by its relationship to depression, closeness to parents also had a direct effect on reducing suicidal ideation.

Other epidemiologic studies support the conclusion that the relationship of a poor quality of family life to adolescent suicidal ideation and behavior is not simply due to the mediating effects of psychiatric disorder. Gould et al. (1996) found that, beyond the risk attributable to psychiatric illness, significant independent psychosocial risk factors for adolescent completed suicide included poor parent–child communication and stressful life events (see also Chapter 4 regarding the difficulty of disentangling the overlap between potentially heritable parental psychopathology and the experiential effects on offspring of a disturbed family environment). In the longitudinal Canterbury study of Australian youngsters, Beautrais (1998; Beautrais et al., 1996) found that poor parental relationship and parental separation, alcohol problems, or imprisonment; poverty; foster care; childhood sexual or physical abuse; and perceived low parental care were associated with serious suicide attempts. Using logistic regression to allow for the intercorrelation of these factors, poor parental relationship, low perceived parental care, and childhood sexual abuse remained predictors of serious suicide attempts, even after controlling for the presence of an Axis I psychiatric disorder. In the MECA study cited above (King et al., 2001), even after adjusting for demographics and the presence of a mood, anxiety, or disruptive disorder, a significant association persisted between suicidal ideation or attempts and poor family environment, low parental monitoring, low youth instrumental competence, sexual activity, recent drunkenness, current smoking, and physical fighting. (Effective parental monitoring is not simply a product of close, active parental surveillance, but also reflects a parent–child relationship that facilitates open communication and child disclosure (Stattin and Kerr, 2000). For a review of studies of family risk factors in child and adolescent suicidal behavior, see Wagner (1997).)

Hurrelmann (1989) suggests at least three mechanisms by which social supports help to moderate the deleterious impact of stress:

1. By decreasing the likelihood of encountering stressful situations (screening effect).
2. By assisting coping with stressful situations through bolstering instrumental competence (buffering effect).
3. Increasing the ability to tolerate the dysphoric affects accompanying stress (tolerance effect).

Paralleling these protective factors are of course the mechanisms whereby the relative absence of social supports increase the adverse effects of stress by increasing exposure to stressful situations, undermining coping efforts, and decreasing the tolerance for negative affects.

Perceived lack of parental support is an important underlying risk factor for adolescent suicidal ideation and attempts, as well as a variety of other difficulties (Dubow et al., 1989). Because various forms of behavioral and psychological difficulties are often highly inter-related, multivariate techniques are helpful in identifying the most significant variables. For example, Simons and Murphy (1985) used path analysis to examine the relation between the absence of parental support, employment problems, school interpersonal difficulties, and suicidal ideation and various potentially mediating variables. Although significant at the zero-order level, self-esteem, hopelessness, and interpersonal problems at school were not related to suicidal ideation when the effects of other variables were controlled for. The most potent predictors of suicidal ideation for girls were involvement in delinquent activities and emotional problems, which in turn were predicted most strongly by perceived absence of parental support.

## Conclusions

This chapter has reviewed extensive research supporting the concept of a "continuum of self-destructiveness" in which suicidality and suicidal tendencies co-occur with other adolescent risk behaviors, such as substance use, aggressive behavior, and high-risk sexual activity. This perspective provides a complementary approach to the more traditional, categorical one in which suicidality is seen as a diagnostic feature of depression or borderline personality disorder. Without contradicting that perspective, the "continuum" perspective, supported by data from numerous cross-sectional and somewhat fewer longitudinal studies, emphasizes the commonality of predisposing factors and suggests interactive processes that unfold over the course of development.

The "syndrome" of problem behaviors, however, is not a neat uniform package (Ensminger, 1990), but rather one "suggesting both co-occurrence and distinctiveness across problem behavior categories" (Barone et al., 1995). Similarly, the heterogeneity of adolescent suicidal behavior, with different subgroups of suicidal adolescents, reflects correspondingly distinctive patterns of predisposing vulnerabilities, diagnostic comorbidity, psychopathology, and attendant risk behaviors.

Such patterns of associations of risk behaviors and suicidality are likely to occur because of shared predisposing conditions. Manifestations of potentially heritable neurobiological substrates, temperamental predispositions, and personality features, such as impulsivity, recklessness, and aggression, interact with life events and family, peer, and broader social/community contexts over the course of development to yield a diathesis toward suicidality. As Jessor notes, modern conceptualizations of adolescent risk behaviors "encompass a wide array of causal domains, from culture and society on one side to biology and genetics on the other; they also convey, at the same time, a hard-earned awareness of complexity and a renewed respect for developmental processes" (Jessor, 1998, p. 1).

Inclusion of suicidality as an additional manifestation of the "syndrome of problem behavior" represents a relatively new approach (Flisher et al., 2000; King et al., 2001). This expansion is in accord with what Jessor (1998) terms the "enlarging perimeter" around problem behavior, which now frequently includes tobacco use, risky driving, and the absence of positive health-maintaining behaviors, as well as the traditional components of delinquency, substance use, and early sexual activity. This trend sets the stage for more sophisticated explanations of the structure and organization of risk behaviors and represents an advancement over single problem thinking (Jessor, 1998).

A corresponding, important theme for future research involves the theoretical and methodological shift from single variable approaches (e.g., low self-esteem) to multi-level, multi-variate explanatory models (Jessor, 1998) that take into account both person and context. While this represents an advance in problem behavior research as a whole, the study of adolescent suicide has not yet seen this transition.

A related methodological concern, as articulated by Cairns et al. (1998), involves the use of person-oriented as opposed to variable-oriented analytic approaches. They note that "behavioral variables rarely function as independent entities that are separable from the web of influences in which they occur" (p. 15). In nature, variables cluster in individuals; however, the current tendency in much of suicide research has been to consider variables as independent entities that take on lives of their own. The emphasis in many studies of adolescent suicidality has been on statistical methods that obscure individual typologies and neglect the interplay of risk and protective factors over time.

To pose these questions is to confront important limitations in the extant literature on youthful suicide. The bulk of this literature is profoundly a-developmental. Most studies are cross-sectional; even those that examine antecedent factors have for the most part done so only retrospectively (e.g., Cohen-Sandler et al., 1982; Yang and Clum, 2000). Prospective studies have only recently become available (e.g., Fergusson et al., 2000; Lewinsohn et al., 2001; Patton et al., 1997; Pfeffer et al., 1993). Also lacking is a life-span perspective, with little exploration of why different vulnerabilities come into prominence in different developmental epochs.

This chapter has suggested that the fields of both problem behavior and suicide research would benefit from considering adolescent suicidality as part of the continuum of risk and self-destructive behavior. While there is considerable empirical support for this perspective, it is also evident that no single typology applies to all suicidal adolescents; hence, distinguishing the developmental characteristics of the various pathways to suicidality will require person-centered, developmental research approaches.

The ultimate goal of this orientation to understanding adolescent suicidality is to apply research findings to prevention and treatment efforts. Relevant findings from this current review include the co-occurrence of problem behaviors, which serve as "flags" for a disposition to self-destructiveness that, given adverse circumstances, may evolve toward suicidality. Much more knowledge is needed about the various developmental trajectories toward suicidality in order to inform prevention, screening, and early treatment interventions. Findings to date also implicate social contexts as conferring risk or protection, as well as providing potential settings for prevention and intervention (Maggs et al., 1997). Current work in the area of risk behavior prevention is also likely to prove highly applicable to the field of suicide prevention. Efforts to link prevention and treatment will ultimately entail comprehensive approaches that include components at the individual, school, family, and community levels (DiClemente et al., 1996).

## REFERENCES

Apter, A., Bleich, A., Plutchik, R., Mendelsohn, S., and Tyano S. (1988). Suicidal behavior, depression, and conduct disorder in hospitalized adolescents. *Journal of the American Academy of Child and Adolescent Psychiatry*, **27**(6), 696–699.

Apter, A., van Praag, H. M., Plutchik, R., Sevy, S., Korn, M., and Brown, S. L. (1990). Interrelationships among anxiety, aggression, impulsivity, and mood: a serotonergically linked cluster? *Psychiatry Research*, **32**(2), 191–199.

Apter, A., Kotler, M., Sevy, S., Plutchik, R., Brown, S. L., Foster, H., Hillbrand, M., Korn, M. L., and van Praag, H. M. (1991). Correlates of risk of suicide in violent and nonviolent psychiatric patients. *American Journal of Psychiatry*, **148**(7), 883–887.

Apter, A., Bleich, A., King, R. A., Kron, S., Fluch, A., Kotler, M., and Cohen, D. J. (1993a). Death without warning? A clinical post-mortem study of 43 Israeli adolescent male suicides. *Archives of General Psychiatry*, **50**, 138–142.

Apter, A., Plutchik, R., and van Praag, H. M. (1993b). Anxiety, impulsivity and depressed mood in relation to suicidal and violent behavior. *Acta Psychiatrica Scandinavica*, **87**(1), 1–5.

Apter, A., Gothelf, D., Orbach, I., Weizman, R., Ratzoni, G., Har-Even, D., and Tyano, S. (1995). Correlation of suicidal and violent behavior in different diagnostic categories in hospitalized adolescent patients. *Journal of the American Academy of Child and Adolescent Psychiatry*, **34**(7), 912–918.

Asarnow, J. R., Carlson, G. A., and Guthrie, D. (1987). Coping strategies, self-perceptions, hopelessness, and perceived family environments in depressed and suicidal children. *Journal of Consulting Clinical Psychology*, **55**, 361–366.

Barone, C., Weissberg, R. P., Kasprow, W. J., Voyce, C. K., Arthur, M. W., and Shriver, T. P. (1995). Involvement in multiple problem behaviors of young urban adolescents. *The Journal of Primary Prevention*, **15**, 261–283.

Beautrais, A. L. (1998). Risk factors for serious suicide attempts among young people: a case control study. In Kosky, R. J. and Eshkevari, H. S., et al. (eds.) *Suicide Prevention: The Global Context* (pp. 167–181). New York, NY: Plenum Press.

Beautrais, A. L., Joyce, P. R., and Mulder, R. T. (1996). Risk factors for serious suicide attempts among youths aged 13 through 24 years. *Journal of the American Academy of Child and Adolescent Psychiatry*, **35**, 1174–1182.

Blatt, S. J. (1995). The destructiveness of perfectionism: implications for the treatment of depression. *American Psychologist*, **50**, 1003–1020.

Brent, D. A. (1997). The aftercare of adolescents with deliberate self-harm. *Journal of Child Psychology and Psychiatry*, **38**, 277–286.

Brent, D. A. (2001). Firearms and suicide. *Annals of the New York Academy of Sciences*, **932**, 225–239. [Discussion; 239–240]

Brent, D. A., Perper, J. A., Moritz, G., Allman, C., Friend, A., Roth, C., Schweers, J., Balach, L., and Baugher, M. (1993a). Psychiatric risk factors for adolescent suicide: a case control study. *Journal of the American Academy of Child and Adolescent Psychiatry*, **32**, 521–529.

Brent, D. A., Perper, J., Moritz, G., Baugher, M., and Allman, C. (1993b). Suicide in adolescents with no apparent psychopathology. *Journal of the American Academy of Child and Adolescent Psychiatry*, **32**(3), 494–500.

Brent, D. A., Johnson, B. A., Perper, J., Connolly, J., Bridge, J., Bartle, S., and Rather, C. (1994). Personality disorder, personality traits, impulsive violence, and completed suicide in adolescents. *Journal of the American Academy of Child and Adolescent Psychiatry*, **33**(8), 1080–1086.

Brent, D. A., Baugher, M., Bridge, J., Chen, T., and Chiappetta, L. (1999). Age- and sex-related risk factors for adolescent suicide. *Journal of the American Academy of Child and Adolescent Psychiatry*, **38**, 1497–1505.

Brodsky, B. S., Oquendo, M., Ellis, S. P., Haas, G. L., Malone, K. M., and Mann, J. J. (2001). The relationship of childhood abuse to impulsivity and suicidal behavior in adults with major depression. *American Journal of Psychiatry*, **158**, 1871–1877.

Cairns, R. B., Cairns, B. D., Rodkin, P., and Xie, H. (1998). New directions in developmental research: models and methods. In Jessor, R. (ed.) *New Perspectives on Adolescent Risk Behavior* (pp. 13–40). Cambridge, UK: Cambridge University Press.

Centers for Disease Control and Prevention (2002). Centers for Disease Control and Prevention (2000). Youth Risk Behavior Surveillance – United States, 2001. *Morbidity Mortality Weekly Review*, **51**, No. SS04; 1–64 (June 28, 2002) **49**, No. SS05;1–104 (June 9, 2000).

Cicchetti, D. and Cohen, D. J. (eds.) (1995). *Developmental Psychopathology*. New York, NY: John Wiley & Sons.

Clark, D. C., and Horton-Deutsch, S. L. (1992). Assessment *in absentia*: the value of the psychological autopsy method for studying antecedents of suicide and predicting future suicides. In Maris, R. W., Berman, A. L., Maltsberger, J. T., and Yufit, R. I. (eds.). *The Assessment and Prediction of Suicide* (pp. 144–182). New York, NY: Guilford Press.

Clark, D. C., Sommerfeldt, L., Schwarz, M., Hedeker, D., and Watel, L. (1990). Physical recklessness in adolescence. Trait or byproduct of depressive/suicidal states? *Journal of Nervous and Mental Diseases*, **178**, 423–433.

Clayton, P. (1998). Editorial: smoking and suicide. *Journal of Affective Disorders*, **50**, 1–2.

Cohen-Sandler, R., Berman, A. L., and King, R. A. (1982). Life stress and symptomatology: determinants of suicidal behavior in children. *Journal of the American Academy of Child and Adolescent Psychiatry*, **21**, 565–574.

DiClemente, R. J., Hansen, W. B., and Ponton, L. E. (1996). New directions for adolescent risk prevention and health promotion research and interventions. In DiClemente, R. J., Hansen, W. B., and Ponton, L. E. (eds.). *Handbook of Adolescent Health Risk Behavior* (pp. 413–420). New York, NY: Plenum Press.

Donovan, J. E., Jessor, R., and Costa, F. M. (1988). Syndrome of problem behavior in adolescence: a replication. *Journal of Consulting and Clinical Psychology*, **56**, 762–765.

Donovan, J. E., Jessor, R., and Costa, F. M. (1993). Structure of health-enhancing behavior in adolescence: a latent-variable approach. *Journal of Health and Social Behavior*, **34**(4), 346–362.

Dryfoos, J. G. (1988). Youth at risk. One in four in jeopardy. Report submitted to the Carnegie Corporation, New York.

Dryfoos, J. G. (1990). *Adolescents at Risk*. New York, NY: Oxford University Press.

Dubow, E. F., Kausch, D. F., Blum, M. C., and Reed, J. (1989). Correlates of suicidal ideation and attempts in a community sample of junior high and high school students. *Journal of Clinical Child Psychology*, **18**, 158–166.

Durant, R. H., Knight, J., and Goodman, E. (1997). Factors associated with aggressive and delinquent behaviors among patients attending an adolescent medicine clinic. *Journal of Adolescent Health*, **21**, 303–308.

Durkheim, E. (1966). Suicide: a study in sociology. New York, NY: Free Press (original work published in 1897).

Engstrom, G., Nyman, G. E., and Traskman-Bendz, L. (1996). The Marke-Nyman Temperament (MNT) Scale in suicide attempters. *Acta Psychiatrica Scandinavica*, **94**, 320–325.

Ensminger, M. E. (1990). Sexual activity and problem behaviors among black, urban adolescents. *Child Development*, **61**, 2032–2046.

Farbstein, I., Dycian, A., King, R., Cohen, D. J., Kron, A., and Apter, A. (2002). A follow-up study of adolescent attempted suicide in Israel and the effects of mandatory general hospital admission. *Journal of the American Academy of Child and Adolescent Psychiatry*, **41**, 1342–1349.

Fergusson, D. M., and Lynskey, M. T. (1995a). Suicidal attempts and suicidal ideation in a birth cohort of 16 year old New Zealanders. *Journal of the American Academy of Child and Adolescent Psychiatry*, **34**, 1308–1317.

Fergusson, D. M., and Lynskey, M. T. (1995b). Antisocial behaviour, unintentional and intentional injuries during adolescence. *Criminal Behavior and Mental Health*, **5**, 312–329.

Fergusson, D. M., Horwood, L. J., and Lynskey, M. T. (1994). The comorbidities of adolescent problem behaviors: a latent class model. *Journal of Abnormal Child Psychology*, **22**, 339–354.

Fergusson, D. M., Woodward, L. J., and Horwood, L. J. (2000). Risk factors and life processes associated with the onset of suicidal behavior during adolescence and early adulthood. *Psychological Medicine*, **30**, 23–39.

Flament, M. F., Cohen, D., Choquet, M., Jeammet, P., and Ledoux, S. (2001). Phenomenology, psychosocial correlates, and treatment seeking in major depression and dysthymia of adolescence. *Journal of the American Academy of Child and Adolescent Psychiatry*, **40**, 1070–1078.

Flisher, A. J., Kramer, R. A., Hoven, C. W., King, R. A., Bird, H. R., Davies, M., Gould, M. S., Greenwald, S., Lahey, B. B., Regier, D. A., Schwab-Stone, M., and Shaffer, D. (2000). Risk behavior in a community sample of adolescents. *Journal of the American Academy of Child and Adolescent Psychiatry*, **39**, 881–887.

Garnefski, N., and Diekstra, R. F. W. (1997). "Comorbidity" of behavioral, emotional, and cognitive problems in adolescence. *Journal of Youth and Adolescence*, **26**, 321–338.

Garrison, C. Z., McKeown, R. E., Valois, R. F., and Vincent, M. L. (1993). Aggression, substance use, and suicidal behaviors in high school students. *American Journal of Public Health*, **83**, 179–184.

Gould, M. S., Fisher, P., Parides, M., Flory, M., and Shaffer, D. (1996). Psychosocial risk factors of child and adolescent completed suicide. *Archives of General Psychiatry*, **53**, 1155–1162.

Gould, M. S., King, R., Greenwald, S., Fisher, P., Schwab-Stone, M., Kramer, R., Flisher, A. J., Goodman, S., Canino, G., and Shaffer, D. (1998). Psychopathology associated with suicidal ideation and attempts among children and adolescents. *Journal of the American Academy of Child and Adolescent Psychiatry*, **37**, 915–923.

Hesselbrock, M. N., and Hesselbrock, V. M. (1992). Relationship of family history, antisocial personality disorder and personality traits in young men at risk for alcoholism. *Journal of Studies on Alcohol*, **53**, 619–625.

Higley, J., Mehlman, P., Higley, S., Fernard, B., Vickers, J., Lindell, S., Tamb, D., Suomi, S., and Linnoila, M. (1996). Excessive mortality in young free-ranging male non-human primates with low cerebrospinal fluid 5-hydroxyindoleacetic acid concentrations. *Archives of General Psychiatry*, **53**, 537–543.

Holinger, P. C. (1979). Violent deaths among the young: recent trends in suicide, homicide, and accidents. *American Journal of Psychiatry*, **136**, 1144–1147.

Horesh, N., Rolnick, T., Iancu, I., Dannon, P., Lepkifker, E., Apter, A., and Kotler, M. (1996). Coping styles and suicide risk. *Acta Psychiatrica Scandinavica*, **93**(6), 489–493.

Horesh, N., Rolnick, T., Iancu, I., Dannon, P., Lepkifker, E., Apter, A., and Kotler, M. (1997). Anger, impulsivity and suicide risk. *Psychotherapy and Psychosomatics*, **66**(2), 92–96.

Horesh, N., Gothelf, D., Ofek, H., Weizman, T., and Apter, A. (1999). Impulsivity as a correlate of suicidal behavior in adolescent psychiatric inpatients. *Crisis: Journal of Crisis Intervention and Suicide*, **20**(1), 8–14.

Hurrelmann, K. (1989). *Human Development and Health*. Berlin: Springer-Verlag.

Jessor, R. (1987). Risky driving and adolescent problem behavior: an extension of problem-behavior theory. *Alcohol, Drugs and Driving*, **3**, 1–12.

Jessor, R. (1991). Risk behavior in adolescence: a psychosocial framework for understanding and action. *Journal of Adolescent Health*, **12**, 597–605.

Jessor, R. (ed.). (1998). *New Perspectives on Adolescent Risk Behavior*. Cambridge UK: Cambridge University Press.

Jessor, R., Turbin, M. S., and Costa, F. M. (1997). Predicting developmental change in risky driving: the transition to young adulthood. *Applied Developmental Science*, **1**, 4–16.

Kahn, J. A., Kaplowitz, R. A., Goodman, E., and Emans, S. J. (2002). The association between impulsiveness and sexual risk behaviors in adolescent and young adult women. *Journal of Adolescent Health*, **30**, 229–232.

Kandel, D. B., Raveis, V. H., and Davies, M. (1991). Suicidal ideation in adolescence: depression, substance use, and other risk factors. *Journal of Youth and Adolescence*, **20**, 289–309.

Kazdin, A. (1995). Conduct disorders in childhood and adolescence (2nd edition). Thousand Oaks, CA: Sage.

King, R. A., and Apter, A. (1996). Psychoanalytic perspectives on youth suicide. *Psychoanalytic Study of the Child*, **51**, 491–511.

King, R. A., Schwab-Stone, M., Flisher, A. J., Greenwald, S., Kramer, R. A., Goodman, S. H., Lahey, B. B., Shaffer, D., and Gould, M. S. (2001). Psychosocial and risk behavior correlates of youth suicide attempts and suicidal ideation. *Journal of the American Academy of Child and Adolescent Psychiatry*, **40**(7), 837–846.

Kingsbury, S., Hawton, K., Steinhardt, K., and James, A. (1999). Do adolescents who take overdoses have specific psychological characteristics? A comparative study with psychiatric and community controls. *Journal of the American Academy of Child and Adolescent Psychiatry*, **38**, 1125–1131.

Koslowsky, M., Bleich, A., Apter, A., Solomon, Z., Wagner, B., and Greenspoon, A. (1992). Structural equation modelling of some of the determinants of suicide risk. *British Journal of Medical Psychology*, **65**, 157–165.

Leadbeater, B. J., Kuperminc, G. P., Blatt, S. J., and Hertzog, C. (1999). A multivariate model of gender differences in adolescents' internalizing and externalizing problems. *Developmental Psychology*, **35**(5), 1268–1282.

Lewinsohn, P. M., Rohde, P., and Seeley, J. R. (1996). Adolescent suicidal ideation and attempts: prevalence, risk factors, and implications. *Clinical Psychology: Science and Practice*, **3**, 25–46.

Lewinsohn, P. M., Rohde, P., Seeley, J. R., and Baldwin, C. L. (2001). Gender differences in suicide attempts from adolescence to young adulthood. *Journal of the American Academy of Child and Adolescent Psychiatry*, **40**(4), 427–434.

Loeber, R., Farrington, D. P., Stouthamer-Loeber, M., Moffitt, T. E., and Caspi, A. (2001). The development of male offending: key findings from the first decade of the Pittsburgh Youth Study. In Bull, R. (ed.). *Children and the Law: The Essential Readings. Essential Readings in Developmental Psychology* (pp. 336–378). Malden, ME: Blackwell Publishers Inc.

Maggs, J. L., Schulenberg, J., and Hurrelmann, K. (1997). Developmental transitions during adolescence: health promotion implications. In Schulenberg, J. Maggs, J. L., et al. (eds.). Health Risks and Developmental Transitions During Adolescence (pp. 522–546). New York, NY: Cambridge University Press.

Martin, C. S., Earleywine, M., Blackson, T. C., Vanyukov, M. M., Moss, H. B., and Tarter, R. E. (1994). Aggressivity, inattention, hyperactivity, and impulsivity in boys at high and low risk for substance abuse. *Journal of Abnormal Child Psychology*, **22**, 177–203.

McGee, L., and Newcomb, M. D. (1992). General deviance syndrome: expanded hierarchical evaluations at four ages from early adolescence ot adulthood. *Journal of Consulting and Clinical Psychology*, **60**, 766–776.

Neeleman, J., Wessely, S., and Wadsworth, M. (1998). Predictors of suicide, accidental death, and premature natural death in a general-population birth cohort. *Lancet*, **351 (9096)**, 93–97.

Olson, S. L., Schilling, E. M., and Bates, J. E. (1999). Measurement of impulsivity: construct coherence, longitudinal stability, and relationship with externalizing problems in middle childhood and adolescence. *Journal of Abnormal Child Psychology*, **27**(2), 151–165.

Orpinas, P. K., Basen-Engquist, K., Grunbaum, J. A., and Parcel, G. S. (1995). The co-morbidity of violence-related behaviors with health-risk behaviors in a population of high school students. *Journal of Adolescent Health*, **16**, 216–225.

Patton, G. C., Harris, R., Carlin, J. B., Hibbert, M. E., Coffey, C., Schwartz, M., and Bowes, G. (1997). Adolescent suicidal behaviours: a population-based study of risk. *Psychological Medicine*, **27**, 715–724.

Perris, C. (1994). Linking the experience of dysfunctional parental rearing with manifest psychopathology: a theoretical framework. In Perris, C., Arrindell, W. A., and Eisemann, M. (eds.). *Parenting and Psychopathology*. Chichester: John Wiley & Sons.

Pfeffer, C. R., Newcorn, J., Kaplan, G., Mizruchi, M. S., and Plutchik, R. (1989). Subtypes of suicidal and assaultive behaviors in adolescent psychiatric inpatients: a research note. *Journal of Child Psychology and Psychiatry*, **30**, 151–163.

Pfeffer, C. R., Klerman, G. L., Hurt, S. W., Kakuma, T., Peskin, J. R., and Siefker, C. A. (1993). Suicidal children grow up: rates and psychosocial risk factors for suicide attempts during follow-up. *Journal of the American Academy of Child and Adolescent Psychiatry*, **32**, 106–113 .

Puig-Antich, J. (1982). Major depression and conduct disorder in prepuberty. *Journal of the American Academy of Child Psychiatry*, **21**(2), 118–128.

Reinherz, H. Z., Giaconia, R. M., Silverman, A. B., Friedman, A., Pakiz, B., Frost, A. K., and Cohen, E. (1995). Early psychosocial risks for adolescent suicidal ideation and attempts. *Journal of the American Academy of Child and Adolescent Psychiatry*, **34**, 599–611.

Renaud, J., Brent, D. A., Birmaher, B., Chiappetta, L., and Bridge, J. (1999). Suicide in adolescents with disruptive disorders. *Journal of the American Academy of Child and Adolescent Psychiatry*, **38**(7), 846–851.

Rotheram-Borus, M. J., Trautman, P. D., Dopkins, S. C., and Shrout, P. E. (1990). Cognitive style and pleasant activities among female adolescent suicide attempters. *Journal of Consulting and Clinical Psychology*, **58**(5), 554–561.

Shaffer, D. (1974). Suicide in childhood and early adolescence. *Journal of Child Psychology and Psychiatry*, **15**, 275–291.

Shaffer, D., and Pfeffer, C. R. (2001). Practice parameter for the assessment and treatment of children and adolescents with suicidal behavior. *Journal of the American Academy of Child and Adolescent Psychiatry*, **40** (supplement), 24S–51S.

Shaffer, D., Garland, A., Gould, M., Fisher, P., and Trautman, P. (1988). Preventing teen-age suicide: a critical review. *Journal of the American Academy of Child and Adolescent Psychiatry*, **27**, 675–687.

Shaffer, D., Gould, M. S., Fisher, P., Trautman, P., Moreau, D., Kleinman, M., and Flory, M. (1996). Psychiatric diagnosis in child and adolescent suicide. *Archives of General Psychiatry*, **53**, 339–348.

Shafii, M., Carrigan, S., Whittinghill, J. R., and Derrick, A. (1985). Psychological autopsy of completed suicide in children and adolescents. *American Journal of Psychiatry*, **142**, 1061–1064.

Simon, T. R., Swann, A. C., Powell, K. E., Potter, L. B., Kresnow, M., and O'Carroll, P. W. (2001). Characteristics of impulsive suicide attempts and attempters. *Suicide and Life-Threatening Behavior*, **32** (supplement), 49–59.

Simons, R. L., and Murphy, P. I. (1985). Sex differences in the causes of adolescent suicide ideation. *Journal of Youth and Adolescence*, **14**, 423–434.

Sosin, D. M., Koepsell, T. D., Rivara, F. P., and Mercy, J. A. (1995). Fighting as a marker for multiple problem behaviors in adolescents. *Journal of Adolescent Health*, **16**, 209–215.

Stattin, H., and Kerr, M. (2000). Parental monitoring: a reinterpretation. *Child Development*, **71**, 1072–1085.

Velez, C., and Cohen, P. (1988). Suicidal behavior and ideation in a community sample of children. *Journal of the American Academy of Child and Adolescent Psychiatry*, **27**, 349–356.

Vermeiren, R., Schwab-Stone, M., Ruchkin, V., King, R. A., van Heeringen C. M. D., and Deboutte, D. (2003). Self-harming behavior and violence in adolescents: a community study. *Journal of American Academy of Child and Adolescent Psychiatry*, **42**, 41–48.

Verona, E., and Patrick, C.J. (2000). Suicide risk in externalizing syndromes: temperamental and neurobiological underpinnings. In Joiner, T. E., and Rudd, M. D. (eds.). *Suicide Science: Expanding the Boundaries* (pp. 137–173). Norwell, MA: Kluwer Academic Publishers.

Vitaro, F., Arseneault, L., and Tremblay, R. E. (1999). Impulsivity predicts problem gambling in low SES adolescent males. *Addiction*, **94**, 565–575.

Wagner, B. M. (1997). Family risk factors in child and adolescent suicidal behavior. *Psychological Bulletin*, **121**, 246–298.

Wagner, B. M., Cole, R. E., and Schwartzman, P. (1996). Comorbidity of symptoms among junior and senior high school suicide attempters. *Suicide and Life-Threatening Behavior*, **26**, 300–307.

Walter, H. J., Vaughan, R. D., Armstrong, B., Krakoff, R. Y., Maldonado, L. M., Tiezzi, L., and McCarthy, J. F. (1995). Sexual, assaultive and suicidal behaviors among urban minority junior high school students. *Journal of the American Academy of Child and Adolescent Psychiatry*, **34**, 73–80.

Wills, T. A., Cleary, S., Filer, M., Shinar, O., Mariani, J., and Spera, K. (2001). Temperament related to early-onset substance use: test of a developmental model. *Preventive Science*, **2**, 145–163.

Woods, E. R., Lin, Y. G., Middleman, A., Beckford, P., Chase, L., and DuRant, R. H. (1997). The associations of suicide attempts in adolescents. *Pediatrics*, **99**, 791–796.

Yang, B., and Clum, G. A. (2000). Childhood stress leads to later suicidality via its effect on cognitive functioning. *Suicide and Life-Threatening Behavior*, **30**(3), 183–198.

# 3

# Adolescent attempted suicide

Alan Apter and Danuta Wasserman

## Introduction

Many young people make nonfatal deliberate attempts to kill themselves. This phenomenon, also known as "parasuicide," is at least ten times more common than suicide; however, the exact prevalence of such acts is unknown. Although the exact relationship between parasuicidal acts and suicide is controversial, it is important to note that the majority of these acts are by adolescents and young adults who constitute a pool from which many of the future suicides are drawn (Diekstra, 1994).

Attempted suicide is relatively rare under 12 years of age, although there may be isolated cases under the age of five. Suicide attempts in young children may well go unrecognized. The rarity of attempted suicides in this age may be because the concept of death develops late in childhood, with full awareness of the implications of death not being gained until early adolescence. Possibly serious impulses toward suicidal behavior do not occur until the concept of death has developed. Other protective factors which have been suggested include the lower rates of depression in young children, their close integration in the family, and the necessity for a marked degree of cognitive maturation before a child can develop feelings such as despair and hopelessness (Hawton and Catalan, 1987).

Although suicide attempts are far more common than completed suicide, the literature on it is far more variable and inconsistent than that on completed suicide. Difficulty in specifying the intent behind a given act and the lack of a consistent definition of attempted suicide have resulted in great variability in estimates of various suicidal behaviors. There is a spectrum of suicidal thoughts and behaviors that begins with ephemeral thoughts about suicide and proceeds to attempted suicide without injury, to attempted suicide with serious injury, and finally to completed suicide. Surveys designed to estimate the incidence or prevalence of suicidal ideation and suicidal behaviors are often difficult to interpret and compare because they simply ask, "have you attempted suicide?" without attempting to elucidate the seriousness of the suicidal intent or the medical outcome of the attempt. This problem is exemplified by the paradoxically higher estimated life time prevalence for younger than older adolescents found in the ECA study (Mosckici et al., 1989). Possible approaches to clarifying what respondents mean when they report having attempted suicide include using more specific definitions of the term "suicide attempt," and specifying the outcome of the attempted suicide through a series of increasingly specific questions. For example, respondents could be asked whether they had specifically "attempted to take their own lives" rather than asking about "attempted suicide." Specific questions about outcome of reported attempts in terms of injury, medical care received, and hospitalization should be asked (Meehan et al., 1992; Ramberg and Wasserman, 2000).

One major difficulty with collecting standardized data on suicide morbidity is thus the measurement of suicidal intent (Moscicki, 1995). Such information is of great importance, however, because self-inflicted injuries that are labeled as attempted suicides range in severity from a "cry for help" to a genuine failed attempt. Another important variable is the medical lethality of the attempt, which some authors feel is an important indicator of intent (Andrews and Lewinsohn, 1992; Brent et al., 1987; Garrison et al., 1993; Meehan et al., 1992).

Important data have come from surveys of psychiatric morbidity in community samples (Andrews and Lewinsohn, 1992; Garrison et al., 1993; Meehan et al., 1992; Tomori and Zalar, 2000) that employed operationally defined questions about suicidal behaviors. However, surveys that depend on subjective reports without objective measures of medical outcome undoubtedly are less reliable and tend to generate a large proportion of false-positives. This is because the majority of attempters do not want to die and the ratio of attempters to completed suicides is considerably higher in adolescents than in older people (Moscicki, 1995).

## Epidemiology

### Population-based data

Population-based data on attempted suicides have not been well investigated in any age group (Moscicki, 1995). Two independently conducted Swedish studies found very high rates of self-reported suicide attempts among 16- and 17-year-olds, ranging from 6.6% (von Knorring and Kristiansson, 1995) to 7.7% (Ramberg and Wasserman, 1995). These figures are considerably higher than the rate for the total Swedish population (Ramberg and Wasserman, 2000), which is around 2.5% to 3.5%, as well as for other populations (Meehan et al., 1992; Paykel et al., 1974).

A population survey found that only half of those adolescents who attempted suicide sought hospital care (Ramberg and Wasserman, 2000). Estimated rates of attempted suicides in U.S. nonpsychiatric, school samples range from 3% in elementary school children to 11% in high-school students and 15% to 18% in college students (Garrison et al., 1989). Most were low lethal attempts for which medical attention was not sought. A survey of Dutch secondary school students found reported lifetime rates of suicide attempts of 2.2% (Kienhorst et al., 1990). Using a similar methodology, Tomori and Zalar (2000) found rates of 7.4% for girls and 3.1% for boys in Slovenia. Studies in the U.S. report low estimates of lethal and/or intentional attempts among adolescents, ranging from 1.6 to 2.5 per 100 (Andrews and Lewinsohn, 1992; Garrison et al., 1993; Meehan et al., 1992).

In the U.S., the Centers for Disease Control's National Youth Risk Behavior Survey (YRBS) (CDC, 2002; Kann et al., 2000; Kolbe et al., 1993) periodically surveys the prevalence of health risk behaviors among high-school youth through comparable national, state, and local surveys. The school-based YRBS used a three-stage sample design to obtain a representative sample of 11 631 students in grades 9–12 in the whole U.S. Students were asked whether they had seriously thought about attempting suicide during the 12 months preceding the survey, whether they had made a specific plan about how they would attempt suicide, how many times they had actually made a suicide attempt, and whether their suicide attempt(s) resulted in an injury or poisoning that had to be treated by a doctor or nurse. For all the 12 months preceding the survey (CDC, 2002) 19.3% of the students reported that they had seriously thought about attempting suicide. Fewer students (14.5%) reported that they had made a specific plan about how they would attempt Suicide. About half the students (8.3%) reported that they had actually attempted suicide, while 2.6% of the students reported that they had made a suicide attempt that required medical attention. Females were significantly more likely than males to report suicidal ideation (24.9 vs. 13.7%); to have made significant plans (10.9 vs. 5.7%); and 2.5% of females and 1.6% of males had made a suicide attempt requiring medical attention but this difference was not statistically significant. Hispanic females were consistently higher than all other ethnic groups in this survey for all forms of suicidal behavior.

The YRBS study is among the few that have attempted to quantify the health import of adolescents' self-reported suicide attempt or to determine whether high-school students' perception of the attempt includes overt injury or other sequelae. The YRBS findings add to the evidence that most self-reported suicide attempts among young adults and adolescents do not result in injury or hospitalization (Smith and Crawford, 1986). These and previous (Ramberg and

Wasserman, 2000) findings suggest that future studies of attempted suicide in adolescents should also assess the medical consequences of the self-reported suicidal behavior (CDC, 2002; Ramberg and Wasserman, 2000).

## Hospital-based (emergency room) data

Studies of subjects referred for treatment of a suicidal act (Beautrais et al., 1996; Schmidtke et al., 1996; Hawton et al., 1997) necessarily suffer from referral biases and may not be generalizable to the general population. Tomori and Zalar (2000) criticized these types of studies, suggesting that they cannot provide the basis for school-based prevention programs. Adolescents who attempt suicide and present at the emergency room appear to differ psychologically from those who are examined in other clinical settings. In addition, there seem to be differences in the nature and type of the attempt in different clinical settings.

Hospital referrals for intentional overdoses or deliberate self-injury have soared in recent years (Diekstra, 1989a), resulting in deliberate self-poisoning becoming the commonest reason for acute hospital admission of adolescent women in many areas. Parasuicide, as measured by subjects referred for treatment, is more common in females than in males (1.5–2.1:1), the sex ratio being highest during adolescence. The highest rates for females are in the age range 15–19 years. In the 1970s, one in 100 girls in Oxford, UK was referred to general hospitals after a suicide attempt (Hawton et al., 1997).

Rates of referred attempted suicide are inversely related to social class. The incidence of attempted suicide is 8- to 12-fold higher in social class V than in social class I. Parasuicidal behavior is also more common in urban, socially deprived, and overcrowded areas (Hawton and Catalan, 1987). Relatively high rates of completed suicide have been found in Oxford and Cambridge University students but this has not been the case for their American counterparts at Yale and Harvard. Rates of attempted suicide were much lower among students of both sexes during term time than among other people of comparable age in the city of Oxford during the same period (Hawton et al., 2000). The very different social class distribution of the students compared with the general population might explain this finding, especially since the reasons for the attempt were similar in both populations, the most important being the breakup of an important relationship.

## The World Health Organization (WHO) study

It has been difficult to obtain comparable cross-national data on adolescent attempted suicide, owing to differences in definitions and difficulties in survey design. Accordingly, the WHO Multicentre Study on Parasuicide (Attempted

Suicide) began in 1989 in 13 European countries and a total of 16 research centers, with the general purpose of preventing suicidal behavior in Europe (Bille-Brahe et al., 1993; Platt et al., 1992; Schmidtke et al., 1996). (The initial countries were Switzerland, France, Italy, Spain, Finland, Austria, the Netherlands, Denmark, the United Kingdom, Sweden, Hungary, Norway, and Germany; additional countries have since joined the project.) To obtain a reliable epidemiological picture of attempted suicide in these European countries, all participant centers use a standardized method of gathering and recording data, including various sociodemographic risk factors and subsequent treatment.

Attempted suicide (parasuicide) is defined in the WHO study as follows: "An act with nonfatal outcome, in which an individual deliberately initiates a nonhabitual behaviour that, without intervention from others, will cause self-harm, or deliberately ingests a substance in excess of the prescribed or generally recognized therapeutic dosage, and which is aimed at realizing changes which the subject desired via the actual or expected physical consequences." The WHO Multicentre Study on Parasuicide (Attempted Suicide) includes both suicidal behavior prompted by a strong intention to die and behavior where there is uncertainty and ambivalence regarding the intention to die, and where the self-destructive act may be designated a cry for help. In the WHO study, only suicide-attempt patients known to health-care services from a defined catchment area are included.

The WHO study – which included 20 325 suicide-attempt patients for the years 1989–95 – thus provides a reliable picture of the European population of suicide attempters who have sought help at various health-care services after their attempt (Platt et al., 1992; Schmidtke et al., 1996).

## Demographics

During the study period 1990–95, the WHO sample included 1965 young people aged 15–19 years who attempted suicide on 2394 occasions, i.e., there were 2394 "suicide-attempt events." The 1415 females and 550 males accounted for 1728 and 666 of the suicide-attempt events respectively. The preponderance of female suicide attempters may possibly be explained by girls' earlier maturation and confrontation with romantic problems, higher rates of depression, and self-poisoning representing a more acceptable coping strategy for girls. Boys in contrast only seem to resort to suicidal behavior in the face of extreme difficulties and may more readily resort to alternative strategies for dealing with stress, such as aggressive behavior or alcohol abuse (Hawton and Catalan, 1987).

Among the young suicide attempters (age 15–19 years) in the WHO study, 3.3% were co-habitating, 2.0% married, and the remaining majority were single;

2.9% already had children of their own. More than half still lived with their parents (59.7%), but a fairly high proportion lived alone (12.0%); the rest lived with relatives, partners or friends or at an institution. The fact that approximately 40% of the 15- to 19-year-old suicide attempters did not live with their parents reflects young suicide patients' difficulties in relationships with their parents and parallels the findings of other studies that many young suicide attempters come from broken homes (Garnefski and Diekstra, 1997; Kotila, 1989) and/or families characterized by psychiatric illness (especially depression and substance abuse) and cumulative negative life events (Pillay and Wassenaar, 1997; Wagner, 1997). In the WHO study group of 15- to 19-year-old attempters, almost 29.2% of the boys and 25.5% of the girls were already working instead of attending school.

Reported youth attempted-suicide rates in the WHO study were highest in England, Hungary, Germany, and Finland; they were intermediate in Denmark, Sweden, Norway, Austria, and Switzerland; and were lowest in Spain, Italy, and the Netherlands. These cross-national differences for youth attempted suicide followed the same pattern as that for adult attempts (Platt et al., 1992; Schmidtke et al., 1996) and both youth and adult completed suicides (Diekstra, 1989a, b; Wasserman et al., 1997) (see also Chapter 7).

**Repetition rates**
The repetition rate for referred attempted suicide may be estimated by the ratio of the number of suicide-attempt events to the number of people involved. For the period 1989–95, this ratio was 1.21 for boys, 1.22 for girls. Repeat suicide attempts may also be measured in terms of the percentage of patients who attempt suicide again within 12 months of the index episode. Of the 1965 young people who attempted suicide, 10.2% – 143 females and 57 males – made a second attempt during the 12-month observation period. Sixty-seven individuals, 3.4%, comprising 48 females and 19 males, made a third attempt within a 12-month period. The majority (27.4%) of 15- to 19-year-old youngsters who repeated their suicide attempts did it within one month after the index suicide attempt.

Another method of estimating repetition risk is to study suicide-attempt patients consecutively admitted to hospital and estimate the proportion that have previously attempted suicide. In the WHO study, more than one-third (34.8%) of the young patients included in the study at the index-attempted suicide had a history of prior attempted-suicide behaviour. First-time suicide attempters made up approximately 65% of both girls and boys in the period 1989–95. Comparisons of subsequent suicide-attempt repetition rates among young people who had and did not have a history of prior suicide attempts on entry to the WHO Multicentre Study on Parasuicide (Attempted Suicide) showed that, in the group of first-time suicide attempters, the repetition rate within 12 months after the index suicide attempt was 6.2% for boys and 7.3% for girls, in comparison to 21.9% for boys and 16.8% for girls who had already attempted suicide previously (Hultén et al., 2001).

These findings suggest that there is a subset of youthful attempters at especially high risk for multiple attempts who warrant intensive follow-up and treatment (see also Chapter 12).

## The Oregon study

Another contrasting body of population-based clinical data comes from a comprehensive survey of suicide attempters seen in emergency rooms that was conducted in the state of Oregon for the years 1988–93, following legislation that mandated reporting of suicide attempts coming to clinical attention. Oregon is a state with a relatively high rate of teenage suicide (15.5 deaths / 100 000 vs. the national average of 11.1). Of the 3783 attempts recorded, 326.4 / 100 000 were made by females vs. 73.4 / 100 000 for males. However, the rate for attempts that were fatal was a hundred-fold higher for males than for females (11.5% vs. 0.1%). Previous attempts were found in 41.5% of cases, especially in those persons whose motivation for the attempt was stated as rape / sexual assault, physical abuse or substance abuse (CDC, 1995).

## The epidemiology of serious suicide attempts – The Canterbury (New Zealand) study

There is a paucity of studies that look at serious suicide attempts in adolescents. The most extensive data in this regard come from the Canterbury (New Zealand) study (Beautrais et al., 1996). The Canterbury Suicide Project is a case–control study of 200 suicide cases, 302 medically serious suicide attempts and 1028 randomly selected control subjects. A medically serious attempt was defined as one requiring treatment in a specialized unit (e.g., the intensive care unit, hyperbaric unit (for CO poisoning), or burn unit); surgery under general anesthesia (e.g., for tendon repair or stab injuries); or medical treatment beyond gastric lavage, activated charcoal or routine neurological observations. Individuals were included in this last category if they required treatment such as antidotes for drug overdose, telemetry, or repeated tests or observations. Also included in the sample were individuals who made suicide attempts with a high risk of fatality, such as hanging or gunshot, and were hospitalized for more than 24 hours. One hundred and twenty-five of the subjects were less than 25 years old. Almost equal numbers of males and females made serious suicide attempts and gender ratio did not differ from those who had completed suicide. Mean age was 19.4 years and ranged from 13 through 24 years. Twice as many females overdosed than males, who predominantly used CO poisoning and hanging. Low income and residential mobility were highly associated with a serious attempt. In addition, childhood sexual abuse, low parental care, and poor parental relationship were significant risk factors as were the presence of mood disorder, substance abuse, and conduct disorder. In addition, interpersonal difficulties, legal problems, work, and financial difficulties made a significant contribution to the risk of a serious suicide attempt (Beautrais, 1998).

## Reasons for suicide attempts

Data from the Stockholm WHO center illustrate reasons for suicide attempts. Among many young suicide attempters seen there, instability in family situation and childhood circumstances was notable. Parental divorce was common, as were parental mental illness or substance abuse. Mental or physical abuse and sexual assault were also frequently reported. These youngsters' suicide attempts may be seen as the outcome of suffering over a long period, and perhaps throughout life, producing vulnerability that the youngster is unable to deal with unaided. The factor triggering the suicide attempt was often acute relationship problems with parents and/or romantic partner. A failure, a quarrel with a parent, or a break-up with a boy- or girlfriend sparked off fury and despair that resonated with losses and disappointments earlier in life. Other immediate reasons cited for suicide attempts included academic failure and financial difficulties.

In the Swedish data, academic difficulty was cited equally often by boys and girls. Suicidal attempts among this group of young people were more often an effort to communicate the pain of a stressful life rather than a genuine wish to die. Relatives of the young people who tried to take their own lives had often failed to notice the youngsters' psychological problems. Only when the suicide attempt had been made did they notice that the child was in distress (Hultén and Wasserman, 1995).

## Methods of attempting suicide

"Active" methods of attempting suicide involve inflicting self-injury, e.g., attempting to hang oneself, throw oneself in front of a vehicle, jump from a height or use a firearm. Intoxications with pills, gas, or liquids are termed "passive" methods.

The Oregon study (CDC, 1995) reported on methods used in that state between 1988 and 1993. Ingestion of drugs accounted for most (75.5%) attempts. Of the attempts involving drugs, analgesics accounted for 47.4% (aspirin and acetaminophen were used most commonly). Cutting and piercing injuries accounted for 11.1% of attempts, of which most were lacerations of the wrists.

Most attempts by multiple methods were lacerations combined with a drug overdose. Drugs were used in 79.8 % of attempts by females compared with 57.4% by males. Male attempters were more likely to use suffocation/hanging, cutting/piercing, or firearms. Of all methods used to attempt suicide, those used most commonly were least likely to result in death (e.g., only 0.4% of drug ingestions were fatal, compared to 78.2% and 35.7% of attempts with firearms or gas poisoning). Most deaths were due to firearms (63.7%) or suffocation/hanging (18.5%) (CDC, 1995).

In the WHO multicenter study, the highest proportion of young people, 35.2%, had attempted to poison themselves with drugs affecting the central nervous system. Roughly 17.7% had used sharp (self-cutting, 21.8% of the boys and 16.2% of the girls) and 2.4% had used herbicides and pesticides to attempt suicide. Intoxication with analgesics, including paracetamol, had been used by 39.8% of the young suicide attempters (42.5% of the girls and 32.5% of the boys). Paracetamol is used especially often by young people since this drug is available without prescription, and young people are often unaware of the dangerousness of overdosing with paracetamol (Hawton et al., 2000). (In the United Kingdom, a major media campaign was launched to warn people of the risk of dying from an overdose of paracetamol.) Other methods, such as jumping from a height and trying to hang, suffocate, drown or shoot oneself, were used by 3.0% of the young people (5.8% of the boys and 1.9% of the girls) who tried to take their own lives.

Alcohol was used as a method of attempting suicide by 2.7% of the boys and 1.6% of the girls in the WHO study. In the Stockholm sample, the frequency of alcohol consumption in conjunction with the suicide attempt was examined. It was found that 37.1% of the boys and 22.7% of the girls were under the influence of alcohol when attempting suicide. The part played by alcohol in relaxing inhibitions is a well known factor in precipitating suicidal behavior (Wasserman, 1993; Wasserman and Värnik, 1998). Since many suicide attempters come from homes in which there is alcohol abuse (Wolk-Wasserman, 1986), effective prevention requires a policy of moulding opinion not only against alcohol abuse, but also against the drinking of alcohol as a remedy for anxiety and depression, or as a means of coping with life's severe crises.

## The prognostic implications of parasuicide and the relationship between attempted suicide and suicide

Although the evaluation and acute management of young people who have made a suicide attempt is a common clinical challenge, knowledge about the natural course of adolescents following suicide attempts is limited (Spirito et al., 1992). On the one hand, there is evidence to show that adolescent suicidal behavior should always be taken very seriously; on the other, some clinicians believe that overtreatment of these cases is not cost-effective and may even be counterproductive (Angle et al., 1983).

A history of suicidal behavior is one of the most significant risk factors for completed suicide among adolescents (Brent et al., 1993). Thus, adolescent suicide completers are far more likely than community controls to have had a history of a suicide attempt (Shaffer et al., 1988; Shafii et al., 1985). Similarly, prospective studies also indicate that the risk of completed suicide is substantially elevated in those who have attempted suicide (Garfinkel et al., 1982; Goldacre and Hawton, 1985).

Although follow-up studies of adolescent suicide attempters have been hampered by the difficulty of re-contacting subjects and other methodological problems, adolescent attempters appear to be at higher risk for nonfatal re-attempts (Spirito et al., 1989; see also Chapter 12). Reported repetition rates range widely from 6.3% (Goldacre and Hawton, 1985) through 51% (Mehr et al., 1982), while the reported risk for eventual completed suicide following an attempt in adolescence ranges from 0% (Hawton et al., 1982; Litt et al., 1983; Mattson et al., 1969; McIntire et al., 1977; Mehr et al., 1982; Morrison and Collier, 1969; Paerregaard, 1975; Pfeffer et al., 1991) through 0.4% (Otto, 1972; Goldacre and Hawton, 1985); 2% (Kotila and Lonnquist, 1988); 5% (Kienhorst et al., 1987); and 9% (Motto, 1984). Lower nonfatal repetition and completed suicide rates are seen in nonpsychiatrically hospitalized samples and in younger suicide attempters (Spirito et al., 1989). Male attempters subsequently complete suicide more often than do female attempters (Motto, 1984).

On the other hand, attempted suicide in adolescence is not necessarily a portent of a poor prognosis, especially in youngsters who have no history of a psychiatric hospitalization (American Academy of Pediatrics, 1980; Dycian et al., 1994; Felice, 1981; Hassanyeh et al., 1989). In Europe, the term "deliberate self harm" has replaced the term "attempted suicide" reflecting a large body of literature distinguishing attempter populations from completer populations (Diekstra, 1989b; ICD 10, 1994). These studies suggest that such attempts are frequently impulsive (Kessel, 1965), the result of an unpredictable acute interpersonal conflict (Kreitman, 1979), and, unlike, completed suicide, often unrelated to illness and symptom severity (Newson-Smith and Hirsch, 1979; Trautman et al., 1991). Zonda (1991) found that Hungarian adolescent attempters were far less likely to re-attempt or to actually commit suicide than adult attempters. Some follow-up studies suggest that approximately half of adolescent suicide attempters improve psychologically following a suicide attempt (Spirito et al., 1989). Angle et al. (1983) reported a favorable outcome for adolescent suicide attempters, irrespective of lethality of intent, parental loss, depression, diagnosis, availability of support systems and specific therapy.

It has also been suggested that suicide attempts in adolescent males have a graver significance than attempted suicide in females (Hawton et al., 1982; Kotila and Lonnquist, 1988; Suokas and Lonnquist, 1991). This was borne out in a population-based follow-up study of Israeli adolescent suicide attempters who had attempted suicide while in early adolescence and were followed up during their subsequent army service. The girls did relatively well, but the boys had great difficulty with many psychiatric and behavioral complications (Farbstein et al., 2002).

## Psychopathological characteristics of adolescent suicide attempters

### Aggression

The relationship between suicide, attempted suicide, and aggression has long been recognized by psychoanalysis, and has been best formulated by Menninger (1933), who proposed that a dynamic triad underlies all aggressive behavior, whether directed inward or outward: the wish to die, the wish to kill, and the wish to be killed.

There are many reports in the daily press of murderers who commit suicide. Roughly one out of four patients with a history of violent actions in the past has made a suicide attempt (Skodal and Karasu, 1978; Tardiff and Sweillam, 1980). Aggressive behavior is an important risk factor for attempted suicide in adults (Skodal and Karasu, 1978), adolescents (Apter et al., 1995) and prepubertal children (Cohen-Sandler et al., 1982; Pfeffer et al., 1983). In a sample of 51 hospitalized adolescents, Inmadar et al. (1982) found that 66.7% had been violent, 43.1% had been suicidal and 27.5% had been both.

For example, Tardiff and Sweillam (1980) found that in a large group of suicidal psychiatric inpatients, 14% of males and 7% of females were assaultive at the time of or just before admission. Female suicide attempters show more hostility and engage in more arguments and friction with friends and relatives than a comparable group of nonsuicidal depressed women. Depressed inpatients with a history of self-destructive acts have been found to have high levels of hostility and violence as measured by their need for seclusion and restraint (Weissman et al., 1973).

In a large group of psychiatric inpatients with mixed diagnoses, about 40% had made a suicide attempt, 42% had engaged in violent behavior in the past, and 23% had histories of both types of behavior (Plutchik et al., 1985). Almost every one of the 30 variables measured in these patients turned out to be a significant predictor of both suicide risk and violence risk. These results strongly support the idea of a close link between suicide risk and violence risk regardless of diagnosis.

Another important finding in this regard is that of Shaffer and Fisher (1981), who found that a combination of **depressive symptoms and antisocial behavior was the most common antecedent of teenage suicide**. Assaultiveness (Pfeffer et al., 1983) and instability of affect as reflected in borderline personality disorder (Apter et al., 1988b) may also be important correlates of adolescent suicidal behavior, especially in combination with depression. Aggressive or violent behavior is highly correlated with suicidal behavior on psychiatric wards (Plutchik and van Praag, 1986), in the histories of psychiatric patients with all kinds of diagnoses (Inmadar et al., 1982; Skodal and Karasu, 1978; Tardiff and Sweillam, 1980) and in all age groups (Pfeffer et al., 1983). A recent study by Plutchik and van Praag (1986) showed that psychometric measures of violence risk were highly correlated with measures of suicide risk.

## Anger

Several authors have indicated that **anger** may be an emotional state that is often associated with adolescent suicide attempts. However, there has been very little empirical investigation of this subject (Spirito et al., 1989). Pfeffer et al. (1988) have described an angry assaultive subtype of childhood suicidal behavior, and angry feelings are common in children referred for psychiatric evaluation including those who are nonsuicidal. Adolescent suicide attempters often exhibit a wide range of aggressive behaviors (Garfinkel et al., 1982).

## Depression

As with suicide completers **depression** is an important risk factor but depression is by no means necessary or sufficient to cause a suicide attempt. Studies conducted in psychiatric hospitals find an association between depression and suicide attempts. Friedman et al. (1983) found that 27 of 28 hospitalized adolescents who had made a suicide attempt had an affective disorder. Robbins and Alessi (1985) also found suicidal behavior to be highly associated with depressed mood in 64 hospitalized adolescents. Carlson and Cantwell (1982) found that 30% of 102 depressed adolescents and children had made a prior suicide attempt in contrast to 18% of the nondepressed children. They also found that severe suicidal ideation correlated with increasingly severe depression, with major depressive disorder diagnosed in 83% of adolescent inpatients with the severest suicidal ideation.

Crumley (1979) reported that 24 (60%) of 40 adolescent suicide attempters seen in a private psychiatric practice were diagnosed as having major affective disorder. One study of black children and adolescents referred for outpatient treatment found that a depressed mood was more common in suicide attempters than in suicide ideators (Bettes and Walker, 1986). The other study found depression to be more common in suicide attempters than in psychiatric controls (Marks and Haller, 1977). When suicide attempters are examined in the emergency room following their attempt, high rates of dysphoria and the associated vegetative symptoms are reported in between 69% and 82% of subjects (Spirito et al., 1989). In studies of nonclinical adult populations, the prevalence of suicidal ideation also increases with the severity of depression scores (Vandivort and Locke, 1979).

However, although depressive symptoms and/or a diagnosis of depressive disorder are common in suicidal children, depression is not a necessary concomitant of either suicidal ideation or attempts, especially in community samples. For example, in the community sample cited above, 41% of the adult subjects who reported suicidal ideation did not report depression (Vandivort and Locke, 1979). Similarly in a nonclinical college sample, about half of the students who admitted making a suicide attempt did not meet the criteria of major depression at any time in their lives (Levy and Deykin, 1989). Among adolescents reporting suicide attempts in a community study using the diagnostic interview schedule for children, Velez and Cohen (1988) found an increasing frequency of depressive symptoms but only a 19% current prevalence of DSM III major affective disorder. Reviewing a variety of reports, Goldney and Pilowsky (1981) concluded that only about 50%- to 75% of suicide attempters were depressed. Similarly, in an inpatient setting Cohen-Sandler et al. (1982) found that 35% of the suicidal child and adolescent patients did not appear to be depressed.

## Impulsivity

**Impulsivity** has frequently been described as a risk factor for suicide and a personality characteristic of adolescent suicide attempters (Crumley, 1979; Kingsbury et al., 1999). Lack of impulse control has been found to distinguish adolescent suicide attempters from adolescents with an acute illness (Slap et al., 1988). However, impulsivity does not seem to characterize all suicide attempters since group comparisons have found no difference between suicidal patients and controls on measures of cognitive impulsivity (Spirito et al., 1989). Instead, impulsivity may be important in identifying high-risk subgroups. A one-year follow-up of suicide attempters showed repeaters to be more impulsive than nonrepeaters. Furthermore, it has been suggested that impulsive suicide attempters come from families where action supersedes verbal mediation and that male attempters may be more impulsive than females (Marks and Haller, 1977). Finally, impulsive suicide attempters have been found to be less depressed and have fewer feelings of hopelessness than nonimpulsive attempters (Williams, 1988). It is surprising how few studies have been conducted on the relationship between impulsivity and teenage suicide given the frequent reference to teenage suicide attempts as impulsive. In those studies that do exist, the distinction between impulsive cognitive style and impulsive attempts must be considered. Another problem is that the measures of impulsivity used in these studies often reflect angry and aggressive behavior as much as behavior suggesting a lack of reflection or planning.

## Anxiety

**Anxiety** has been identified as an important risk factor for suicidal behavior in adults. A follow-up study of patients with major affective disorder (Fawcett et al., 1990) found that anxiety symptoms were strongly related to completed suicide within one year of assessment. There have also been studies that indicate that anxiety disorders are associated with an increased risk of suicidal behavior (Allgulander and Lavori, 1991; Mannuzza et al., 1992; Massion et al., 1993; Weissman et al., 1989). Studies with adolescents have shown mixed results. Taylor and Stansfeld (1984) found that suicide attempters when compared to psychiatric outpatients seemed to exhibit higher levels of anxiety (38% vs. 22%); however, the difference was not significant. Another study (Kosky et al., 1986) reported that depressed suicidal ideators (of whom 39% had attempted suicide) manifested high levels of anxiety (76.4%), but these levels were not significantly different from those of depressed nonsuicidal adolescents. Interestingly, Bettes and Walker (1986) found in a large sample of disturbed youth (inpatients and outpatients) that male adolescents who express suicidal thoughts in the absence of acts were more likely to be rated as anxious as compared to suicide attempters. The authors interpreted this finding by suggesting that engaging in suicidal acts may serve to reduce symptoms, and this might account for the lower rate of anxiety among males who engage in such acts. Consistent with the above, Andrews and Lewinsohn (1992) found a significant association between anxiety disorders and suicide attempts in males, but not in females in a large community sample of adolescents.

Most research on anxiety as a risk factor for suicidal behavior has focused on the measurement of state anxiety. This may not be a fruitful method if state anxiety is significantly reduced following a suicide attempt. Ideally, risk factors used for predictive purposes should be stable (Hawton and Catalan, 1987). As such, research on the relationship between anxiety and suicidal behavior might benefit by focusing on the measurement of anxiety as a trait rather than as a state. In fact, recently, Apter and his colleagues (Apter et al., 1990, 1993a,b) found that adult psychiatric inpatient suicide attempters had significantly higher levels of trait anxiety than inpatient nonattempters, whereas state anxiety did not discriminate between the two groups. Moreover, trait anxiety was highly associated with a self-report scale of suicide risk. Another study (Oei et al., 1990) found that adult depressed patients with suicidal ideation had significantly higher levels of state and trait anxiety than depressed patients with no suicidal ideation. A study of Dutch adolescent high-school students (De Wilde et al., 1993) found that suicide attempters exhibited significantly higher levels of state and trait anxiety than nondepressed nonattempters.

### Conduct disorder, substance abuse, and borderline personality disorder

As with completed suicide, attempted suicide and suicidal ideation are also associated with diagnoses other than affective disorders, in particular **conduct disorder**, **drug and alcohol abuse**, and **borderline personality disorder** (BPD) (Pfeffer et al., 1988). The frequent association between conduct disorder, substance and alcohol abuse, and BPD (especially in clinical samples where selection bias may play a role) makes it difficult to tease out their relative contributions to suicidality; indeed suicidality appears to increase with co-morbidity (Apter et al., 1988a). However, the link between these disorders and suicidality is at least in part independent of any co-existing depression. For example, in a sample of child and adolescent patients, 18% had suicidal ideation accompanied by low depression scores. Most of these patients were diagnosed as having a behavior disorder (Carlson and Cantwell, 1982).

## Patterns of care after a suicide attempt

The extensive material from the WHO study on attempted suicide provides available information on the provision of aftercare treatment recommendations made to young people aged 15–19 following attempted suicide.

Major differences were reported between individual European centers regarding the care offered to (but not necessarily accepted by) young people after a suicide attempt. No aftercare was apparently recommended to 28.5% of the boys and 25.5% of the girls. It is difficult to determine whether these young patients were not offered aftercare or whether they refused such offers. A negative attitude towards care and treatment staff is not unusual among young people, and such an attitude may be partially connected with the phase of development they are in, when the desire for autonomy is strong; thus, the offer of care may be interpreted as a means of control and threat to independence, and arouse anxiety

(Hultén et al., 2000). It is also common not only for adults, but also for young people, to deny suicide acts with great vehemence (Spirito, 1996). Parents' lack of involvement, ignorance of the suicide attempt, or desire to trivialize the suicide attempt may be other factors that make it easier for a teenager to turn down an offer of treatment.

The results of several surveys (Mehlum, 1994; Otto, 1972) show that previous suicide attempts are an important indicator for repeated suicide attempts and future suicide, and also that males who have used violent methods of attempting suicide show the highest risk of completed suicide.

In the WHO Multicenter Study on Parasuicide (Attempted Suicide), girls who had attempted suicide previously were offered aftercare more often (81%) than boys who had attempted suicide previously (76%). The proportion of male prior suicide attempters offered care was remarkably low, considering that boys are a high-risk group for repeated suicide attempts and die from suicide more often than girls. The fact that males who had previously attempted suicide were offered care to a lesser extent than their female counterparts may be explained by the fact that boys with borderline and antisocial personality disorders and adjustment disorders are usually hard to motivate for care unless it is specially adapted for them (Spirito, 1996). In the practice of child and youth psychiatry, relatively little attention has been paid hitherto to young people's noncompliance in conjunction with care after attempted suicide in spite of the research findings (Mattson et al., 1969; Piacentini et al., 1995; Spirito, 1996; Trautman et al., 1993).

The nine European centers studied (Hulten et al., 2000) also lack a joint action policy for recommending aftercare to young people who used comparable methods in their suicide attempts. Some centers recommended aftercare more often to young people who had used medicines in their suicide attempt than to those who had used violent methods, whereas at other centers it was the other way round.

The same variability appears in the patterns of care recommended after a suicide attempt with reference to gender. Although girls had a greater chance than boys of being offered aftercare at six of the nine centers investigated, boys proved to have a greater chance in Germany, Spain, and Switzerland.

These findings show that uniform policies regarding treatment recommendations for young suicide-attempt patients are lacking across the health-care facilities surveyed in Europe and that this care is subject to varying priorities in different countries.

Guidelines for treatment of suicide-attempt patients should be adapted to gender and to various psychiatric and personality diagnoses. It seems particularly important to give individually adapted care to boys and young men who repeat their suicide attempts, since this group has an elevated risk of mortality from future suicide.

## REFERENCES

Allgulander, C., and Lavori, P. W. (1991). Excess mortality among 3302 patients with "pure" anxiety neurosis. *Archives of General Psychiatry*, **48**, 599–602.

American Academy of Pediatrics. (1980). Committee on adolescence. Teenage suicide. *Pediatrics*, **66**(1), 144–146.

Andrews, J. A., and Lewinsohn, P. M. (1992). Suicidal attempts among older adolescents: prevalence and co-occurrence with psychiatric disorders. *Journal of the American Academy of Child and Adolescent Psychiatry*, **31**, 655–662.

Angle, C. R., O'Brien, T. P., and McIntire, M. S. (1983). Adolescent self poisoning. A nine year follow up. *Developmental and Behavioral Pediatrics*, **4**, 83–87.

Apter, A., Bleich, A., Plutchik, R., Mendelsohn, S., and Tyano, S. (1988a). Suicidal behavior, depression, and conduct disorder in hospitalized adolescents. *Journal of the American Academy of Child and Adolescent Psychiatry*, **27**, 696–699.

Apter, A., Bleich, A., and Tyano, S. (1988b). Psychotic and affective psychopathology in hospitalized adolescents. *Journal of the American Academy of Child and Adolescent Psychiatry*, **27**, 116–120.

Apter, A., van Praag, H. M., Plutchik, R., Serg, S., Korn, M., and Brown, S. (1990). Interrelationships among anxiety, aggression, impulsivity, and mood: a serotonergically linked cluster? *Psychiatry Research*, **32**, 191–199.

Apter, A., Bleich, A., King, R. A., Kron, S., Fluch, A., Kotler, M., and Cohen, D. J. (1993a). Death without warning? A clinical postmortem study of suicide in 43 Israeli adolescent males. *Archives of General Psychiatry*, **50**, 138–142.

Apter, A., Plutchik, R., and van Praag, H. M. (1993b). Anxiety, impulsivity and depressed mood in relation to suicidal and violent behavior. *Acta Psychiatrica Scandinavica*, **87**, 1–5.

Apter, A., Gothelf, D., Orbach, I., Har-Even, D., Weizman, R., and Tyano, S. (1995). Correlation of suicidal and violent behavior in different diagnostic categories in hospitalized adolescent patients. *Journal of the American Academy of Child and Adolescent Psychiatry*, **34**(7), 912–918.

Beautrais, A. L. (1998). Risk factors for serious suicide attempts among young people: a case control study. In Kosky, R. J., Eshkevari, H. S., et al. (eds.) *Suicide Prevention: The Global Context* (pp. 167–181). New York, NY: Plenum Press.

Beautrais, A. L., Joyce, P. R., and Mulder, R. T. (1996). Risk factors for serious suicide attempts among youths aged 13 through 24 years. *Journal of the American Academy of Child and Adolescent Psychiatry*, **35**, 1174–1182.

Bettes, B. A., and Walker, E. (1986). Symptoms associated with suicidal behavior in children and adolescence. *Journal of Abnormal Child Psychology*, **14**(4), 591–604.

Bille-Brahe, U., Bjerke, T., Crepet, P., De Leo, D., Haring, C., Hawton, K., Kerkhof, A., Lönnqvist, J., Michel, K., Philippe, A., Pommereau, X., Querejeta, I., Salander-Renberg, E., Schmidtke, A.,

Temesváry, B., Wasserman, D., and Sampaio-Faria, J. G. (1993). *WHO/EURO Multicentre Study on Parasuicide. Facts and Figures.* Copenhagen: WHO Regional Office for Europe.

Brent, D. A., Perper, J. A., and Allman, C. J. (1987). Alcohol, firearms, and suicide among youth. Temporal trends in Allegheny County. Pennsylvania, 1960 to 1983. *Journal of the American Medical Association,* **257**(24), 3369–3372.

Brent, D. A., Johnson, B., Bartle, S., Bridge, J., Rather, C., Matta, J., Connolly, J., and Constantine, D. (1993). Personality disorder, tendency to impulsive violence and suicidal behavior in adolescents. *Journal of the American Academy of Child and Adolescent Psychiatry,* **32**(1), 69–75.

Carlson, C. A., and Cantwell, D. P. (1982). Suicidal behavior and depression in children and adolescents. *Journal of the American Academy of Child Psychiatry,* **21**, 361–368.

Center for Disease Control (1995). Suicide among children, adolescents and young adults. Morbidity and Mortality Weekly Report, **44**(15), 289.

Center for Disease Control (2002). *Morbidity and Mortality Weekly Report,* **50**(31), 657–630.

Cohen-Sandler, R., Berman, A. L., and King, R. A. (1982). A follow-up study of hospitalized suicidal children. *Journal of the American Academy of Child and Adolescent Psychiatry,* **21**(4), 398–403.

Crumley, F. E. (1979). Adolescent suicide attempts. Journal of the American Medical Association, **241**(22), 2404–2407.

Crumley, F. E. (1981). Adolescent suicide attempts and borderline personality disorder: clinical features. *Southern Medical Journal,* **74**, 546–549.

De Wilde, E. J., Kienhorst, I. C. W. M., Diekstra, R. F. W., and Wolters, W. H. G. (1993). The specificity of psychological characteristics of adolescent suicide attempters. *Journal of the American Academy of Child and Adolescent Psychiatry,* **32**, 51–59.

Diekstra, R. F. W. (1989a). Suicidal behavior in adolescents and young adults: the international picture. *Crisis,* **10**, 16–35.

Diekstra, R. F. W. (1989b). Suicide and the attempted suicide: an international perspective. Acta *Psychiatrica Scandinavica,* **80** (suppl. 354), 1–24.

Diekstra, R. (1994). On the burden of suicide. In Kelleher, M. (ed.) *Divergent Perspectives on Suicidal Behavior* (pp. 2–27). Cork: O'Leary Ltd.

Dycian, A., Fishman, G., and Bleich, A. (1994). Suicide and self inflicted injuries. *Aggressive Behavior,* **20**, 16–19.

Farbstein, I., Dycian, A., King, R., Cohen, D. J., Kron, A., and Apter, A. (2002). A follow-up study of adolescent attempted suicide in Israel and the effects of mandatory general hospital admission. *Journal of the American Academy of Child and Adolescent Psychiatry.* **41**, 1342–1349.

Fawcett, J., Scheftner, W. A., Fogg, L., Clark, D. C., Young, M. A., Hedeker, D., and Gibbons, R. (1990). Time-related predictors of suicide in major affective disorder. *American Journal of Psychiatry,* **147**, 1189–1194.

Felice, M. E. (1981). Letter to the editor. *Pediatrics,* **67**, 934–935.

Friedman, R. C., Arnoff, M. S., and Charkin, J. F. (1983). History of suicidal behavior in depressed borderline adolescent inpatients. *American Journal of Psychiatry,* **140**, 1023–1026.

Garfinkel, B., Froese, A., and Hood, J. (1982). Suicide attempts in children and adolescents. *American Journal of Psychiatry,* **139**, 1257–1261.

Garnefski, N., and Diekstra, R. F. W. (1997). Adolescents from one parent, stepparent and intact families: emotional problems and suicide attempts. *Journal of Adolescence*, **20**, 201–208.

Garrison, C. Z. (1983). The study of suicidal behavior in schools. *Suicide and Life-Threatening Behavior*, **19**(1), 120–130.

Garrison, C. Z., Schlucter, M. D., Schoenbach, V. J., and Kaplan, B. K. (1989). Epidemiology of depressive symptoms in young adolescents. *Journal of the American Academy of Child and Adolescent Psychiatry*, **28**, 343–351.

Garrison, C. Z., McKeown, R. E., Valois, R. F., and Vincent, M. L. (1993). Aggression, substance use and suicidal behavior in high school students. *American Journal of Public Health*, **83**(2), 179–184.

Goldacre, M., and Hawton, K. (1985). Repetition of self poisoning and subsequent death in adolescents who take overdose. *British Journal of Psychiatry*, **146**, 395–398.

Goldney, R. D., and Pilowsky, I. (1981). Depression in young women who have attempted suicide. *Australian and New Zealand Journal of Psychiatry*, **14**, 203–211.

Hassanyeh, F., O'Brien, G., Holton, A. R., Hurren, K., and Watt, L. (1989). Repeat self harm: an 18-month follow-up. *Acta Psychiatrica Scandinavica*, **79**, 265–267.

Hawton, K., and Catalan, J. (1987). *Attempted Suicide. A Practical Guide to its Nature and Management.* Oxford: Oxford University Press.

Hawton, K., O'Grady, J., Osborn, M., and Cole, D. (1982). Adolescents who take overdoses: their characteristics, problems and contacts with helping agencies. *British Journal of Psychiatry*, **140**, 118–123.

Hawton, K., Fagg, J., Simkin, S., Bale, E., and Bond, A. (1997). Trends in deliberate self-harm in Oxford, 1985–1995. Implications for clinical services and the prevention of suicide. *British Journal of Psychiatry*, **171**, 556–560.

Hawton, K., Fagg, J., Simkin, S., Bale, E., and Bond, A. (2000). Deliberate self-harm in adolescents in Oxford, 1985–1995. *Journal of Adolescence*, **23**(1), 47–55.

Hultén, A. (2000). Suicidal behaviour in children and adolescents in Sweden and some European countries. Epidemiological and clinical aspects. Doctoral Dissertation, Karolinska Institut, Stockholm. ISBN: 91– 628– 4254–4.

Hultén, A., and Wasserman, D. (1995). Suicide and attempted suicide among children and adolescents. In Beskow, J. (ed.) *Right to Life; Lust for Life. Suicidal Behavior in the Child and Adolescent Population.* Stockholm: Forskningsrådsnämnden, Rapport 95:4.

Hulten, A., Wasserman, D., Hawton, K., Jiang, G. X., Salander-Renberg, E., Schmidtke, A., Bille-Brahe, U., Bjerke, T., Kerkhkof, A., Michel, K., and Querejeta, I. (2000). Recommended care for young people (15–19 years) after suicide attempts in certain European countries. *European Child and Adolescent Psychiatry*, **9**(2), 100–108.

Hultén, A., Wasserman, D., Jiang, G.K., Hawton, K., Hjelmeland, H., Deleo, D., Ostamo, A., Salander–Renberg, E., and Schmidtke, A. (2001). Repetition of attempted suicide among teenagers in Europe; frequency, timing, and risk factors, *European Child and Adolescent Psychiatry*, **10**, 161–169.

ICD 10, Geneva, WHO, 1994.

Inmadar, S. E., Lewis, D. O., Siomopolous, G., Shanock, S. S., and Lamella, M. (1982). Violent and suicidal behavior in psychotic adolescents. *American Journal of Psychiatry*, **139**(7), 932–935.

Kann, L., Kinchen, S. A., Williams, B. I., Ross, J. G., Lowry, R., Grunbaum, J. A., and Kolbe, L. J. (2000). Youth Risk Behavior Surveillance – United States, 1999. State and local YRBSS Coordinators. *Journal of School Health*, **70**(7), 271–285.

Kienhorst, C. W. M., Wolters, W. H. G., Diekstra, R. F. W., and Otte, E. (1987). A study of the frequency of suicidal behavior in children aged 5 to 14. *Journal of Child Psychology and Psychiatry*, **28**, 153–165.

Kienhorst, C. W., de Wilde, E. J., Van den Bont, J., Diekstra, R. F., and Wolters, W. H. (1990). Characteristics of suicide attempters in a populaion-based sample of Dutch adolescents. *British Journal of Psychiatry*, **156**, 243–248.

Kingsbury, S., Hawton, K., Steinhardt, K., and James, A. (1999). Do adolescents who take overdoses have specific psychological characteristics? A comparative study with psychiatric and community controls. *Journal of the American Academy of Child and Adolescent Psychiatry*, **38**(9), 1125–1131.

Kolbe, L. J., Kann, L., and Collins, J. L. (1993). Overview of the Youth Risk Behavior Surveillance System. *Public Health Reports*, **108** (supplement 1), 2–10.

Kosky, R., Silburn, S., and Zubrick, S. R. (1986). Symptomatic depression and suicidal ideation: a comparative study with 628 children. *Journal of Nervous and Mental Disease*, **174**, 523–528.

Kotila, L. (1989). Age-specific characteristics of attempted suicide in adolescence. *Acta Psychiatrica Scandinavica*, **79**, 436–443.

Kotila, L., and Lonnquist, J. (1988). Adolescent suicide attempts: sex differences predicting suicide. *Acta Psychiatrica Scandinavica*, **77**, 264–270.

Kreitman, N. (1979). Reflections on the management of parasuicide. *British Journal of Psychiatry*, **135**, 275.

Levy, J. C., and Deykin, E. Y. (1989). Suicidality, depression and substance abuse in adolescence. *American Journal of Psychiatry*, **146**, 1462–1467.

Litt, I. F., Cuskey, W. R., and Rudd, S. (1983). Emergency room evaluation of the adolescent who attempts suicide: Compliance with follow-up. *Journal of Adolescent Health Care*, **4**, 106–108.

Mannuzza, S., Aronowitz, B., Chapman, T., Klein, D. F., and Fyer, A. J. (1992). Panic disorder and suicide attempts. *Journal of Anxiety Disorders*, **6**, 261–274.

Marks, P. A., and Haller, D. L. (1977). Now I lay down for keeps: a study of adolescent suicide attempts. *Journal of Clinical Psychology*, **33**, 390–400.

Massion, A. O., Warshaw, M. G., and Keller, M. B. (1993). Quality of life and psychiatric morbidity in panic disorder and generalized anxiety disorder. *American Journal of Psychiatry*, **150**, 600–607.

Mattson, A., Seese, L. R., and Hawkins, J. W. (1969). Suicidal behavior as a child psychiatric emergency. *Archives of General Psychiatry*, **20**, 100–109.

McIntire, M. S., Angle, C. R., Wikoff, R. L., and Schlicht, M. L. (1977). Recurrent adolescent suicidal behavior. *Pediatrics*, **60**, 605–608.

Meehan, P. J., Lamb, J. A., Saltzman, L. E., and O'Carroll, P. W. (1992). Attempted suicide among young adults. Progress toward a meaningful estimate of prevalence. *American Journal of Psychiatry* **149**, 41–44.

Mehlum, L. (1994). Young male suicide attempters 20 years later: the suicide mortality rate. *Military Medicine*, **159**(2), 138–141.

Mehr, M., Zeltzer, L. K., and Robinson, R. (1982). Continued self destructive behaviors in adolescent suicide attempters, part II. *Journal of Adolescent Health Care*, **2**, 183–187.

Menninger, K. (1933). *Man Against Himself*. New York, NY: Harcourt Brace.

Morrison, G. C., and Collier, J. G. (1969). Family treatment approaches to suicidal children and adolescents. *Journal of the American Academy of Child and Adolescent Psychiatry*, **8**, 140–153.

Moscicki, E. K. (1995). Epidemiology of suicide. *Suicide and Life Threatening Behavior*, **25**(1), 22–35.

Moscicki, E. K., Locke, B. Z., Rae, D. S., and Boyd, J. H. (1989). Depressive symptoms among Mexican Americans: the Hispanic Health and Nutrition Examination Survey. *American Journal of Epidemiology*, **130**(2), 348–360.

Motto, J. A. (1984). Suicide in male adolescents. In Sudak, H. S., Ford, A. B., and Rushforth, N. B. (eds.) *Suicide in the Young* (pp. 224–244). Boston, MA: John Wright PSG, Inc.

Newson-Smith, J. G., and Hirsch, S. R. (1979). Psychiatric symptoms in self-poisoning patients. *Psychological Medicine*, **9**(3), 493–500.

Oei, T. I., Verhoeven, W. M. A., Westenberg, H. G. M., Zwart, F. M., and van Ree, J. M. (1990). Anhedonia, suicide ideation and dexamethasone non-suppression in depressed patients. *Journal of Psychiatry Research*, **24**, 25–35.

Otto, U. (1972). Suicidal acts by children and adolescents: a follow-up study. *Acta Psychiatrica Scandinavica Supplementum*, **233**, 5–123.

Paerregaard, G. (1975). Suicide among attempted suicides: a 10-year follow-up. *Suicide*, **5**(3), 140–144.

Paykel, E. S., Myers, J. K., Lindenthal, J. J., and Tanner, J. (1974). Suicidal feelings on the general population: a prevalence study. *British Journal of Psychiatry*, **142**, 460–469.

Pfeffer, C. R., Plutchik, R., and Mizruchi, S. (1983). Suicidal and assaultive behavior in children, classification, measurement and interrelation. *American Journal of Psychiatry*, **140**, 154–157.

Pfeffer, C. R., Newcorn, J., Kaplan, G., Mizruchi, M. S., and Plutchik, R. (1988). Suicidal behavior in adolescent psychiatric inpatients. *Journal of the American Academy of Child and Adolescent Psychiatry*, **27**(3) 357–361.

Pfeffer, C. R., Klerman, G. L., Hurt, S. W., Lesser, M., Peskin, J. R., and Siefker, C. A. (1991). Suicidal children grow-up: demographic and clinical risk factors for adolescent suicide attempts. *Journal of the American Academy of Child and Adolescent Psychiatry*, **30**(4), 609–616.

Piacentini, J., Rotheram-Borus, M. J., Gillis, J. R., Graae, F., Trautman, P., Cantwell, C., Garcia-Leeds, C., and Shaffer, D. (1995). Demographic predictors of treatment attendance among adolescent suicide attempters. *Journal of Consulting and Clinical Psychology*, **63**(3), 469–473.

Pillay, A. L., and Wassenaar, D. R. (1997). Family dynamics, hopelessness and psychiatric disturbance in parasuicidal adolescents. *Australian and New Zealand Journal of Psychiatry*, **31**, 227–230.

Platt, S., Bille-Brahe, U., Kerkhof, A., et al. (1992). Parasuicide in Europe: the WHO/EURO Multi-centre Study on Parasuicide. Introduction and preliminary analysis. *Acta Psychiatrica Scandinavica*, **85**, 97–104.

Plutchik, R., and van Praag, H. M. (1986). The measurement of suicidality, aggressivity and impulsivity. Paper presented at the International College of Neuropsychopharmacology, 1986.

Plutchik, R., van Praag, H. M., and Conte, H. R. (1985). Suicide and violence risk in psychiatric patients. In Shagass, C. (ed.) *Biological Psychiatry*. New York, NY: Elsevier.

Ramberg, I.L., and Wasserman, D. (1995). Suicidal thoughts, attempted suicide and attitudes towards suicidal behaviour among high school students. In Beskow, J. (ed.) *Right to Life; Lust for Life. Suicidal Behavior in the Child and Adolescent Population*. Stockholm: Forskningsrådsnämnden, Rapport 95:4.

Ramberg, I. L., and Wasserman, D. (2000). Prevalence of reported suicidal behaviour in the general population and mental health-care staff. *Psychological Medicine*, **30**(5), 1189–1196.

Robbins, D. R., and Alessi, N. E. (1985). Depressive symptoms and suicidal behavior in adolescents. *American Journal of Psychiatry*, **142**, 588–592.

Schmidtke, A., Bille-Brahe, U., De Leo, D., Kerkhof, A., Bjerke, T., Crepet, P. et al. (1996). Attempted suicide in Europe: rates, trends and sociodemographic characteristics of suicide attempters during the period 1989–1992. Results of the WHO/EURO Multicentre Study on Parasuicide. *Acta Psychiatrica Scandinavica*, **93**, 327–328.

Shaffer, D., and Fisher, P. (1981). The epidemiology of suicide in children and young adolescents. *Journal of the American Academy of Child Psychiatry*, **20**, 545–565

Shaffer, D., Garland, A., Gould, M., Fisher, P., and Trautman, P. (1988). Preventing teenage suicide: a critical review. *Journal of the American Academy of Child and Adolescent Psychiatry*, **27**(6), 675–687.

Shafii, M., Carrigan, S., Whittinghill, J. R., and Derrik, A., (1985). Psychological autopsy of completed suicide in children and adolescents. *American Journal of Psychiatry*, **142**, 1061–1064.

Skodal, A. E., and Karasu, T. B. (1978). Emergency psychiatry: the assault of patients. *American Journal of Psychiatry*, **135**, 202–205.

Slap, G., Vorters, D., Chaudhuri, S., and Centor, R. (1988). Risk factors for attempted suicide during adolescence. Poster presented at the American Society for Adolescent Medicine, New York.

Smith, K., and Crawford, S. (1986). Suicidal behavior among "normal" high school students. *Suicidal and Life-Threatening Behavior*, **16**, 313–325.

Spirito, A. (1996). Improving treatment compliance among adolescent suicide attempters. *Crisis*, **17**(4), 152–154.

Spirito, A., Brown, L., Overholzer, J., and Fritz, G. (1989). Attempted suicide in adolescence: a review and critique of the literature. *Clinical Psychological Review*, **9**, 335–363.

Spirito, A., Plummer, B., Gispert, M., Levy, S., Kurkjan, J., Levander, W., Hagberg, S., and Devost, L. (1992). Adolescent suicide attempts: outcomes at follow up. *American Journal of Orthopsychiatry*, **62**(3), 464–468.

Suokas, J., and Lonnquist, J. (1991). Outcome of attempted suicide and psychiatric consultation: risk factors and suicide mortality during a five-year follow-up. *Acta Psychiatrica Scandinavica*, **84**, 545–549.

Tardiff, K., and Sweillam, A. (1980). Assault suicide, and mental illness. *Archives of General Psychiatry*, **37**, 164–169.

Taylor, E. A., and Stansfeld, S. A. (1984). Children who poison themselves: I. A clinical comparison with psychiatric controls. *British Journal of Psychiatry*, **145**, 127–132.

Tomori, M., and Zalar, B. (2000). Characteristics of suicide attempters in a Slovenian high school population. *Suicide and Life-Threatening Behavior*, **30**(3), 222–238.

Trautman, P. D., Rotheram-Borus, M. J., Dopkins, S., and Lewin, N. (1991). Psychiatric diagnoses in minority female adolescent suicide attempters. *Journal of the American Academy of Child and Adolescent Psychiatry*. 30(4), 617–622.

Trautman, P., Stewart, M., and Morishima, A. (1993). Are adolescent suicide attempters noncompliant with outpatient care? *Journal of the American Academy of Child and Adolescent Psychiatry*, **32**, 89–94.

Vandivort, D. S., and Locke, B. Z. (1979). Suicide ideation; its relation to depression, suicide and suicide attempt. *Suicide and Life-Threatening Behavior*, **9**, 205–218.

Velez, C., and Cohen, P. (1988). Suicidal behavior and ideation in a community sample of children. *Journal of the American Academy of Child and Adolescent Psychiatry*, **27**, 349–356.

von Knorring, A.-L., and Kristiansson, G. (1995). Depression och självmordsbeteende hos ungdomar (Depression and suicidal behavior in young people). In Beskow, J. (ed.) *Rätt till liv lust till liv. Om självmordsbeteende bland barn och ungdomar*. Stockholm: Forskningsrådsnämnden, Rapport 95:4:35–43. ISSN 0348-3991.

Wagner, B. M. (1997). Family risk factors for child and adolescent suicidal behavior. *Psychological Bulletin*, **121**(2), 246–298.

Wasserman, D. (1993). Alcohol and suicidal behaviour. *Nordic Journal of Psychiatry* (Nordisk Psykiatrisk Tidskrift), **47**(4), 265–271.

Wasserman, D., and Värnik, A. (1998). Suicide-preventive effects of perestroika in the former USSR: the role of alcohol restriction. *Acta Psychiatrica Scandinavica, Supplementum*, **394**, 1–4.

Wasserman, D., Dankowicz, M., Värnik, A., and Olsson, L. (1997). Suicide trends in Europe, 1984–1990. In Botsis, A. J., Soldatos, C. R., and Stefanis, C. N. (eds.) *Suicide: Biopsychosocial Approaches*. Amsterdam: Elsevier Science.

Weissman, M., Fox, K., and Klerman, G. L. (1973). Hostility and depression associated with suicide attempts. *American Journal of Psychiatry*, **130**, 450–455.

Weissman, M. M., Klerman, G. L., Markowitz, J. S., and Ouellette, R. (1989). Suicidal ideation and suicide attempts in panic disorder and attacks. *New England Journal of Medicine*, **321**, 1209–1214

Williams, B. A. (1988). Reinforcement and response strength. In *Steven's Handbook of Experimental Psychology*, vol. 2. New York, NY: Wiley.

Wolk-Wasserman, D. (1986). *Attempted Suicide–The Patient's Family, Social Network and Therapy* [Doctoral dissertation]. Stockholm: Graphic Systems. ISBN 91–7900–118.

Zonda, T. (1991). A longitudinal follow-up study of 583 attempted suicides, based on Hungarian material. *Crisis*, **12**(1), 48–57.

## 4

# Familial factors in adolescent suicidal behavior

David A. Brent and J. John Mann

## Overview

This chapter will examine both genetic and family-environmental factors associated with suicide and suicidal behavior, with an emphasis on youthful suicidal behavior. Described herein is a model for the familial transmission of suicidal behavior that includes both genetic and nongenetic components. To conclude, the research and clinical implications of the extant literature on familial factors in suicide will be delineated.

There are several lines of evidence supporting the importance of familial factors in suicidal behavior. First, there is evidence that suicidal behavior aggregates in families from twin, adoption, and family studies. Second, while the majority of suicide victims and suicide attempters are psychiatrically ill, most psychiatrically ill patients neither attempt nor complete suicide. This suggests that a psychiatric diagnosis may be necessary, but not sufficient to explain the phenomenon of suicidal behavior. Individuals who make suicide attempts also have a diathesis for suicidal behavior. That diathesis may be subject to familial transmission, and the familial transmission of the diathesis may be distinct from the familial transmission of psychiatric disorders. Finally, many studies have noted the prevalence of a disordered family environment in suicide attempters and completers, suggesting a familial, if not a genetic, contribution to suicidal risk. Each of these categories of studies will be reviewed in turn.

## Adoption studies

The classic adoption study on suicide was performed in Denmark by Schulsinger et al. (1979), comparing the rates of suicide among the biological and adoptive relatives in adoptees who committed suicide and in a matched living adoptee control group. The sixfold higher rate of suicide in the biological relatives of the suicide adoptees and the *absence* of suicide among the adopted relatives of the suicide versus control adoptees supports a genetic rather than environmental

**Table 4.1.** Adoption studies: rates of suicide in biological vs. adoptive relatives of adoptees who committed suicide and live adoptee controls

|  | Index cases | Suicide/biological relatives | Suicide/adopted relatives |
|---|---|---|---|
| Adopted |  |  |  |
|   Suicide | 57 | 12/269* | 0/148 |
|   Controls | 57 | 2/269 | 0/150 |

*Source:* Schulsinger et al. (1979).

* $p < 0.01$.

**Table 4.2.** Incidence of suicide in biological relatives of depressive and control adoptees*

| Diagnosis in adoptee | Incidence of suicide in biological relative | $p$ |
|---|---|---|
| Affective reaction | 5/66 (7.6%) | 0.0004** |
| Neurotic depression | 3/127 (2.4%) | 0.056 |
| Bipolar depression | 4/75 (5.3%) | 0.0036 |
| Unipolar depression | 3/139 (2.2%) | 0.067 |
| No mental illness | 1/360 (0.3%) |  |

*Source:*

*Abstracted from Kety (1986).

**Compared with biological relatives of control adoptees with no known history of mental illness.

effect (see Table 4.1). However, due to the nature of the study, it was not possible to determine if this effect was attributable to the transmission of major psychiatric disorders or a suicide diathesis *per se*. However, the rate of suicide was higher in the biological relatives of suicide adoptees regardless of whether the adoptees were psychiatric patients or not.

Wender et al. (1986) reported on an adoption study of affective disorder, also using the Danish adoption registry. The highest suicide rates in the biological relatives of the affectively ill adoptees were in those with a diagnosis known as "affective reaction," which roughly translates to the impulsive-unstable personality disorders or so-called Cluster B disorders (see Table 4.2). This finding, in turn, suggests a familial link between impulsive aggression and suicide. Moreover, the 15-fold excess of suicide among the relatives of the adoptees with affective disorders supports the role of affective disorder in suicide.

**Table 4.3.** Twin studies (Roy et al., 1991). Concordance for suicide in monozygotic vs. dizygotic twins

|  | No. of pairs | No. of pairs concordant | Percentage (%) |
| --- | --- | --- | --- |
| Monozygotic | 62 | 7 | 11.3 |
| Dizygotic | 114 | 2 | 1.8 |

## Twin studies

Tsuang (1977) reviewed the extant world's literature on twin concordance for suicidal behavior. He found that there was a higher rate of concordance for suicide among monozygotic than among dizygotic twins, supportive of a genetic effect. However, the rate of concordance even among monozygotic twins was low (17.7%), perhaps because the definition of concordance was restricted to suicide, rather than including a broader spectrum of suicidal behavior. Of the nine twin pairs concordant for suicide, case records were available on four, indicating concordance for psychopathology as well as for suicide. The drop-off in concordance from monozygotic to dizygotic twins suggests that multiple genes are involved in suicide, not surprising in light of the complexity of this behavior.

In a more recent review of twin studies, Roy et al. (1991) also found a much higher concordance rate for monozygotic than for dizygotic twins (11.3% vs. 1.8%) (Table 4.3). In a subsequent study, Roy et al. (1995) found a high concordance rate for suicide attempt in the surviving monozygotic twin of the co-twin's suicide (38%). In a large representative sample of almost 3000 Australian twin pairs, if a monozygotic twin attempted suicide, his/her co-twin had a 17.5-fold increased risk of having made an attempt (Statham et al., 1998). In controlling for other risk factors for suicide, such as mood disorder, substance abuse, trauma, personality problems, and life events, a family history of a suicide attempt still conveyed a fourfold increased risk for the co-twin making an attempt. There was no evidence that the attempts among twins clustered in time, which tends to rule out a suicide in one twin being an imitation of, or modeled on, the suicide of the other twin. The heritability of a serious suicide attempt was estimated at 55%.

These results have been replicated in a twin study of adolescent girls (Glowinski et al., 2001). In a representative sample of 3416 female adolescent Missouri twins, the odds of a suicide attempt if a co-twin had attempted was 11.6 for monozygotic twins, and 4.2 for dizygotic twins. The genetic and shared environmental influences together accounted for between 35% and 75% of the variance.

**Table 4.4.** Family studies: suicide probands. Risk of suicidal behavior in relatives of suicide probands vs. relatives of controls

| Author | Year | Index | OR |
|--------|------|-------|-----|
| Tsuang | 1983 | Patient suicides | 3.8 |
| Egeland and Sussex | 1985 | Amish suicides | 4.6 |
| Gould et al. | 1996 | Adolescent suicides | 4.4–4.7[*] |
| Brent et al. | 1996a | Adolescent suicides | 4.3[*] |
| Cheng et al. | 2000 | Adult suicide | 5.0[*] |

[*]Adjusted OR, controlling for familial rates of psychopathology.

In a study of suicidal ideation and attempts in 3372 male twin pairs from the Vietnam Era Twin registry, both suicidal ideation and suicide attempt showed additive genetic effects (36% and 17%, respectively (Fu et al., 2002).

## Family studies

There have been several family studies that compare the risk for suicide or suicide attempt in the first-degree relatives of probands who have completed suicide, compared to the rate among relatives of control probands. Although the methodology varies, the results are remarkably consistent insofar as the risk of suicidal behavior in the relatives of suicide probands is increased around four-fold compared to the relatives of control probands (see Table 4.4). Tsuang (1983), in a family study, found a nearly fourfold higher rate of suicide in relatives of patients who committed suicide compared with the relatives of patients who did not commit suicide. They examined the rates of suicide among the first-degree relatives of 195 schizophrenics, 100 manic-depressives, and 225 depressives, of whom 29 had committed suicide. The morbid risk for suicide was 7.9% in the relatives of the patient suicides, 2.1% in the relatives of the nonsuicide patients, and 0.3% in the relatives of a nonpatient control group. This suggests two components to the familial risk of suicide: patient status (i.e., psychiatric disorder) and status as a suicide victim. Thus, this study was one of the first to suggest that the familial transmission of suicide was partly distinct from the familial transmission of psychopathology.

Egeland and Sussex (1985) surveyed all suicides ascertained for a 100-year period in the Old Order Amish, using a combination of family history and family study methodologies, and found that 73% of the suicides occurred in

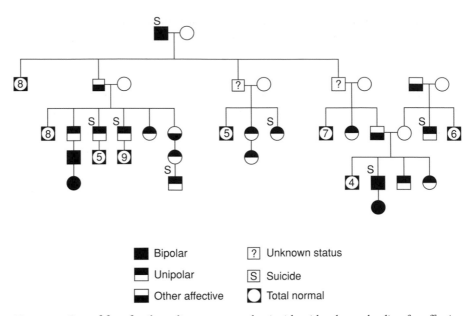

Figure 4.1 One of four family pedigrees among the Amish with a heavy loading for affective disorder and suicide. All seven suicides were found among individuals with a definite affective disorder. Adapted from "Suicide and family loading for affective disorders" by J. Egeland and J. Sussex (1985) *Journal of the American Medical Association*, **254**, 915–918.

just 16% of the sample, yielding an approximate odds ratio of 4.6. While over 90% of the suicides had an affective illness, this study is of interest because there were some pedigrees that were both loaded for affective disorder and for suicide (see Figure 4.1), whereas others were equally laden for affective disorder without as much as a single suicide. One explanation for this finding is that the familial transmission of suicide included a diathesis for suicidal behavior that was transmitted either additively with, or independently of, affective disorder. An alternative explanation is that two different forms of affective illness were being transmitted, with one form more likely to result in suicide.

Mitterauer (1990) reported on a series of studies conducted in Salzburg. The pattern of familial transmission of psychosis and of suicide was examined in the 65 families of patients with endogenous psychosis (not defined) who committed suicide. The patterns of transmission of these two conditions were found to be distinct, although these pedigrees were not subjected to formal segregation analysis. In a second study, family genetic analysis of 110 pedigrees of patients with endogenous psychosis with ($n = 60$) and without suicide ($n = 50$) in the proband showed that the familial loading of endogenous psychosis was the same in both sets of pedigrees, supporting independence of transmission of suicide and endogenous psychosis. In a third related study, 342 manic-depressive probands with a family history of suicide were compared to 80 manic-depressives without such a family history. Several symptoms were more common in the family-history-positive probands including: suicidal tendencies, suicide attempts, hypochondriasis, rage, "angry mania," and delusions associated with mania or depression. While the higher rate of suicide attempts in the probands with a family history of suicide is consistent with the distinct familial transmission of suicidal behavior, the association of other, "core" symptoms of manic-depressive illness with this transmission suggests that what may be transmitted is the *nature* or a more virulent form of the illness rather than a diathesis for suicidal behavior. Of interest is that two of the symptoms, "rage" and "angry mania," could relate to the impaired regulation of aggression, noted also in Wender et al. (1986), cited above, again suggesting that aggressive behavior is part of the diathesis for suicidal behavior that is transmitted independently of the major psychiatric disorder and contributes to the familial transmission of suicide.

Three studies compared the risk of suicidal behavior (both attempts and completion) in the relatives of suicide probands, compared to community control probands, while controlling for differences between the proband and relative groups, including differences in family psychopathology (Brent et al., 1996a; Cheng et al., 2000; Gould et al., 1996). Since the higher rate of suicidal behavior in the relatives of suicide probands persists after this statistical control, this supports the view that the familial transmission of suicidal behavior occurs above and beyond the transmission of psychiatric disorders alone.

Gould et al. (1996), in a family history study, reported over a fourfold excess of suicidal behavior in the relatives of 120 adolescent suicide victims compared to 147 community controls, which persisted even after adjusting for other significant family risk factors, including maternal mood problems, paternal problems with the police, and poor parent–child communication. This result is significant because it suggests that the spectrum of suicidal behavior that is familially transmitted includes both attempts and completions, and also suggests that this transmission is *not* mediated solely by parental psychopathology or the parent–child relationship.

Brent et al. (1996a) conducted a family study of 58 adolescent suicide victims and 55 community controls. The rates of attempted and completed suicide were higher in the relatives of the completers than of the controls (see Table 4.5). Moreover, this difference persisted in first-degree relatives, even after controlling for differences in relative and proband psychopathology, supporting the view that the familial transmission of suicidal behavior is independent or interactive with psychopathology (adjusted odds ratio = 4.3, 95% confidence interval, 1.1–16.6).

**Table 4.5.** Rates of suicidal attempts and completers in relatives of adolescent suicides vs. relatives of controls[+]

| Relationship 95% CI | Relatives of: | | OR |
| --- | --- | --- | --- |
| | Completers | Controls | |
| First-degree relatives | 11.6 | 2.4[**] | 5.3 (2.0–14.3) |
| Mothers | 18.2 | 3.6[*] | 5.9 (1.2–28.3) |
| Fathers | 5.7 | 1.8 | 3.2 (0.3–32.2) |
| Siblings | 11.0 | 2.1[*] | 5.9 (1.2–27.9) |
| Second-degree relatives | 4.9 | 1.4[**] | 3.7 (1.6–8.7) |

[*] $p < 0.01$.
[**] $p < 0.001$.
[+]Brent et al. (1996a).

**Table 4.6.** Risks of familial suicidal ideation in relatives of adolescent suicides vs. relatives of controls (OR (95% CI))[+]

| | Uncontrolled | Controlling for familial psychopathology |
| --- | --- | --- |
| First-degree relatives | 1.9 (1.0–3.7) | 1.6 (0.5–5.1) |
| Second-degree relatives | 1.8 (1.0–3.0) | 1.0 (0.4–2.3) |

[+]Brent et al. (1996a).

There was a twofold excess of first-degree relatives of completers with suicidal ideation (see Table 4.6). However, after controlling for the differences in rates of psychopathology between the relatives of the two groups, this difference was no longer significant. This suggests that suicidal ideation is related to psychopathology, but that the tendency to *act* upon suicidal ideation is the core liability to suicidal behavior that is familially transmitted. In addition, these data provide some clues as to the specific nature of this liability; namely, the tendency to impulsive violence. If our completers were subdivided by the presence or absence of aggressive behavior, the familial aggregation of suicidal behavior was much greater in the first-degree relatives of aggressive vs. nonaggressive completers (15.6% vs. 2.9%). This finding in turn is consistent with studies relating alterations in serotonergic neurotransmission to both impulsive aggression and suicidal behavior (Coccaro et al., 1989; Mann et al., 1992).

There have also been several family studies that have compared the rate of suicide or suicidal behavior among the relatives of suicide attempters compared to the relatives of psychiatric or community controls (see Table 4.7).

**Table 4.7.** Family studies: attempted suicide probands. Rates of suicide or suicidal behavior in relatives of suicide attempters vs. relatives of controls

| Author | Year | Index | OR |
|--------|------|-------|-----|
| Garfinkel et al. | 1982 | Adolescent attempters | 5.4 |
| Linkowski et al. | 1985 | Inpatient adult attempters | 2.0–3.5 |
| Roy | 1983 | Inpatient adult attempters | 3.4 |
| Pfeffer et al. | 1994 | Prepubertal attempters | 4.3 |
| Malone et al. | 1995 | Inpatient adult attempters | 7.6 |
| Bridge et al. | 1997 | Adolescent attempters | 12.1* |
| Johnson et al. | 1998 | Inpatient adolescent attempters | 2.3* |
| Roy | 2000 | Alcoholic attempters | 3.5 |
| Roy | 2001 | Cocaine-abusing attempters | 4.5 |

*Adjusted OR, controlling for familial rates of psychopathology.

The methodology varies significantly in this set of studies from chart review (Garfinkel et al., 1982; Roy, 1983, 2000) to family history (Linkowski et al., 1985; Malone et al., 1995), to formal family history study with direct interview of several first-degree relatives (Bridge et al., 1997; Johnson et al., 1998; Pfeffer et al., 1994). Despite some differences in methodology, all studies report a higher risk for suicide attempt or completion in the relatives of attempters compared to the relatives of controls, while the range of odds ratios or association is more variable; the median odds ratio of around 4 is similar to that reported by family studies of completed suicide.

Garfinkel et al. (1982), in a chart review study, found a markedly elevated rate of suicide attempts and completions among the relatives of 505 adolescent suicide attempters seen in an emergency department compared to an equal number of demographically matched emergency room controls. Moreover, greater lethality of attempt in the adolescent was associated with a greater probability of a family history of suicidal behavior.

In the only reported family study of a prepubertal sample, Pfeffer et al. (1994) found an increased rate of suicide attempts in the relatives of 25 attempters, but not in those of 28 suicide ideators, or of 16 inpatient psychiatric controls, compared to the relatives of 54 normal children. This indicates some degree of specificity of familial transmission of suicidal behavior. Relatives of attempters also had higher rates of substance abuse and assaultive behavior (particularly in male relatives), suggesting a link between the familial transmission of impulsive aggression and of suicidal behavior.

Both Roy (1983) and Linkowski et al. (1985) found a higher prevalence of family history of suicide among the relatives of attempter vs. nonattempter inpatients. Roy (1983) conducted a chart review of adult inpatients, comparing 243 patients with a family history of suicide to 5602 inpatients with no family history of suicide. A family history of suicide was associated with a higher rate of suicide attempts in patients with a wide variety of disorders, including schizophrenia, unipolar and bipolar disorder, "depressive neurosis," and personality disorders. These findings support the view that the tendency to suicide behavior is transmitted independently of psychiatric disorders, although one cannot rule out the possibility that it is the *severity or subtype* of disorder that conveys the risk that is being transmitted. Similar results have been reported in studies of alcoholics and cocaine abusers, respectively (Roy, 2000, 2001). Linkowski et al. (1985) used the family history method to show that a family history of suicide (mainly violent suicide) was associated with violent suicidal behavior (i.e., most suicide methods other than superficial cutting and overdose) in a sample of 73 unipolar depressed or bipolar patients, again supporting a linking between the familial transmission of violence and that of suicide. This effect was particularly strong in male patients, where a family history of suicide increased the odds of violent vs. nonviolent attempts nearly 15-fold. These findings, along with those of Garfinkel et al. (1982), suggest that more serious suicidal behavior may be more likely to be familially transmitted.

Malone et al. (1995) also found an increased prevalence of a positive family history of suicide attempt among 100 depressed suicide inpatient attempters compared to an equal number of depressed, nonattempting inpatient controls. A higher rate of suicide attempts was found in the parents of attempters than in the parents of controls, but no difference in the rate of parental depression was found, again supporting the view that the familial transmission of suicidal behavior occurs separately from that of affective disorder.

These family studies provide strong evidence for the familial aggregation of suicide and suicidal behavior, but were not designed to address the question of whether the familial transmission of suicidal behavior could be attributed to the transmission of psychopathology. Moreover, most of the previous literature with the notable exception of Pfeffer et al. (1994), focused exclusively on the family history of suicide, rather than examining a broader spectrum of suicidal behavior.

These results, in family studies where the proband has completed suicide, are consistent with family studies conducted on both referred and nonreferred samples of adolescent suicide attempters, compared to psychiatric and community controls, respectively (Bridge et al., 1997; Johnson et al., 1998). In the first family study, the relatives of 62 clinically referred adolescent attempters and 70 never-suicidal psychiatric controls were compared (Johnson et al., 1998). There was a twofold elevation of suicide attempts in the attempter probands (odds ratio = 2.1, 95% confidence interval, 1.04–4.3), which persisted after controlling for Axis I and Axis II psychopathology in relatives and in the probands. In addition, the rate of familial avoidant personality disorder was 4.4 times greater in the relatives of the suicide attempters. Similar to the study of adolescent completers, there was a 2.3-fold higher rate of suicide attempts in the relatives of the aggressive vs. nonaggressive attempters. In the community study (Bridge et al., 1997), which must be regarded as preliminary, the relatives of three attempters were compared to those of 55 nonattempters, and, remarkably, there was a 12-fold excess in attempts that persisted after controlling for differences in relative and proband psychopathology (Bridge et al., 1997). In a high-risk study Brent et al. (2002) compared 141 offspring of 83 mood-disordered attempters and 88 offspring of 58 mood-disordered nonattempters. The risk of attempt in the offspring of attempters was 6.2 times higher than the rate of attempts in offspring of nonattempters, despite similar rates of psychopathology in both offspring groups. An increased risk of attempt in offspring was associated with sexual abuse in parents and in offspring, with impulsive aggression in parent and offspring, and with both mood and substance abuse disorders in offspring. The pattern of parent and offspring attempts was *not* consistent with imitation.

Two studies found that the greater the medical lethality of the proband attempt, the greater the familial loading of suicide (Garfinkel et al., 1982; Linkowski et al., 1985), whereas this was not found in one other study (Johnson et al., 1998). A higher family loading for suicide attempt was associated with greater aggression in the proband, similar to other reports noted above (Johnson et al., 1998). Pfeffer et al. (1994) showed that suicidal behavior in the proband was associated with greater family loading for both suicidal and assaultive behaviors. Increased family loading for suicidal behavior persisted even after controlling for increased risk of psychopathology in the relatives of suicide attempters (Bridge et al., 1997; Johnson et al., 1998). This group of studies shows a relationship between impulsive aggression and familial transmission of suicidal behavior, leading to the conclusion that suicidal behavior appears to be familially transmitted above and beyond the liability for specific psychiatric disorders. Studies also demonstrate that there is an increase in family loading for suicide among suicide attempters with various primary diagnoses, including schizophrenia, bipolar disorder, unipolar depression, and substance abuse (Roy, 1983; Roy et al., 2000, 2001). Finally, the rates of completed suicide are elevated in the relatives of attempted suicide victims, and the familial rates of attempted suicide are elevated in suicide victims, supporting the view that the phenotype being familially transmitted includes both attempted and completed suicide.

## Candidate gene studies

Candidate gene studies involve comparing the prevalence of different genetic variants (polymorphisms) of genes in cases vs. controls. These studies have been criticized because they may be vulnerable to cryptic interrelationships among cases, or differential stratification among cases and controls that could lead to spurious results. Two variants on the candidate gene approach have been developed to address these issues. The first approach uses a family-based control methodology, in which the differential transmission of alleles is compared in cases with two available biological parents (Spielman et al., 1993). The advantage of this approach is that it is not vulnerable to problems of population stratification; the main disadvantages are recruitment and efficiency, since the method requires assessing both the case and two biological parents. Moreover, bias may enter into such studies, especially if the unavailability of both biological parents may be related to the trait under study, such as may be the case in impulsive aggression. The second approach is called genomic control (GC; Devlin and Roeder, 1999; Devlin et al., 2000). The sampling involves cases and controls, much like classical association studies, but then several genes thought to be uninvolved in the disease in question are sampled at random, to rule out, within a certain confidence interval, the possibility that an apparent association of the disease with the candidate gene is attributable to spurious association.

The choice of candidate genes to examine in studying the etiology of suicide is made easier by the extensive and rather consistent findings from post-mortem studies of suicide victims, and *in vivo* studies of suicide attempters. A consistent association between alteration in central serotonin metabolism and both completed and attempted suicide has been demonstrated (Mann, 1998) (see also Chapter 5). This association cuts across diagnostic categories, has both discriminant and predictive validity, and is related to suicide and to impulsive aggression (Coccaro, 1989; Coccaro et al., 1989; Linnoila and Virkkunen, 1992; Mehlman et al., 1994; Virkkunen et al., 1989). Moreover, there is evidence that levels of 5-hydroxyindoleacetic acid (5-HIAA), a metabolite of serotonin measured in cerebrospinal fluid (CSF), is under genetic control with about 40% of the variance estimated to be genetic (Clark et al., 1995; Mehlman et al., 1994). Therefore, it is logical to focus on genetic variation in genes related to serotonin metabolism and receptor response.

## Tryptophan hydroxylase

The most extensive studies have been on tryptophan hydroxylase (TPH), the rate-limiting enzyme in the synthesis of serotonin. Two polymorphisms have been studied, A779C and the A218C, which are in tight disequilibrium with one another, and therefore will be discussed together. The sampling and choice of controls in the study of this gene have been quite variable: Finnish alcoholic offenders (Nielsen et al., 1994, 1998; Rotondo et al., 1997), personality-disordered individuals (New et al., 1998), mood-disordered patients (Bellivier et al., 1998; Buresi et al., 1999; Furlong et al., 1998; Kunugi et al., 1999a; Mann et al., 1997; Tsai et al., 1999), schizophrenics (Paik et al., 2000), suicide attempters (Buresi et al., 1999; Geijer et al., 2000) suicide victims (Bennett et al., 2000; Turecki et al., 2001), and community volunteers (Jonsson et al., 1997; Manuck et al., 1999). The contrasts reported have usually been attempters vs. nonattempters, within diagnostic category, with the exceptions of the comparison of suicide attempters or suicide victims with controls.

One set of studies investigated whether there was any functional significance associated with this polymorphism. Two studies using community volunteers and one studying alcoholic offenders found a relationship between an allelic form of TPH and CSF 5-HIAA or fenfluramine challenge. In a community sample, a blunted response to serotonin release was associated with the A allele, but noted in males only (Manuck et al., 1999). In healthy volunteers, Jonsson et al. (1997) found lower CSF 5-HIAA in association with the A allele. Thus these two studies are in agreement. Manuck et al. (1999) also found that aggressive behavior was associated with a blunted serotonergic responsiveness and with the A allele. In the study of Finnish alcoholic criminal offenders (all male), lower central serotonin activity was related to the C allele, although this was not replicated in a larger but similar sample (Nielsen et al., 1998). New et al. (1998) and Mann et al. (1997) in very small samples of psychiatric patients found no statistically significant relationship of fenfluramine-stimulated prolactin release or CSF 5-HIAA with this TPH allele.

In the studies that examined alcoholic offenders, an association between the C allele and suicide attempt was reported in the impulsive group of Finnish criminal offenders, with the classification of "impulsive" not clearly specified but related to the nature of their most recent crime (Nielsen et al., 1994). This association was confirmed with a discordant sibling linkage analysis that showed a relationship of the TPH C allele not only to suicide attempt, but also to alcoholism and a personality trait on the Karolinska Personality Scale (KPS) termed "socialization" (Nielsen et al., 1998). In a study of personality-disordered patients, the C allele was related to measures of impulsive aggression in males only (New et al., 1998). Another genetic variant, on the TPH promoter (TPH-P, A6526G, A form), was found to be related to suicide attempt, particularly in impulsive alcoholic offenders, as was the haplotype of the C allele of the A779C and the A allele of the A6526G of the TPH-P (Rotondo et al., 1999).

Studies of mood-disordered patients have found an association between suicide attempt and the A allele in depressed patients in two studies (Mann et al., 1997; Tsai et al., 1999), whereas no association was found in two other studies (Furlong et al., 1998; Kunugi et al., 1999a). Among bipolar patients, no association between TPH variants and suicidal behavior has been reported (Bellivier et al., 1998; Furlong et al., 1998; Kirov et al., 1999). The latter study utilized a family-based control approach. Associations have been reported with bipolar disorder, depression, and borderline personality disorder (Bellivier et al., 1998; Mann et al., 1997).

One study found an association between the C allele and suicide attempt in schizophrenics (Paik et al., 2000).

Three studies have compared suicide attempters with unspecified diagnoses to community controls. One found an association between attempt and the A allele (Buresi et al., 1999). A second study reported a statistically nonsignificant association in the same direction (Geijer et al., 2000). The latter combined their sample with that of Buresi and colleagues and confirmed a statistically significant association with the A allele. A third study, which used a family-based method, found no association between TPH allele frequencies and suicide attempt, but did find a relationship with depression (Zalsman et al., 2001a).

Four studies have compared suicide victims (diagnoses unspecified) to controls. Turecki et al. (2001) found no association with individual alleles, but a greater frequency of the haplotype 6526G, 5806T, and 218C in completers. Ono et al. (2000) found no association with either the A6526G polymorphism of the serotonin transporter or the A218C polymorphism of the TPH gene, and could not haplotype the sample because the two genes were not in linkage disequilibrium in this Japanese sample. Bennett et al. (2000) found no association of suicide with either A218C or A779C. Roy et al. (2001), in examining the surviving identical twin of suicide victims and comparing them to controls, found an association with the C form of the TPH allele.

In a study of community volunteers, an association between impulsive aggressive traits and the A form of the TPH allele was reported, particularly in men (Manuck et al., 1999).

Thus, it is not clear whether the TPH A218C polymorphism is associated with lower serotonin function or suicidal behavior. Most studies have involved sample sizes that were too small or perhaps were too heterogeneous in terms of ethnicity to permit sufficient statistical power.

## Serotonin transporter studies

The serotonin transporter upstream or 5′ flanking promoter region has two allelic variants, a short form and a long form. The short form of the promoter region has been shown *in vitro* in transformed lymphoblastoid cell lines to have a lower level of expression (Greenberg et al., 1999). There have been six studies reported in the literature. Three compared suicide victims and controls (Bondy et al., 2000; Du et al., 1999; Mann et al., 2000), two compared suicide attempters and controls (Geijer et al., 2000; Zalsman et al., 2001b), one examined correlates of suicide attempt within a mood-disordered sample (Bellivier et al., 2000), and one examined the relationship of the serotonin transporter (5-HTTLPR) polymorphism to attempt in an alcohol-dependent sample (Gorwood et al., 2000).

Mann et al. (2000) compared suicide victims and controls and found that the 5-HTTLPR allele was not associated with suicide. An association was found with depression due to the presence of more heterozygotes. No relationship between binding to the 5-HTTLPR and this polymorphism was found. Du et al. (1999) compared depressed suicide victims to controls and also found an association with the L allele. Bondy et al. (2000) found an association between suicide and the S (short) form.

Like the Mann et al. (2000) study of suicide completers, Geijer et al. (2000), in a comparison of attempters and controls (not matched for diagnosis), found no difference between the two groups. Zalsman et al. (2001b) also found no relationship between the serotonin transporter, polymorphisms, and suicide attempt in a family-based control study. However, homozygosity for the L allele was associated with a tendency to violence. Roy et al. (2001) found no relationship between serotonin transporter alleles and suicide in the surviving co-twins of monozygotic twins who committed suicide.

Bellivier et al. (2000), in a comparison within a sample of mood-disordered individuals, found that the S form was associated with violent suicide attempt.

Gorwood et al. (2000) found that the S allele was associated with multiple and more medically serious attempts in a sample of alcohol-dependent patients. The S allele also was associated with depression in this sample.

Thus it is not clear that the 5-HTTPRL locus is related to suicidal behavior or even to differences in 5-HTT binding.

## HTR2A studies

There have been seven reported studies of the relationship of suicidal behavior to the HTR2A receptor. All have examined the T102C polymorphism; two other polymorphisms have also been reported upon (His 452Tyr, A1438G). Two have compared suicide victims to control (Du et al., 1999; Turecki et al., 1999), three have compared suicide attempters to controls (Geijer et al., 2000; Kunugi et al., 1999b; Zhang et al., 1997), one has examined suicide attempt with mood disorders (Tsai et al., 1999), and one has examined suicidal ideation within most disorders (Du et al., 2000).

Both case–control studies comparing suicide victims and controls found no relationship between HTR2A polymorphisms (T102C in both studies, A1438G for Turecki et al., 2001; His452Tyr for Du et al., 1999). In one study, the 102T/1438A haplotype was associated with greater 5HT2A receptor binding (Turecki et al., 2001).

In the three studies comparing suicide attempters and controls, two found no effect (Geijer et al., 2000; Kunugi et al., 1999a), and one found an association between attempt and the 102C form (Zhang et al., 1997).

Tsai et al. (1999) compared attempters and nonattempters within a sample of mood-disordered patients and found no effect with respect to the T102C polymorphism.

Du et al. (2000) found a relationship between ideation and the 102C allele in a sample of depressives. Suicidal behavior itself was not reported upon.

Thus, there seems to be no clear agreement as to the association of the T102C polymorphism with suicidal behavior.

## Monoamine oxidase A studies

In a study of community volunteers, Manuck et al. (2000) studied four haplotypes of monoamine oxidase A (MAOA) and found an association between the types 2 or 3 haplotype and impulsive aggression in men. This haplotype was also associated with less enzyme activity. The relationship between this haplotype and suicidal behavior has not yet been studied.

There are several issues raised by these studies, relating to the functional significance of the polymorphisms, the influence of sex and ethnicity, the design of the studies, the characterization of the samples with regard to psychiatric disorder, the assessment of possible "endophenotypes," the importance of assessing traumatic experiences such as sexual abuse, and the statistical issues involved in looking at multiple genes simultaneously.

## Functional significance

Relatively few studies have reported on the functional significance of the polymorphisms. With regard to TPH, the results are inconsistent, but within one sample quite informative, insofar as sex effects were observed both for the functional significance of the polymorphism (blunted response to serotonin release by fenfluramine), and the phenotype (impulsive aggression). It is unclear why associations in different directions would be reported (e.g., 218A in some reports, 218C in others), but it is possible that one allele is problematic under certain circumstances (e.g., depression), where the complementary allelic form is problematic when the individual is violent, personality disordered, or alcoholic.

## Sex difference

Sex effects on the significance of two sets of polymorphisms (TPH and MAOA) were reported, with effects observed only in men (Manuck et al., 1999, 2000; New et al., 1998). Some studies included only men (Manuck et al., 2000; Nielsen et al., 1994, 1998; Rotondo et al., 1997), or consisted mainly of males (e.g., all studies of completed suicide). It would seem particularly important to stratify samples by sex.

## Ethnic differences

Ethnic differences are also an important consideration, and may explain why studies in clinically similar samples differ (e.g., a positive study in depressed Caucasians (Mann et al., 1997) vs. a negative one in Japanese mood-disordered patients (Kunugi et al., 1999a)). However, there has also been a failure to replicate the findings of Mann et al. (1997) in another Caucasian population (Furlong et al., 1998), whereas Mann et al.'s results *were* replicated in a Taiwanese sample (Tsai et al., 1999) and a French sample (Buresi et al., 1999). Particularly when studying haplotypes, there are likely to be significant ethnic differences, with a finding of linkage disequilibrium between haplotypes in a Caucasian sample, but not in a Japanese one (Ono et al., 2000; Turecki et al., 2001).

## Characterization of clinical phenotypes

The characterization of psychiatric disorder and other clinical characteristics could result in differences in outcome. For example, in the study of Nielsen et al. (1998), a differentiation was made on the basis of whether an offender was "impulsive" or "nonimpulsive." This turned out to be a critical differentiation since the associations were found to be much stronger in the impulsive subgroup. This differentiation was made on the basis of the most recent crime, so that a person could actually be reclassified from impulsive to nonimpulsive, which goes against the view that impulsivity is a trait characteristic. Most studies did not ascertain Axis II conditions, except Mann et al. (1997) who did find a significant association between borderline personality disorder and TPH.

A related issue is that there may be an "endophenotype" associated with suicidal behavior, namely impulsive aggression, yet most studies did not assess this, even though it appeared to be related to both TPH and MAOA (but only in males, Manuck et al., 1999, 2000; New et al., 1998).

The assessment of a reported history of physical or sexual trauma may be critical to disentangling the role of genetic factors in suicidal behavior. Trauma (e.g., sexual abuse) may interact with genetic risk, or may override it, and thereby introduce phenocopies into a sample that will make it difficult to find a genetic effect.

Finally, relatively few studies have examined more than one gene simultaneously. When more than one gene was examined at the same time, the usual approach was to examine the relationship between a condition and a particular haplotype. However, it also may be that, particularly if multiple genes are examined, one or more polymorphisms could convey risk in a dose–response relationship.

## Family-environmental studies

There is a consistent literature linking family discord with suicidal behavior (see Table 4.8). Taylor and Stansfeld (1984) compared 50 youthful suicide attempters and 50 psychiatric controls. More frequent disturbances of both mother–child and father–child relationships were reported, with relatively few other differences noted, thereby highlighting the role of family difficulties in differentiating attempter and nonattempter patient populations. They also noted that more of the attempters were postpubertal, which may have contributed to the increased frequency of conflict with patients.

Kosky et al. (1986) compared 481 depressed, nonsuicidal children aged 15 and younger with 147 depressed, suicidal children. The two groups were very similar with respect to symptomatic presentation, and were mainly differentiated by a greater frequency of family difficulties in the suicidal depressed group. Specifically, the suicidal depressed group had more frequent problems with the father–child relationship, the sibling–child relationship, family discord, and abuse.

**Table 4.8.** Family environmental stressors and suicidal behavior

| Author | Sample | Variable | OR |
|---|---|---|---|
| Taylor and Stansfeld (1984) | Attempters vs. psychiatric controls | Family discord | 2.6 |
| Kosky et al. (1986) | Ideators vs. psychiatric controls | Family discord | 2.2 |
| Kosky et al. (1990) | Attempters vs. ideators | Family discord | 1.2 |
| Roberts and Hawton (1980) | – | Abuse of children and suicide attempts in mothers | 2.6–5.2 |
| Pfeffer et al. (1994) | Prepubertal attempters vs. controls<br><br>Attempters vs. depressed ideators | Assaultive behavior in relatives | 2.8 |
| Wagner et al. (1995) | – | Abuse | 2.0 |
|  |  | Running away | 7.0 |
|  |  | Not living with biological parent | 3.5 |
| Fergusson and Lynskey (1995) | Community sample of attempters and nonattempters | Low income | 2.8 |
|  |  | Low maternal emotional response | 3.6 |
|  |  | Family conflict | 2.4 |
|  |  | ≥4 changes in school | 3.3 |
| Fergusson et al. (1996) | Community sample of attempters and nonattempters | Noncontact sexual abuse | 1.0 |
|  |  | Contact abuse/nonintercourse | 2.9 |
|  |  | Intercourse | 11.8 |
| Molnar et al. (2001) | Community sample | Females |  |
|  |  | Rape | 2.5 |
|  |  | Molestation | 1.8 |
|  |  | Males |  |
|  |  | Rape | 3.7 |
|  |  | Molestation | 3.5 |

Kosky et al. (1990) then addressed whether children and adolescents with suicidal ideation could be differentiated from those who actually attempted suicide. From a series of consecutive referrals, 258 ideators were compared to 82 attempters. The two groups showed a very similar symptomatic presentation, with one exception – attempters were more likely to have abused substances. Family discord was more common in the attempters, with discord including "hostility, quarreling, scapegoating, and verbal and physical abuse." Interpersonal loss was an additional risk factor for boys but not for girls.

Kienhorst et al. (1992) compared 48 adolescents who recently attempted suicide to 66 nonattempting depressed adolescents. Half the subjects were clinically referred, and half obtained through screening a large community sample. While the two groups were comparable in depressive severity, the attempter group showed greater degrees of cognitive distortion and hopelessness. Multiple indicators of family dysfunction were more common or more severe in the attempter group, including physical and sexual abuse, running away from home, change in caretaking parent, conflict with mother, and conflicts between parents. The attempter group were also more likely to know someone who had attempted or completed suicide, but did not specify if these contacts were familial or nonfamilial. Kienhorst et al. (1992) presented a model in which a problematic family environment interacted with a cognitive and affectively vulnerable adolescent to lead to a suicide attempt.

Wagner et al. (1995) reported on a large community survey of 1050 adolescents drawn from 10 rural public schools in a Mid-Atlantic State. Those who reported a lifetime history of a suicide attempt ($n = 147$) were compared to those who were either suicide ideators or depressed ($n = 261$) and to the remainder ($n = 642$). The depressed/ideator group had slightly higher depression scores than the attempter group, both were higher than the "normal" group. Attempters were more likely to have been physically abused by parents, to have run away from home, and to be living with other than a biological parent than either depressed/ideators or "normals." Attempters were also more likely to have known someone who completed suicide, although the nature of the relationship was not specified.

Gould et al. (1996), in the above-noted comparison of adolescent suicide victims and controls, found an association between poor parent–child communication and suicide, especially between fathers and suicide victims. As noted above, family history of suicidal behavior persisted as a risk factor even after adjusting for poor parent–child communication. Gould et al. (1996), like Kosky et al. (1990), found loss to be a more potent risk factor for suicidal behavior in boys than in girls.

Brent et al. (1994), in a comparison of the families of 67 adolescent suicide victims and 67 demographically matched community controls, found that family discord was five times more common in the victims, but that this effect disappeared if one controlled for both parental and proband psychopathology. This suggests that some of the discord was secondary to psychopathology with parent and child and is consistent with Gould et al. (1996), who did not find discord to be significant in multivariate analyses. In the study of Brent et al. (1994), parental depression also conveyed an increased risk for suicide, even after controlling for proband diagnosis, suggesting that the association of parental depression and suicide was in part environmentally mediated, since this risk was conveyed above and beyond that due to the transmission of psychiatric disorder *per se*.

Fergusson and colleagues (1995, 1996, 2000) have shown that several family characteristics are associated with adolescent and young adult suicide attempts, including low income, low maternal responsiveness, family conflict, parental alcoholism, residential instability, and sexual abuse.

Other studies have shown a specific relationship between family violence and suicidal behavior (see Table 4.7). Roberts and Hawton (1980) reviewed a case-registry of parents who had abused their children, and cross-checked this against general hospital ledgers for suicide attempts. Overall, 114 families, with 114 mothers and 105 fathers, were studied. The rates of suicide attempts in these above mothers and fathers were over five and three times the rate in the general population, respectively. In general, the reasons for the attempts in the abusing group were related to difficulties with their domestic partner. Moreover, those abusive mothers who attempted suicide were about three times more likely than other nonbusive suicide attempters to re-attempt within the year. This study highlights the complexities in attributing a particular "cause" of suicidal behavior to either environment or heredity. The abuse may be an environmental stressor that predisposes the child to suicidal behavior in the future, but that child may also be at risk for suicidal behavior by virtue of inheriting genes from the mother related to poor regulation of affect and aggression. Pfeffer et al. (1994), in their family study, also found a relationship between assaultive behavior in relatives and suicidal behavior in prepubertal offspring.

Finally, the importance of sexual abuse as a contributor to suicidal risk cannot be overemphasized. Fergusson et al. (1996), in a large community study, showed that the population-attributable risk of sexual abuse for suicide attempts in adolescents was estimated to be 19.5%, with much greater risk for suicidal behavior associated with more serious sexual abuse, such as intercourse. Subsequent follow-up of this sample shows that the main effect of sexual abuse on suicidal behavior is mediated through an increased risk for psychopathology (Fergusson et al., 2000). Molnar et al. (2001) also showed a strong relationship between sexual abuse and suicide attempt, with sexual abuse being associated with a much earlier onset of suicide attempt. Brown et al. (1999) found the population-attributable risk of sexual abuse for suicide attempt to be 16.6%, and that sexual abuse conveyed a much greater risk for attempted suicide than physical abuse. Romans et al. (1995) also showed a very strong association between sexual abuse and suicide attempts in young adult women, with the risk for attempt increasing with the severity and frequency of the abuse, and the closeness of the relationship between the perpetrator and the victim (i.e., father or stepfather). Victims of abuse who attempted suicide were more likely to suffer other psychosocial disadvantages, including "affectionless control" from parents, physical abuse, exposure to parental marital discord and separation, and placement out of the home. Furthermore, those who were sexually abused and later attempted suicide were more likely to have been physically assaulted by a sexual partner, experienced a sexual assault, and to have experienced earlier intercourse, cohabitation, and pregnancy. Therefore, sexual abuse occurs in the matrix of psychosocial disadvantage and may initiate, or at least be part of, a complex cascade of risk factors for suicidal behavior.

## Exposure to suicide and suicidal behavior

One possible mechanism to explain the clustering of suicide in families is through exposure and imitation. For example, if a parent attempts or completes suicide, this may serve as a model for a child and in some way lower the threshold for suicidal behavior to take place. The evidence to support this is mixed and the methodology of certain studies does not always distinguish between exposure to suicide and to suicidal behavior, and between familial and nonfamilial exposure.

Gould et al. (1990) has demonstrated that a small but statistically significant number of adolescent suicide completions occur in time-space clusters, consistent with contagion and imitation. However, Brent et al. (1993a, 1996b) found no evidence of an increased incidence of suicidal behavior in siblings or parents exposed to the suicide of an adolescent family member, compared to the relatives of a community control group. In fact, even the close friends of adolescent suicide victims do not appear to be at increased risk of suicidal behavior over a three-year follow-up (Brent et al., 1993b, 1996c). Hazell and Lewin (1993) also found that 68 adolescents exposed to an adolescent suicide did not show an increased rate of suicidal behavior, compared to 552 unexposed adolescent controls. However, one large school survey, by Wagner et al. (1995), showed adolescents who had a history of a suicide attempt were about three times more likely to have known someone who completed suicide, whether compared to depressed/ideator or less pathological adolescent controls. However, the nature of the relationship (e.g., familial or nonfamilial) and the timing of the exposure were not reported.

Exposure to suicidal behavior may be a marker for assortative friendships, since friends with risk factors for suicidal behavior may be more likely to be in the same social network. Exposure to suicidal behavior, as compared to suicide completion alone, may have more of an impact, although the data are less clear as to whether this is mediated by primarily intra-familial mechanisms. Brent et al. (1990) compared 42 affectively ill suicidal (ideation with a plan or attempter) adolescent inpatients with a comparison group of 14 affectively ill, never-suicidal patients, and found that a higher proportion of the suicidal group had been exposed to suicidality within the family. Moreover, the exposure was a more powerful risk factor for suicidality in the index subjects than was family history (odds ratios of 2.4 vs. 1.4). Several other studies have indicated that knowing someone who has attempted suicide is associated with a suicide attempt. Lewinsohn et al. (1996), in a large community study of adolescent psychopathology, found that adolescent attempters were over four times more likely to have had a recent exposure to a friend's suicide attempt than were nonattempters, even after controlling for the influence of depression. Hazell and Lewin (1993), in a prospective study, found that exposure of an adolescent to an adolescent attempt was associated with an increased incidence of suicide attempts, when compared to adolescents who were exposed to an adolescent completion, or to unexposed, control adolescents. Shafii et al. (1985), in a psychological autopsy study of 20 adolescent suicide victims and 17 controls, who were also friends of the victims, found completers were more likely to have been exposed to an aggregate of familial and nonfamilial suicidality (ranging from ideation to completion). Two studies of familial suicidal behavior showed no evidence of time clustering of relative's attempts (Brent et al., 2002; Statham et al., 1998). However, it is very difficult to reject the hypothesis that a family member's suicidal behavior served as a model for another relative's suicide attempt, even many years later.

In conclusion, the bulk of the evidence suggests that exposure to completed suicide, even within a family, is not associated with an increased risk of suicidal behavior, although time-space clustering of teen suicide does occur. However, there is more extensive support demonstrating that exposure to a peer's attempted suicide may increase the risk for suicidal behavior, although only one study has specifically identified exposure to familial suicidal ideation and behavior as a risk factor for adolescent suicidality. Therefore, it is plausible, although far from proven, that imitation may explain in part the intra-familial clustering of suicidal behavior.

## Parental loss

Another possible mechanism by which suicide in a parent could increase the risk of suicidal behavior in their offspring is via parental loss. One of the difficulties in the literature has been that loss has been defined to mean a relationship disruption, parental divorce or separation, or actual death, so that it is difficult to compare across studies. Nevertheless, diverse studies have shown a relationship between early parental death (e.g., before the age of 12) and attempted suicide. Malone et al. (1995), in a comparison of adult inpatient depressed attempters and nonattempters, found a higher rate of early parental loss in the attempter group. Lewinsohn et al. (1996), in a large community study of adolescents, found that parental death before the age of 12 was over three times more likely to occur among attempters as among nonattempters. Cohen-Sandler et al. (1982) compared prepubertal suicidal inpatients to nonsuicidal depressed and nondepressed inpatients, and found an increased incidence of a wide variety of family-related life events, particularly separation and divorce, in the suicidal group, both in early and in later childhood. Two studies suggest that the relationship between divorce and suicidal behavior is mediated by the increased rate of psychopathology in parents whose marriages end in divorce (Brent et al., 1994; Gould et al., 1998).

Adam et al. (1982) compared 98 adult attempters to 102 controls. In this study, parental loss could occur through death, divorce, or separation, but, in contradistinction to many studies in the literature, the contribution of type of loss to suicidal risk was analyzed separately. A higher incidence of loss, globally defined, was noted in the attempters. The differences due to divorce and separation were highly significant, whereas those due to parental death were not. When paternal death was analyzed separately, there was a higher proportion of attempters with this history. Parental death was more frequent in the period before ten years of age; the same was true with respect to the increased prevalence of divorce and separation in the attempter sample. Family instability was much more common in the attempter group, both before and, in the long run, after the loss. Although multivariate statistical techniques were not applied, the data seem to suggest that at least part of the effect of parental loss was mediated by family instability.

These studies suggest that parental loss in general, and perhaps due to completed suicide, could increase the risk for suicidal behavior in offspring, particularly if the loss occurs when the child is less than the age of 12. However, the adoption study of Schulsinger et al. (1979) does show that mechanisms other than loss or imitation are likely to be involved.

## Model for the familial transmission of suicidal behavior

On the basis of the extant literature, we propose a model for the familial development of suicidal behavior (see Figure 4.2). A parent who is a suicide attempter most likely has at least two sets of liabilities: difficulties with regulation of aggression and the presence of a mood disorder or other type of psychopathology. If both liabilities are transmitted, then the liability first manifested in the

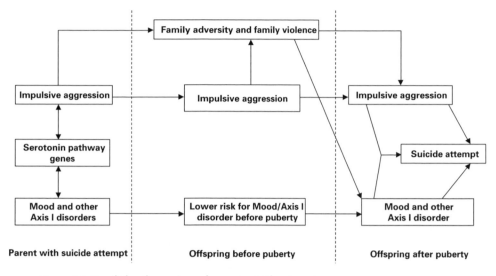

Figure 4.2 Familial pathways to early-onset suicide attempt.

prepubertal child will be difficulty with impulsive violence. Prior to puberty, the incidence of mood and other psychiatric disorders is low, so this suicidality will not be manifested in most children until after puberty. After puberty, both sets of liabilities will manifest themselves, making the likelihood of a suicide attempt the greatest. In addition, the difficulty with impulsive aggression in the parent will serve as an environmental stressor by increasing the likelihood of exposure to family discord, family violence, and abuse. On the basis of previous investigations (e.g., Coccaro, 1989; Coccaro et al., 1989; Mann et al., 1992, 2001; Nielsen et al., 1994, 1998) we further hypothesize that the genes related to impulsive regulation are also involved in serotonergic neurotransmission. Other influences, such as poor parental care, parental loss, and imitation, may also play a role in the familial transmission of suicidal behavior, but both for the sake of simplicity and because the empirical data are less complete, these other potential influences are not depicted in this model.

## Conclusions

There is fairly conclusive evidence demonstrating the familial aggregation of suicidal behavior. The familial transmission of suicidal behavior appears to be independent or interactive with the familial transmission of psychopathology. The familial transmission of suicidal behavior includes both attempts and completions, but suicidal ideation appears to be transmitted along with psychiatric disorders (Brent et al., 1996a). Instead, it is the tendency to *act* on suicidal impulses that appears to be transmitted. There appears to be a strong relationship between the transmission of suicidal behavior and transmission of the tendency to impulsive aggression. In turn, these findings provide further support for the relationship between impulsive violence and suicidal behavior, with both being related to disordered neurotransmission of serotonin. Some of the candidate gene studies of suicidal behavior and aggression herein are consistent with this hypothesis. High-risk studies to elucidate the behavioral precursors of suicidal behavior, additional candidate gene studies, and affected relative-pair studies to study the genetics of suicidal behavior are all indicated.

These data also have important clinical implications. The relatives of attempters and completers are at increased risk for both suicide and suicide attempts. If one is treating a suicide-attempting adolescent, it is vital to also examine the parents for psychopathology and suicidal risk. Affective illness in a parent appears to increase the risk for suicide in the offspring but only when the parent has a history of attempted suicide. The identification and treatment of parental psychopathology may lower suicidal risk in the adolescent because parental depression is a risk factor even in the absence of depression in the offspring (Brent et al., 1994), although other factors, such as sexual abuse and family history of suicidal behavior, may be more potent risk factors (Brent et al., 2002). Conversely, if one is dealing with a suicidal or depressed adult, the offspring of this patient should also be assessed, because of the greatly increased risk of suicidal behavior in the children of these adult patients. Finally, these results suggest that the complete treatment of suicidal behavior involves treating both the primary psychiatric disorder and the tendency to impulsive aggression. Traditionally, treatment has tended to focus on the former. However, if our proposed model of suicidal behavior is correct, then more complete prophylaxis and treatment of suicidal risk can be achieved by simultaneously addressing both sets of liabilities.

## Acknowledgements

This work was supported by NIMH grants MH 43366, 55123, and 56612, 56390 and 62185. The expert assistance of Stephanie Costa in preparation of the manuscript is appreciated.

## REFERENCES

Adam, K. S., Bouckoms, A., and Streiner, D. (1982). Parental loss and family stability in attempted suicide. *Archives of General Psychiatry*, **39**, 1081–1085.

Bellivier, F., Leboyer, M., Courtet, P., Buresi, C., Beaufils, B., Samolyk, D., Allilaire, J., Feingold, J., Mallet, J., and Malafosse, A. (1998). *Archives of General Psychiatry*, **55**, 33–37.

Bellivier, F., Szoke, A., Henry, C., Lacoste, J., Bottos, C., Nosten-Bertrans, M., Hardy, P., Rouillon, F., Launay, J. M., Laplanche, J.-L., and Leboyer, M. (2000). Possible association between serotonin transporter gene polymorphism and violent suicidal behavior in mood disorders. *Biological Psychiatry*, **48**, 319–322.

Bennett, P. J., McMahon, W. M., Watabe, J., Achilles, J., Bacon, M., Coon, H., Grey, T., Keller, T., Tate, D., Tcaciuc, I., and Gray, D. (2000). Tryptophan hydroxylase polymorphisms in suicide victims. *Psychiatry and Genetics*, **10**, 13–17.

Bondy, B., Erfurth, A., de Jonge, S., Kruger, M., and Meyer, H. (2000). Possible association of the short allele of the serotonin transporter promoter gene polymorphism (5-HTTLPR) with violent suicide. *Molecular Psychiatry*, **5**, 193–195.

Brent, D. A., Kolko, D. J., Goldstein, C. E., Allan, M. J., and Brown, R. V. (1990). Suicidality in affectively disordered adolescent inpatients. *Journal of the American Academy of Child and Adolescent Psychiatry*, **29**, 586–593.

Brent, D. A., Perper, J. A., Moritz, G., Liotus, L., Schweers, J., Roth, C., Balach, L., and Allman, C. (1993a). Psychiatric impact of the loss of an adolescent sibling to suicide. *Journal of Affective Disorders*, **28**, 249–256.

Brent, D. A., Perper, J. A., Moritz, G., Allman, C., Schweers, J., Roth, C., Balach, L., Canobbio, R., and Liotus, L. (1993b). Psychiatric sequelae to the loss of an adolescent to suicide. *Journal of the American Academy of Child and Adolescent Psychiatry*, **32**, 509–517.

Brent, D. A., Perper, J. A., Moritz, G., Liotus, L., Schweers, J., Balach, L., and Roth, C. (1994). Familial risk factors for adolescent suicide: a case–control study. *Acta Psychiatrica Scandinavica*, **89**, 52–58.

Brent, D. A., Bridge, J., Johnson, B. A., and Connolly, J. (1996a). Suicidal behavior runs in families: a controlled family study of adolescent suicide victims. *Archives of General Psychiatry*, **53**, 1145–1152.

Brent, D. A., Moritz, G., Bridge, J., Perper, J., and Canobbio, R. (1996b). The impact of adolescent suicide on siblings and parents: a longitudinal follow-up. *Suicide and Life-Threatening Behavior*, **26**, 253–259.

Brent, D. A., Moritz, G., Bridge, J., Perper, J., and Canobbio, R. (1996c). Long-term impact of exposure to suicide: a three year controlled follow-up. *Journal of the American Academy of Child and Adolescent Psychiatry*, **35**, 646–653.

Brent, D. A., Oquendo, M. A., Birmaher, B., Greenhill, L., Kolko, D. J., Stanley, B., Zelazny, J., Brodsky, B. S., Bridge, J., Ellis, S. P., Salazar, O., and Mann, J. J. (2002). Familial pathways to early-onset suicide attempts: a high-risk study. *Archives of General Psychiatry* **59**: 801–807.

Bridge, J. A., Brent, D. A., Johnson, B., and Connolly, J. (1997). Familial aggregation of psychiatric disorders in a community sample of adolescents. *Journal of the American Academy of Child and Adolescent Psychiatry*, **36**, 628–636.

Brown, J., Cohen, P., Johnson, J. G., and Smailes, E. M. (1999). Childhood abuse and neglect: specificity of effects on adolescent and young adult depression and suicidality. *Journal of the American Academy of Child and Adolescent Psychiatry*, **38**, 1490–1496.

Buresi, C., Courtet, P., Leboyer, M., Feingold, J., and Malafosse, A. (1999). Association between suicide attempt and the tryptophane hydroxylase. *American Journal of Human Genetics, Supplement*, **61**, A270.

Cheng, A. T., Chen, T. H. H., Chen, C. C., and Jenkins, R. (2000). Psychosocial and psychiatric risk factors for suicide: case–control psychological autopsy study. *British Journal of Psychiatry*, **177**, 360–365.

Clark, C. P., Gillin, J. C., and Golshan, S. (1995). Do differences in sleep architecture exist between depressives with comorbid simple phobia as compared with pure depressives? *Journal of Affective Disorders*, **33**, 251–255.

Coccaro, E. F. (1989). Central serotonin and impulsive aggression. *British Journal of Psychiatry*, **155**, 52–62.

Coccaro, E., Siever, L., Klar, H. M., Maurer, G., Cochrane, K., Cooper, T. B., Mohs, R. C., and Davis, K. L. (1989). Serotonergic studies in patients with affective and personality disorders. *Archives of General Psychiatry*, **46**, 587–599.

Cohen-Sandler, R., Berman, A. L., and King, R. A. (1982). Life stress and symptomatology: determinants of suicidal behavior in children. *American Academy of Child Psychiatry*, **21**, 178–186.

Devlin, B., and Roeder, K. (1999). Genomic control for association studies. *Biometrics*, **55**, 997–1004.

Devlin, B., Roeder, K., and Wasserman, L. (2000). Genomic control for association studies: a semiparametric test to detect excess-haplotype sharing. *Biostatistics*, **1**, 369–387.

Du, L., Faludi, G., Palkovits, M., Demeter, E., Bakish, D., Lapierre, Y., Sotonyi, P., and Hrdina, P. (1999). Frequency of long allele in serotonin transporter gene is increased in depressed suicide victims. *Biological Psychiatry*, **46**, 196–201.

Du, L., Bakish, D., LaPierre, Y. D., Ravindran, A., and Hrdina, P. D. (2000). Association of polymorphism of serotonin 2A receptor gene with suicidal ideation in major depressive disorder. *American Journal of Medical Genetics*, **96**, 56–60.

Egeland, J. A., and Sussex, J. N. (1985). Suicide and family loading for affective disorders. *Journal of the American Medical Association*, **254**, 915–918.

Fergusson, D. M., and Lynskey, M. T. (1995). Childhood circumstances, adolescent adjustment, and suicide attempts in a New Zealand birth cohort. *Journal of the American Academy of Child and Adolescent Psychiatry*, **34**, 612–622.

Fergusson, D. M., Lynskey, M. T., and Horwood, L. J. (1996). Childhood sexual abuse and psychiatric disorder in young adulthood: II. Psychiatric outcomes of childhood sexual abuse. *Journal of the American Academy of Child and Adolescent Psychiatry*, **34**, 1365–1374.

Fergusson, D. M., Woodward, L. J., and Horwood, L. J. (2000). Risk factors and life processes associated with the onset of suicidal behavior during adolescence and early adulthood. *Psychological Medicine*, **30**, 23–39.

Fu, Q., Heath, A. C., Bucholz, K. K., Nelson, E. C., Glowinski, A. L., Goldberg, J., Lyons, M. J., Tsuang, M. T., Jacob, T., True, M. R., and Eisen, S. A. (2002). A twin study of genetic and environmental influences on suicidality in men. *Psychological Medicine*, **32**, 11–24.

Furlong, R. A., Ho, L., Rubinsztein, J. S., Walsh, C., Paykel, E. S., and Rubinsztein, D. C. (1998). No association of the tryptophan hydroxylase gene with bipolar affective disorder, unipolar affective disorder, or suicidal behavior in major affective disorder. *American Journal of Medical Genetics*, **81**, 245–247.

Garfinkel, B. D., Froese, A., and Hood, J. (1982). Suicide attempts in children and adolescents. *American Journal of Psychiatry*, **139**, 1257–1261.

Geijer, T., Frisch, A., Persson, M.-L., Wasserman, D., Rockah, R., Michaelovsky, E., Apter, A., Jonsson, E. G., Nothen, M. M., and Weizman, A. (2000). Search for association between suicide attempt and serotonergic polymorphisms. *Psychiatric Genetics*, **10**, 19–26.

Glowinski, A. L., Bucholz, K. K., Nelson, E. C., Fu, Q., Madden, P. A. F., Reich, W., Madden, P. A. F., and Heath, A. C. (2001). Suicide attempts in an adolescent female twin sample. *Journal of the American Academy of Child and Adolescent Psychiatry*, **40**(11), 1300–1307.

Gorwood, P., Batel, P., Ades, J., Hamon, M., and Boni, C. (2000). Serotonin transporter gene polymorphisms, alcoholism, and suicidal behavior. *Biological Psychiatry*, **48**, 259–264.

Gould, M. S., Wallenstein, S., and Kleinman, M. (1990). Time-space clustering of teenage suicide. *American Journal of Epidemiology*, **131**, 71–78.

Gould, M. S., Fisher, P., Parides, M., Flory, M., and Shaffer, D. (1996). Psychosocial risk factors of child and adolescent completed suicide. *Archives of General Psychiatry*, **53**, 1155–1162.

Gould, M. S., Shaffer, D., Fisher, P., and Garfinkel, R. (1998). Separation/divorce and child and adolescent completed suicide. *Journal of the American Academy of Child and Adolescent Psychiatry*, **37**, 155–162.

Greenberg, B. D., Tolliver, T. J., Huang, S., Li, Q., Bengel, D., and Murphy, D. L. (1999). Genetic variation in the serotonin transporter promoter region affects serotonin uptake in human blood platelets. *American Journal of Medical Genetics*, **88**, 83–87.

Hazell, P., and Lewin, T. (1993). Friends of adolescent suicide attempters and completers. *Journal of the American Academy of Child and Adolescent Psychiatry*, **32**, 76–81.

Johnson, B. A., Brent, D. A., Bridge, J., Connolly, J., Matta, J., Constantine, D., Rather, C., and White, T. (1998). The familial aggregation of adolescent suicide attempts. *Acta Psychiatrica Scandinavica*, **97**, 18–24.

Jonsson, E. G., Goldman, D., Spurlock, G., Gustavsson, J. P., Nielsen, D. A., Linnoila, M., Owen, M. J., and Sedvall, G. C. (1997). Tryptophan hydroxylase and catechol-*O*-methyltransferase gene polymorphisms: relationships to monoamine metabolite concentrations in CSF of healthy volunteers. *European Archives of Psychiatry and Clinical Neuroscience*, **247**, 297–302.

Kety, S. (1986). Genetic factors in suicide. In Roy, A. (ed.) *Suicide*. Baltimore, MD: Williams & Wilkins.

Kienhorst, C. W. M., de Wilde, E. J., Diekstra, R. F. W., and Wolters, W. H. G. (1992). Differences between adolescent suicide attempters and depressed adolescents. *Acta Psychiatrica Scandinavica*, **85**, 222–228.

Kirov, G., Owen, M. J., Jones, I., McCandless, F., and Craddock, N. (1999). Tryptophan hydroxylase gene and manic-depressive illness. *Archives of General Psychiatry*, **56**, 98–99.

Kosky, R., Silburn, S., and Zubrick, S. (1986). Symptomatic depression and suicidal ideation: a comparative study with 628 children. *Journal of Nervous and Mental Disease*, **174**, 523–528.

Kosky, R., Silburn, S., and Zubrick, S. R. (1990). Are children and adolescents who have suicidal thoughts different from those who attempt suicide? *Journal of Nervous and Mental Disease*, **178**, 38–43.

Kunugi, H., Ishida, S., Kato, T., Tatsumi, M., Sakai, T., Hattori, M., Hirose, T., and Nanko, S. (1999a). A functional polymorphism in the promoter region of monoamine oxidase-A gene and mood disorders. *Molecular Psychiatry*, **4**, 393–395.

Kunugi, H., Ishida, S., Kato, T., Sakai, T., Tatsumi, M., Hirose, T., and Nanko, S. (1999b). No evidence for an association of polymorphisms of the tryptophan hydroxylase gene with affective disorders or attempted suicide among Japanese patients. *American Journal of Psychiatry*, **156**, 774–776.

Lewinsohn, P. M., Rohde, P., and Seeley, J. R. (1996). Adolescent suicidal ideation and attempts: prevalence, risk factors, and clinical implications. *Clinical Psychology: Science and Practice*, Spring, 25–46.

Linkowski, P., de Maertelaer, V., and Mendlewicz, J. (1985). Suicidal behavior in major depressive illness. *Acta Psychiatrica Scandinavica*, **72**, 233–238.

Linnoila, V. M. I., and Virkkunen, M. (1992). Aggression, suicidality, and serotonin. *Journal of Clinical Psychiatry*, **53**, 10, 46–51.

Malone, K. M., Haas, G. L., Sweeney, J. A., and Mann, J. J. (1995). Major depression and the risk of attempted suicide. *Journal of Affective Disorders*, **34**, 173–185.

Mann, J. J. (1998). The neurobiology of suicide. *Nature Medicine*, **4**, 25–30.

Mann, J. J., McBride, P. A., Brown, R. P., Linnoila, M., Leon, A. C., DeMeo, M., Mieczkowski, T., Myers, J. E., and Stanley, M. (1992). Relationship between central and peripheral serotonin indexes in depressed and suicidal psychiatric inpatients. *Archives of General Psychiatry*, **49**, 442–446.

Mann, J. J., Malone, K. M., Nielsen, D. A., Goldman, D., Erdos, J., and Gelernter, J. (1997). Possible association of a polymorphism of the tryptophan hydroxylase gene with suicidal behavior in depressed patients. *American Journal of Psychiatry*, **154**, 1451–1453.

Mann, J. J., Huang, Y.-Y., Underwood, M. D., Kassir, S. A., Oppenheim, S., Kelly, T., Dwork, A. J., and Arango, V. (2000). A serotonin transporter gene promoter polymorphism (5-HTTLPR) and prefrontal cortical binding in major depression in suicide. *Archives of General Psychiatry*, **57**, 729–738.

Mann, J. J., Brent, D. A., and Arango, V. (2001). The neurobiology and genetics of suicide and attempted suicide: a focus on the serotonergic system. *Neuropsychopharmacology*, **24**, 467–477.

Manuck, S. B., Flory, J. D., Ferrell, R. E., Dent, K. M., Mann, J. J., and Muldoon, M. F. (1999). Aggression and anger-related traits associated with a polymorphism of the tryptophan hydroxylase gene. *Biological Psychiatry*, **45**, 603–614.

Manuck, S. B., Flory, J. D., Ferrell, R. E., Mann, J. J., and Muldoon, M. F. (2000). A regulatory polymorphism of the monoamine oxidase-A gene may be associated with variability in aggression, impulsivity, and central nervous system serotonergic responsivity. *Psychiatry Research*, **95**, 9–23.

Mehlman, P. T., Higley, J. D., Faucher, B. A. et al. (1994). Low CSF 5-HIAA concentrations and severe aggression and impaired impulse control in nonhuman primates. *American Journal of Psychiatry*, **151**, 1485–1491.

Mitterauer, B. (1990). A contribution to the discussion of the role of the genetic factor in suicide, based on five studies in an epidemiologically defined area (Province of Salzburg, Austria). *Comprehensive Psychiatry*, **31**, 557–565.

Molnar, B. E., Buka, S. L., and Kessler, R. C. (2001). Child sexual abuse and subsequent psychopathology: results from the National Comorbidity Survey. *American Journal of Public Health*, **91**, 753–760.

New, A. S., Gelernter, J., Yovell, Y., Trestman, R. L., Nielsen, D. A., Silverman, J., Mitropoulou, V., and Siever, L. J. (1998). Tryptophan hydroxylase genotype is associated with impulsive-aggression measures: a preliminary study. *American Journal of Medical Genetics*, **81**, 13–17.

Nielsen, D. A., and Goldman, D. (1996). TPH replication study: not! *Archives of General Psychiatry*, **53**, 964–965.

Nielsen, D. A., Goldman, D., Virkkunen, M., Tokola, R., Rawlings, R., and Linnoila, M. (1994). Suicidality and 5-hydroxyindoleacetic acid concentration associated with a tryptophan hydroxylase polymorphism. *Archives of General Psychiatry*, **51**, 34–38.

Nielsen, D. A., Virkkunen, M., Lappalainen, J., Eggert, M., Brown, G. L., Long, J. C., Goldman, D., and Linnoila, M. (1998). A tryptophan hydroxylase gene marker for suicidality and alcoholism. *Archives of General Psychiatry*, **55**, 593–602.

Ono, H., Shirakawa, O., Nishiguchi, N., Nishimura, A., Nushida, H., Ueno, Y., and Maeda, K. (2000). Tryptophan hydroxylase gene polymorphisms are not associated with suicide. *American Journal of Medical Genetics*, **96**, 861–863.

Paik, I., Toh, K., Kim, J., Lee, C., and Lee, C.-U. (2000). TPH gene may be associated with suicidal behavior, but not with schizophrenia in the Korean population. *Human Heredity*, **50**, 365–369.

Pfeffer, C. R., Normandin, L., and Tatsuyuki, K. (1994). Suicidal children grow up: suicidal behavior and psychiatric disorders among relatives. *Journal of the American Academy of Child and Adolescent Psychiatry*, **33**, 1087–1097.

Roberts, J., and Hawton, K. (1980). Child abuse and attempted suicide. *British Journal of Psychiatry*, **137**, 319–323.

Romans, S. E., Martin, J. L., Anderson, J. C., Herbison, G. P., and Mullen, P. E. (1995). Sexual abuse in childhood and deliberate self-harm. *American Journal of Psychiatry*, **152**, 1336–1342.

Rotondo, A., Nielsen, D. A., Nakhai, B., Hulihan-Giblin, B., Bolos, A., and Goldman, D. (1997). Agonist-promoted down-regulation and functional desensitization in two naturally occurring variants of the human serotonin 1A receptor. *Neuropsychopharmacology*, **17**, 18–26.

Rotondo, A., Schuebel, K. E., Bergen, A. W., Aragon, R., Virkkunen, M., Linnoila, M., Goldman, D., and Nielsen, D. A. (1999). Identification of four variants in the tryptophan hydroxylase promoter and association to behavior. *Molecular Psychiatry*, **4**, 360–368.

Roy, A. (1983). Family history of suicide. *Archives of General Psychiatry*, **40**, 971–974.

Roy, A. (1999). Suicidal behavior in depression: relationship to platelet serotonin transporter. *Neuropsychobiology*, **39**, 71–75.

Roy, A. (2000). Relation of family history of suicide to suicide attempts in alcoholics. *American Journal of Psychiatry*, **157**, 2050–2051.

Roy, A. (2001). Characteristics of cocaine-dependent patients who attempt suicide. *American Journal of Psychiatry*, **158**, 8.

Roy, A., Segal, N. L., Centerwall, B. S., and Robinette, D. (1991). Suicide in twins. *Archives of General Psychiatry*, **48**, 29–32.

Roy, A., Segal, N. L., and Sarchiapone, M. (1995). Attempted suicide among living co-twins of twin suicide victims. *American Journal of Psychiatry*, **152**, 1075–1076.

Roy, A., Rylander, G., Forslund, K., Asberg, M., Mazzanti, C. M., Goldman, D., and Nielsen, D. (2001). Excess tryptophan hydroxylase 17 779C allele in surviving cotwins of monozygotic twin suicide victims. *Neuropsychobiology*, **43**(4), 233–236.

Schulsinger, F., Kety, S. S., Rosenthal, D., and Wender, P. H. (1979). A family study of suicide. In Schou, M., and Stromgren, E. (eds.) *Origin, Prevention and Treatment of Affective Disorder* (pp. 277–287). London: Academic Press.

Shafii, M., Carrigan, S., Whittinghill, J. R., and Derrick, A. (1985). Psychological autopsy of completed suicide in children and adolescents. *American Journal of Psychiatry*, **142**, 1061–1064.

Spielman, R. S., McGinnis, R. E., and Ewens, W. J. (1993). Transmission test for linkage disequilibrium: the insulin gene region and insulin-dependent diabetes mellitus (IDDM). *American Journal of Human Genetics*, **52**, 506–516.

Statham, D. J., Heath, A. C., Madden, P. A. F., Bucholz, K. K., Bierut, L., Dinwiddie, S. H., Slutske, W. S., Dunne, M. P., and Martin, N. G. (1998). Suicidal behavior: an epidemiological and genetic study. *Psychological Medicine*, **28**, 839–855.

Taylor, E. A., and Stansfeld, S. A. (1984). Children who poison themselves: I. A clinical comparison with psychiatric controls. *British Journal of Psychiatry*, **145**, 127–132.

Tsai, S. J., Hong, C. J., and Wang, Y. C. (1999). Tryptophan hydroxylase gene polymorphism (A218C) and suicidal behavior. *NeuroReport*, **18**, 3773–3775.

Tsuang, M. T. (1977). Genetic factors in suicide. *Diseases of the Nervous System*, **38**, 498–501.

Tsuang, M. T. (1983). Risk of suicide in the relatives of schizophrenics, manics, depressives, and controls. *Journal of Clinical Psychiatry*, **44**, 396–400.

Turecki, G., Briere, R., Dewar, K., Antonetti, T., Lesage, A. D., Seguin, S., Cawky, N., Vanier, C., Alda, M., Joober, R., Benkelfat, C., and Rouleau, G. A. (1999). Prediction of level of serotonin 2A receptor binding by serotonin receptor 2A genetic variation in postmortem brain samples from subjects who did or did not commit suicide. *American Journal of Psychiatry*, **156**, 1456–1458.

Turecki, G., Zhu, Z., Tzenova, J., Lesage, A., Seguin, M., Tousignant, M., Chawky, N., Vanier, C., Lipp, O., Alda, M., Joober, Benkelfat, C., Rouleau, G. A. (2001). TPH and suicidal behavior: a study in suicide completers. *Molecular Psychiatry*, **6**, 98–102.

Virkkunen, M., DeJong, J., Bartko, J., and Linnoila, M. (1989). Psychobiological concomitants of history of suicide attempts among violent offenders and impulsive fire setters. *Archives of General Psychiatry*, **46**, 604–606.

Wagner, B. M., Cole, R. E., and Schwartzman, M. S. (1995). Psychosocial correlates of suicide attempts among junior and senior high school youth. *Suicide and Life-Threatening Behavior*, **25**, 358–372.

Wender, P. H., Kety, S. S., Rosenthal, D., Schulsinger, F., Ortmann, J., and Lunde, I. (1986). Psychiatric disorders in the biological and adoptive families of adopted individuals with affective disorders. *Archives of General Psychiatry*, **43**, 923–929.

Zalsman, G., Frisch, A., King, R. A., Pauls, D. L., Grice, D. E., Gelernter, J., Alsobrook, J., Michaelovsky, E., Apter, A., Tyano, S., Weizman, A., and Leckman, J. F. (2001a). Case control and family-based studies of tryptophan hydroxylase gene A218C polymorphism and suicidality in adolescents. *American Journal of Medical Genetics*, **105**, 451–457.

Zalsman, G., Frisch, A., Bromberg, M., Gelernter, J., Michaelovsky, E., Campino, A., Erlich, Z., Tyano, S., Apter, A., and Weizman, A. (2001b). Family-based association study of serotonin transporter promoter in suicidal adolescents: no association with suicidality but possible role in violence traits. *American Journal of Medical Genetics*, **105**, 239–245.

Zhang, H.-Y., Ishigaki, T., Tani, K., Chen, K., Shih, J. C., Miyasato, K., and Ohara, K. (1997). Serotonin 2A receptor gene polymorphism in mood disorders. *Biological Psychiatry*, **41**, 768–773.

# 5

# Biological factors influencing suicidal behavior in adolescents

## Alan Apter

The dearth of biological studies of child and adolescent suicide necessitates that this chapter reviews the general situation, pointing out those areas that have the most relevance to adolescent suicidal behavior. The emphasis of this review also reflects the author's view that suicidal behavior in the young is strongly related to aggression and impulsivity (Oquendo and Mann, 2000; van Praag, 2000).

## Serotonin and suicide

### Psychopathology and suicide

One of the main obstacles to reducing the suicide rate in adolescents is a relative inability to identify youth who are at risk of suicide attempts and completions. A related problem is our lack of understanding of the mechanisms that predispose adolescents to suicidal behavior. One consistent theme in the literature, however, is that suicide and suicidal behavior are linked to a wide variety of psychiatric disorders, including affective illness, substance abuse, conduct disorder, and schizophrenia (Brent et al., 1993). Over 90% of adolescent and adult suicide victims appear to have at least one major psychiatric disorder (Brent, 1989). However, since the majority of patients with psychiatric disorders do not commit or attempt suicide, it appears that a psychiatric disorder may be a necessary, but not a sufficient, risk factor for suicide. Therefore, one of the most pressing clinical research areas in the field of adolescent suicidality is to identify those factors, other than psychiatric disorder, that predispose to suicide. Some investigations have suggested a connection with hereditary personality traits that are related to impulsivity, aggression, and lack of emotional stability in the face of stress from life events. These personality factors seem to be related to serotonergic dysfunction. (Apter et al., 1993; van Praag, 1996).

## Serotonin system functioning and risk for suicide

There appears to be an intimate relationship between the serotonergic parameters of aggression, anxiety, impulsivity, and suicidal behavior, especially in young
people (Apter et al., 1990). In 1993, Brent et al. reported that adolescent suicide
completers had more impulsive aggressive personality disorders than did controls and that they had higher aggression ratings, as assessed by a parent questionnaire. This seems to hold true for suicide attempters and for the families of
adolescent suicide completers and attempters. Apter et al. (1995) also showed
that adolescents with aggression and conduct disorder may be suicidal, even in
the absence of depression. Suicidal adolescent inpatients also show a range of
interrelated psychological behaviors (aggression, impulsivity, and anxiety) that
are related to serotonergic functioning.

Therefore, a compelling argument can be made that further biological and
molecular psychiatric research is needed in order to emphasize the different
dimensions or components of behavior that contribute to psychopathology,
without regard to specific categorical nosology. This, especially, appears to be
the case concerning suicidality (Apter et al., 1990; van Praag, 1996). Currently, the
biological system most plausibly implicated in suicidality, impulsive violence, and
anxiety is the serotonergic system (Apter et al., 1990, 1991). Finally, it is relevant
to point out that serotonergic activity has been shown to be familial, both in
humans and in nonhuman primates (Coccaro et al., 1994; Sedvall et al., 1980).

## Familial clustering of suicide and suicide attempts

The familial clustering of suicide and suicide attempts is well known (for a detailed
description, see Chapter 4). Relatives of suicide completers show high rates of
attempts and completions, compared to relatives of community controls, friends
(Brent et al., 1994), nonsuicidal controls (Tsuang, 1983), and adoptive relatives
(Garrison et al., 1991). Family studies of Amish people indicate that 73% of the
suicides were clustered in 16% of the pedigrees. In addition, patients who attempt
suicide have been found to have much higher rates of attempts in their relatives
than medical, psychiatric or normal controls (Brown et al., 1979; Pfeffer et al.,
1994). Later family studies of adolescent suicide completers (Brent, 1997) have
shown that their first-degree relatives display more suicide attempts, affective disorder, conduct disorder, antisocial personality disorder, and impulsive violence.
Similar results have been shown for adolescent suicide attempters (Brent, 1997).
Both studies showed that the transmission of suicidal behavior was independent
of the transmission of psychiatric disorder. Although it is plausible that familial
transmission occurs to some extent through psychosocial and environmental

influences, such as imitation, exposure to psychosocial adversity and dysfunctional family processes, adoption studies suggest that familial transmission can
occur without exposure to a suicide model and, conversely, that exposure to an
adoptive relative's suicide does not lead to suicidal behavior.

## Genetic serotonin studies of suicide risk

### Serotonin transporter gene polymorphism

One candidate gene that may be a potential influence on aggressive suicidal
behavior is the serotonin transporter (5-HTT) gene (Furlong et al., 1988a). This
gene codes for the serotonin transporter, which is localized in the outer membrane of the presynaptic serotonergic neurons (Heilis et al., 1997; Ramamoorthy
et al., 1993).

The serotonin transporter is sodium-dependent and has high affinity for serotonin. It has an important role in controlling serotonin availability, functioning in
the synapse by regulating the re-uptake of serotonin. 5-HTT is the major target
of erotonin re-uptake inhibitor medications (Heilis et al., 1997; Sanders-Bush
and Mayer, 1996). Some drugs are aggregated in the serotonergic neurons by
the 5-HTT gene (Lesch et al., 1993).

The gene encoding the 5-HTT protein gene (SLC6A4) was mapped on the
proximal long arm of chromosome 17, close to 17q12 (Gelernter et al., 1997;
Lesch et al., 1993; Ramamoorthy et al., 1993). In 1994, Lesch et al. showed that
the 5-HTT gene has 14 exons and 12 introns. In the second intron, there is a
region of variable number tandem repeats (VNTR) of 17 base pairs (bp) with
three major alleles. Another polymorphism found in the promoter region is the
"5-HT-linked polymorphic region" (5-HTTLPR), which consists of two common
alleles, short ("S") and long ("L") variants, that differ by repeats of 20–23GC44
bp (Heilis et al., 1996).

Lesch et al. (1995) showed that there are no differences in the amino acid
sequence order between probands who are ill with affective mood disorder
and a healthy population. No major mutation was found in the 5-HTTSLC6A4
coding area region, either in psychiatrically affected probands, or in control
group subjects (Di Bella et al., 1996). Since no constructive structural protein
sequential changes were found in the gene encoding the 5-HTT protein, it was
assumed that a dysfunction or alteration changes in the expression of the gene
might be found in serotonin-related psychopathologies.

In some studies, alcohol dependency and ethanol tolerance were also found
to have an association with the "S" allele (Turker et al., 1998), while other studies
showed no association (Gelernter et al., 1997). Hallikainen et al. (1999) found an
association between the "S" allele and type 2 alcoholism and habitual impulsive

violent behavior. With regard to autism, there are contradictory findings (Cook et al., 1997). Some evidence has been found in connection to Alzheimer disease (Lesch and Mossner, 1998; Li et al., 1997).

The role of the 5-HTTLPR polymorphism in suicidal behavior was studied by Russ et al. (2000) and Geijer et al. (2000). In both case–control studies, there was no significant difference in the frequencies of the 5-HTTLPR5-HTT promoter alleles between Caucasian European patients who attempted suicide and the control group. However, Du et al. (1999) reported a modest association between the "L" allele of the 5-HTTLPR and suicidality in depressed patients, while Bondy et al. (2000) found a possible association of the "S" allele with violent suicide victims.

Zalsman et al. (2001a) examined the association of 5-HTTLPR with suicidal behavior and related traits in Israeli suicidal adolescent inpatients using the haplotype relative risk (HRR) method that controls for artifacts caused by population stratification. Forty-eight inpatient adolescents who had recently attempted suicide were assessed by structured interviews. Detailed clinical history, diagnoses, suicide intent, suicide risk, impulsivity, violence, and depression were all noted. Blood samples were collected and deoxyribonucleic acid (DNA) extracted from patients and their biological parents. The 5-HTTLPR allele frequencies were tested for association with suicidality by the HRR method. In addition, the relationship between genotypes and the phenotypic severity of several clinical parameters was analyzed. No significant allelic association of the 5-HTTLPR polymorphism with suicidal behavior was found (chi square $= 0.023$, $p = 0.88$). Analysis of variance of the suicide-related trait measures for the three genotypes demonstrated a significant difference in violence measures between patients carrying the LL and LS genotypes ($9.50 \pm 4.04$ vs. $5.36 \pm 4.03$; $p = 0.029$). This study suggested that the 5-HTTLPR polymorphism is unlikely to have major relevance to the pathogenesis of suicidal behavior in adolescence but may contribute to violent behavior in this population. Such an association has also been found with violence traits, as measured by the Past Feelings and Acts of Violence Scale (PFAVS). This questionnaire has been found to be highly sensitive and reliable in detecting aggression and violence (Plutchik and van Praag, 1990) – two important factors in the evaluation of suicidal adolescents (Apter et al., 1993, 1995; Coccaro 1989; Coccaro et al., 1989; Gould et al., 1992). The PFAVS significantly discriminated between psychiatric inpatients with and without violent behavior (Plutchik and van Praag, 1986). In a former study, a subgroup of violent patients showed a higher suicide risk and impulsivity, compared with a nonviolent subgroup (Apter et al., 1995). However, it should be noted that two studies (Coccaro, 1989; Coccaro et al., 1989) emphasized that impulsiveness and aggressive behavior, which are essential parts of suicidality, tend to correlate with dysregulation of suicidality in central serotonin activity studies. In these studies, an association between the serotonergic genotype and aggressive behavior was observed but there was no such association with impulsivity – a finding which is not supported in this genetic study.

If the LL genotype (but not the LS and SS genotypes) occurs significantly more frequently in the high-risk group of aggressive suicidal adolescents, then the mechanism of inheritance of suicidality is apparently more complex than a Mendelian recessive or co-dominance model.

### The tryptophan hydroxylase gene polymorphism

Based on genetic studies and findings relating serotonin to suicidal behavior, some researchers have suggested that the gene coding for the rate-limiting enzyme in serotonin metabolism, tryptophan hydroxylase (TPH), is a candidate gene for suicidal behavior.

Nielsen et al. (1992) placed the human TPH gene in the linkage map on chromosome 11. Using the single-strand conformational polymorphism (SSCP) technique, they identified a polymorphism in intron 7, and designated the alleles "U" and "L," depending on their SSCP migration. In a study of impulsive violent alcoholics, the same group (Nielsen et al., 1994) reported an association between the TPH genotype and the cerebrospinal fluid (CSF) levels of 5-hydroxyindoleacetic acid (5-HIAA) levels. The polymorphism was found to be associated with a history of suicide attempts and the number of suicide attempts independent of psychiatric diagnosis, impulsivity, or 5-HIAA levels. The "L" polymorphic allele was significantly associated with suicidality (Abbar et al. 1995), suggesting that these data were not sufficient to support the existence of an association between the TPH gene and suicidal behavior, criticized these findings.

Different results were reported by Mann et al. (1997), who found a possible association of the U allele but not the L allele in 52 American Caucasian, nonimpulsive, major depressed inpatients with and without a history of suicide attempts.

Several years later, however, Nielsen et al. (1997, 1998) replicated their own results in another group of Finnish patients, using polymerase chain reaction-restriction fragment length polymorphism (PCR-RFLP) assays for, essentially, the same polymorphic system. They demonstrated that the SSCP polymorphism (U/L) that they had identified previously corresponded to two single nucleotide polymorphisms (SNPs), A218C and A779C in intron 7. The studies, using the PCR-RFLP method to detect what was originally described as an SSCP polymorphism, actually detected the two SNP polymorphisms, A218C and A779C (Nielsen et al., 1997). TPH 779A and 218A correspond to the U TPH allele and TPH 779C and 218C correspond to the L TPH allele (Nielsen et al., 1992). Paralleling their earlier findings, Nielsen et al. (1998) found that the TPH 779C allele was link-associated to suicidality. This study also used a sib-pair analysis (369 sib-pairs), which yielded a significant linkage to suicidal behavior and severe suicide attempts.

Several other groups have reported results that were either mixed or negative. Also using RFLP, a Swiss-French group (Bellivier et al., 1998) reported an association between the TPH gene and bipolar disorder in the intron 7 polymorphism, but no association between the A218C polymorphism and suicidal behavior. Later, they published a re-analysis of their data in an extension of the original sample, suggesting that the association they reported between bipolar affective disorder and the TPH gene A218C polymorphism was due to a subgroup of patients with a history of suicidal behavior. In their study, the A allele frequency was even higher in a subgroup of patients who had made a violent suicide attempt. Thereafter, the same group performed a case–control study of 236 suicide attempters matched with 161 controls, and found an association with the A allele of the A218C polymorphism (Buresi et al., 1997).

Furlong et al. (1998b) failed to link-associate the TPH gene with suicide in patients with affective disorder. Manuck et al. (1999) reported a significantly higher score for the TPH U allele on measures of aggression and anger – traits that are thought to be connected to suicidal behavior. Kunugi et al. (1999), in a Japanese population, reported no evidence of an association between the TPH A218C and A779C polymorphisms and suicidal behavior in 46 suicide attempters and 208 healthy controls. Abbar et al. (1995), in a case–control association study of a French population, compared 62 suicide attempters with 52 healthy controls. They noted no association between the TPH polymorphism and suicide attempts, but, since they studied a different polymorphism (an RFLP recognized by *Ava* II), their results cannot be compared directly to those of Nielsen, nor any of the other studies discussed here (Nielsen, 1996). Zalsman et al. (2001b) failed to demonstrate the association of the TPH polymorphism A218C to suicidality, aggression or impulsivity in a Jewish population. Nolan et al. (2000) found an association of the TPH "L" allele to violence in schizophrenic males.

## Neurochemical studies of serotonin and suicidality

Serotonergic neurotransmission is a complex mechanism involving pre- and post-synaptic events and distinct 5-HT receptor subtypes. Serotonin (5-HT) receptors have been classified into several categories: 5-HT1, 5-HT2, 5-HT3, 5-HT4,

5-HT5, 5-HT6, and 5-HT7 receptors. 5-HT1 receptors have A–F subtypes and 5-HT2 receptors have A–C subtypes. Of these, the 5-HT2A receptor has been the most widely studied with respect to suicide. Studies include platelet receptor studies, fenfluramine challenge and prolactin response, postmortem brain studies and CSF metabolites of serotonin.

Buchsbaum et al. (1976) reported finding a correlation between low platelet monoamine oxidase (MAO) activity in students and suicidal behavior in relatives. This may be related to the catabolism of serotonin. Suicide attempters have been shown to have lower responsiveness and sensitivity of their platelet 5-HT2 receptors than nonattempters (Mann et al., 1992; McBride et al., 1994). There appears to be a high correlation between the medical damage resulting from a suicide attempt and the number of 5-HT receptors; results with phosphoinositide hydrolysis mediated by the 5-HT2 receptor have indicated blunted signal transduction in high-lethality suicide attempters (Mann et al., 1992). Arora and Melzer (1993) showed similar results in schizophrenic suicide attempters. Pandey et al. (1995) also found a significant correlation between the number of platelet 5-HT2A receptors (B max) and suicidal behavior which was independent of psychiatric diagnosis, and suggested the potential usefulness of platelet 5-HT2A receptors as a biological marker for identifying suicide-prone patients. Reduced [$^{3}$H]imipramine binding and 5-HT uptake in platelets may be related to hypo-functioning presynaptic serotonergic mechanisms in suicidal behavior (Marazzati et al., 1995). Low platelet MAO activity may be a biological characteristic of patients who attempt suicide (Tripodianakis et al., 2000). Some authors have also found low levels of tryptophan and serotonin in suicidal individuals (Almeida-Montes et al., 2000; Spreux-Varoquax et al., 2001).

There are now an impressive number of studies relating a blunted prolactin response to fenfluramine challenge with suicidal behavior, especially the more lethal suicide attempts, regardless of psychiatric diagnosis (Correa et al., 2000; Malone et al., 1995, 1996; Mann et al., 1992). These findings may be especially marked in young depressed patients (Mann et al., 1995) and in patients with a personality disorder (New et al., 1997), although Correa et al. (2000) feel that this is a trait marker of suicidality that is unrelated to depression.

## Neuroimaging studies

Recently developed neuroimaging techniques, such as single-photon emission tomography (SPET) offer the unique possibility of studying in vivo the characteristics of the serotonin system in suicidal patients. Audenaert et al. (2001) found that deliberate self-harm patients had significantly reduced 5-HT2a receptor binding, especially when violent methods were used. For a review see Mann et al. (1996b).

## Postmortem binding studies

Postmortem investigations of the cerebral cortex of suicide victims have shown increased 5-HT1a receptor binding in the ventrolateral prefrontal cortex and increased binding of 5-HT2a receptors in the frontal cortex (Arango et al., 1995; Mann and Arango, 1992). Mann et al. (1996a) also reported lower [$^3$H]paroxetine binding in suicides, mainly due to the presence of significantly fewer high-affinity nontransporter sites. This finding was replicated by Pacheco et al. (1996) in the hippocampal area of schizophrenic suicide attempters. Teenage suicide victims also show evidence of 5-HT2A postreceptor dysregulation, which was indicated by altered protein kinase C binding (Pandey et al., 1997). To date, no association has been found between suicide and 5-HT3 receptors (Mann et al., 1996a), 5-HT1A receptors (Lowther et al., 1997) or 5-HIAA concentrations (Arranz et al., 1997). Recently, Mann et al. (2000) have found fewer serotonin transporter sites in the ventral prefrontal cortex of suicide victims.

## Cerebrospinal fluid studies

Low baseline and postprobenecid CSF 5-hydroxyindoleacetic acid (5-HIAA) is thought to be indicative of lowered 5-HT metabolism in the central nervous system (van Praag, 1986a). The finding of decreased levels of baseline and post-probenecid CSF 5-HIAA in most, but not all, studies of depressed individuals provides strong evidence that suggests disordered 5-HT metabolism in depressive disorder.

Further investigation of these CSF 5-HIAA findings led to the hypothesis that the 5-HT disturbance is not related to a particular subtype of depression, but rather to particular psychopathological dimensions that are often associated with depression. One dimension that was initially the focus of much attention was suicidality (van Praag, 1986a).

The risk of suicide attempts in depressed patients is not evenly distributed. Some depressed patients resort to suicide, but the majority does not, and there seems to be no direct relationship between degree of depression and degree of suicidality, suggesting potentially different biological markers for depression and suicidality. This is supported by the fact that, in a group of depressed patients with a lifetime history of at least one suicide attempt, the attempt frequency is skewed, with a minority of patients being responsible for the majority of attempts. Thus, a subgroup of depressed patients attempts suicide frequently, while the majority does so infrequently, or not at all. The group of depressed multiple suicide attempters also appears most likely to have decreased CSF 5-HIAA.

Decreased CSF 5-HIAA has been demonstrated in depressed patients after admission for a suicide attempt (Oreland et al., 1981; van Praag, 1982a,b). It has also been found in patients with a lifetime history of suicidal behavior (Agren, 1980), as well as in subjects with suicidal ideation (Agren, 1983). It should be noted, however, that one study has reported both increased and decreased CSF 5-HIAA levels in patients with suicidal ideation (Agren, 1983).

CSF 5-HIAA also appears to provide prospective information. Traskman et al. (1981) followed 46 inpatients admitted for a suicide attempt, 30 of whom had shown low CSF 5-HIAA levels at index admission. One year after discharge, six of these patients had committed suicide. All six individuals had shown lowered 5-HIAA levels. Commensurate with this, increased relapse rates were also reported in depressives with low levels of CSF 5-HIAA (Traskman et al., 1981). In 1989, Roy et al. also found that a low 5-HIAA level in CSF is a strong predictor of subsequent suicide or completed suicides in these patients – a finding replicated by Nordstrom et al. (1994).

Three negative studies have been published, all regarding samples containing a significant number of bipolar subjects. Two studies were of the same group of subjects and reported low CSF homovanillic acid (HVA) but normal CSF 5-HIAA in depressed patients with a history of suicide attempts (Roy et al., 1986). Moreover, 5-HIAA levels in the CSF were much lower than those reported by Asberg's group (van Praag, 1986a). In the third negative study (Vestergaard et al., 1978), a mixed group of unipolar, bipolar, and first-time depressives was studied and the criterion for suicidality was not reported. None of these studies examined the issue of violent versus nonviolent suicide.

Further evidence suggesting a correlation between low CSF 5-HIAA and suicidality, rather than between low CSF 5-HIAA and depression, comes from the fact that nondepressed suicide attempters have also been shown to have low CSF 5-HIAA. Patients with personality disorders (Brown et al., 1979, 1982a,b) who have attempted suicide show low CSF 5-HIAA, as do schizophrenics who were ordered to commit suicide by "voices" (Ninan et al., 1984). Similarly, Traskman et al. (1981) reported on a group of suicidal patients with anxiety disorders, all of whom had low CSF-5-HIAA. Oreland et al. (1981) confirmed these findings in suicidal patients with minor depressive illness, anxiety states, personality disorder, and drug or alcohol addiction. No negative studies have been reported in nondepressed suicide attempters. There also may be a relationship between low CSF 5-HIAA and greater medical lethality and/or planning of the suicide attempt (Mann and Malone, 1997; Mann et al., 1992).

## The serotonin (5-HT) system and aggression

In general, data from studies of the role of 5-HT in human aggression suggest that aggression and hostility are associated with a decreased level of 5-HT and its metabolite 5-HIAA. Brown et al. (1979) investigated 26 military men with personality disorders who were being evaluated for suitability for further service. CSF 5-HIAA showed a significant negative correlation with past history of aggressive behavior, while CSF 3-methoxy-4-hydroxy-phenylglycol (MHPG) showed a significant positive correlation with such behavior. In a second study, Brown et al. (1982a,b) demonstrated significant negative correlations between CSF 5-HIAA and aggression scores on the Minnesota Multiphasic Personality Inventory, as well as with a history of suicide attempts in 12 individuals diagnosed as having borderline personality disorder. These data support the concept of decreased 5-HT levels in aggression, and indicate the possibility of increased norepinepherine (NE) levels in these aggressive individuals.

Similarly, Lidberg et al. (1984) reported the case histories of three individuals who demonstrated aggression towards family members, eventually murdering a child. All three had low 5-HIAA levels. In 1985, Lidberg et al. compared 16 men who had committed homicide, with 22 men who had attempted suicide and 39 controls. CSF 5-HIAA levels were reduced in the suicidal men, especially in those who had used violent means, and in those who had killed a sexual partner (i.e., crimes of passion involving impulsivity and intense affect). Linnoila et al. (1983) found that impulsive murderers had lower CSF 5-HIAA levels than nonimpulsive murderers, and multiple murderers had lower CSF 5-HIAA levels than single murderers. Other monoamine metabolites were also decreased in these impulsive murderers, but not significantly. These studies also presented evidence that it may not be the aggressive behavior, *per se*, but rather a lack of impulse control that constitutes the behavioral correlate of deficient 5-HT metabolism. Bioulac et al. (1980) found that criminals with the 47,XYY syndrome showed a significant correlation between high aggression scores and decreased CSF 5-HIAA. Treatment with 5-HT led to clinical improvement. Decreased CSF 5-HIAA has also been demonstrated in mentally retarded individuals who exhibit aggression directed towards others and in patients with aggression who were not suicidal (Stanley et al., 2000).

Coccaro et al. (1989) found a prolactin response to fenfluramine challenge that was inversely related to impulsive aggressiveness, suggesting a net decrease in serotonergic functioning. These findings have been repeated in a sample of adolescent subjects (McCay et al., 1993).

O'Neil et al. (1986) reported a case study of a retarded man with Cornelia de Lange syndrome, intense aggressive behavior towards others, and low blood 5-HT levels, in whom treatment with trazodone and tryptophan resulted in an increase of blood 5-HT levels and a decrease of aggressive behavior. In 1995, Virkkunen et al. reviewed a series of studies supporting the idea that most impulsive offenders who have a tendency to behave aggressively while intoxicated have a low brain serotonin turnover rate. (The impulsive violent offenders with the lowest CSF 5-HIAA concentrations also had disturbed diurnal activity rhythms and were also prone to hypoglycemia after an oral glucose challenge.) Finally, in contrast to the above results, it should be noted that Pliszka (1987) reported that violent delinquent boys have higher whole – blood 5-HT levels than nonviolent offenders and depressed/anxious adolescents.

Animal studies have also provided a preponderance of evidence demonstrating that potentiation of 5-HT function decreases aggression in mice and muricidal rats, while decreasing 5-HT function increases aggression in mice (Sheard et al., 1976). This suggests the importance of serotonergic mechanisms in mediating aggression in these animal models (Valzelli, 1984). Similarly, Reissner et al. (1966) reported that reduced serotonergic function is associated with impaired impulse control and aggressive behavior in dogs. Similar findings have been shown in monkeys (Botchin et al., 1993; Kyes et al., 1995). Other animal studies have suggested that when a critical balance between the monoaminergic systems is disturbed, animals exhibit specific types of aggressive behavior (Valzelli, 1984).

## The serotonin system as a biological link between suicidality and aggression

Oquendo and Mann (2000) have recently reviewed this topic. Abnormalities of 5-HT and noradrenergic functioning have been implicated in aggressive impulsivity, self-injurious behavior and suicidal behavior. In 1996, van Praag proposed that, in a subset of cases of depression, the primary symptoms are in fact outwardly and inwardly directed aggression and anxiety. These symptoms appear to be related to a disturbance of the serotonin system.

In 1976, Asberg et al. reported on 44 patients with endogenous depression and 24 patients with reactive depression, demonstrating a high correlation between decreased CSF 5-HIAA, the primary metabolite of 5-HT, and a history of suicide attempts, particularly those that involved a violent component, during the index illness. This finding has been confirmed by a number of other researchers (Banki and Arato, 1983; Oreland et al., 1981; Traskman et al., 1981). Agren (1980) also reported that low CSF 5-HIAA correlated not only with suicidal ideation, but also with overt anger. He suggested that this might provide evidence in support of the hypothesis that depressives with low CSF 5-HIAA are more prone to violent suicidal acts than depressives without low CSF 5-HIAA.

Depressives with low CSF 5-HIAA appear to be not only more suicidal, but also more aggressive (van Praag, 1986b). Two groups of melancholic patients were compared on several aggression measures, as well as on CSF 5-HIAA levels. The depressives were divided into two groups, one with normal and the other with low postprobenecid CSF 5-HIAA levels. The latter group had made more suicide attempts and demonstrated higher hostility ratings on several measures than the former group.

Interestingly, van Praag (1983) and Ninan et al. (1984) have reported significantly lower concentrations of CSF 5-HIAA in suicidal schizophrenics, with a correlation between recent suicide attempts and lower 5-HIAA, thus suggesting that the psychopathological correlate of decreased CSF 5-HIAA might involve suicidality across psychiatric diagnoses. However, it should be noted that Roy et al. (1985) could not repeat these findings, nor could Pickar et al. (1986), although they did show a relationship between lower CSF 5-HIAA and higher drug-free hostility and uncooperativeness ratings in these schizophrenics. In addition, Brown et al. (1982b) reported that history of aggressive behavior, history of suicide attempts and low CSF 5-HIAA were all significantly positively correlated among patients with personality disorders. Rydin et al. (1982) showed that depressed and/or suicidal patients with low CSF 5-HIAA had higher hostility scores and a lower anxiety tolerance than their counterparts with normal CSF 5-HIAA values, as determined by Rorschach responses.

Low CSF 5-HIAA has been shown to be predictive of violent suicide attempts and completed suicide, suggesting that these measures represent trait, rather than state, measures (Traskman-Bendz and Asberg, 1986). It has also been found that low CSF 5-HIAA is related to higher lifetime lethality and more planning of suicide attempts in depressed attempters (Mann and Malone, 1997). Self-directed aggression, whether in the form of nonsuicidal self-mutilation or suicidal behavior, is a prominent feature of personality disorder. Such patients show blunted prolactin and cortisol responses to challenge with fenfluramine (New et al., 1997).

One interesting, clinical, aspect of the suicide/aggression hypo-serotonergic story is the fact that a small, still poorly defined, group of patients receiving fluoxetine and other selective serotonin re-uptake inhibitors (SSRIs) experience a spectrum of side-effects, ranging from restless extreme agitation to aggressive behavior with self-destructive impulses and behaviors. One plausible, but still unproven, mechanism for such adverse effects occurring early in treatment may be an acute decrease in serotonergic functioning as a result of the SSRI's marked effect on 5-HT neuronal firing rates (Anderson et al., 1995).

## Serotonin and the developmental psychopathology of suicidal behavior

Regardless of the etiology of suicidal behavior in young people, suicide attempts and suicide are extremely rare before puberty. Ryan et al. (1992) reported altered prolactin and cortisol responses to L-5-HTP in prepubertal, depressed children but did not find any correlation with either aggression or suicidality. Kruesi et al. (1990) examined correlates of low CSF 5-HIAA and did not find any correlation with aggression in preadolescent boys. However, on follow-up, when the boys were around 14 years of age, a strong correlation was noted (Kruesi et al., 1992). Brent (1997) suggested that aggression, particularly impulsive or reactive aggression, predates suicidal behavior, but that until the child enters puberty and becomes at risk for other pathological conditions, such as depression or substance abuse, the risk for suicidal behavior remains latent.

Fenfluramine challenge also yields different results at different ages. Thus, young aggressive boys have higher sensitivity to fenfluramine than young nonaggressive boys, however, this difference does not hold for older boys (Halperin et al., 1997).

## Catecholamines and suicidal behavior

To date, little work has been done in this area and the findings are not clearcut (see reviews by van Praag (1986c), Roy and Linnoila (1988), and Oquendo and Mann (2000)). Traskman et al. (1981) and Roy et al. (1986) found that CSF homovanillic acid (HVA), the primary metabolite of dopamine (DA), was lowered in depressed, but not in nondepressed, suicide attempters. Other investigators, however, were not able to confirm this finding (van Praag, 1986c).

Some investigators have also reported a relationship between suicidality and decreased CSF 3-methoxy-4-hydroxy-phenylglycol (MHPG), the major metabolite of CNS norepinephrine (NE), but this finding has not been confirmed by others either (van Praag, 1986c). Ostroff et al. (1982) found low NE/epinephrine ratios in the urine of three patients who eventually committed suicide. In addition, reduced platelet MAO activity has been found in alcoholic suicides (reviewed by van Praag, 1986c). A blunted growth hormone response after clonidine (an alpha-2-agonist) challenge has been found in depressed suicidal patients (Pichot et al., 1995).

In postmortem studies, an increased binding to alpha-1-adrenergic sites (Arango et al., 1993), and an increased number of alpha-1-adrenergic sites (de Parmentier et al., 1997) has been reported. Inconsistent findings regarding alterations in cortical beta-adrenergic receptor densities have been described (Little et al., 1995). In addition, a significant loss of pigmented locus coerulus (LC) neurones was found in the postmortem brains of suicides (Arango et al., 1996). Similarly, low brain inositol levels in suicide victims may also indicate dysfunction in catecholamine second messenger precursors (Shimon et al., 1997). Reduced levels of tyrosine hydroxylase, the rate-limiting enzyme in NE and DA synthesis, in the LC have been reported by some authors (Biegon and Fieldlust, 1992), but not by others (Ordway et al., 1994). Concentrations of the three monoamines (5-HT, NA, and DA) and their metabolites were simultaneously measured in the frontal cortex, gyrus cinguli, and hypothalamus of suicide victims and controls. No differences were found (Arranz et al., 1997). Finally, a tetranucleotide repeat polymorphism in the first intron of the tyrosine hydroxylase locus was found to be infrequent in suicide attempters in whom there was a diagnosis of adjustment disorder (Persson et al., 1997).

It has been hypothesized that suicidality may be more related to the ratio between CSF HVA and CSF 5-HIAA than to the concentration of CSF 5-HIAA itself (Roy and Linnoila, 1988). Therefore, in the future, the relationships between the 5-HT-ergic, the DAergic, and the NEergic systems may be a fruitful line for further inquiry.

Finally, there is evidence that abnormalities in the DA system are related to self-injurious behavior in patients with borderline personality disorder and depression (Oquendo and Mann, 2000).

## Cholesterol in suicidal and aggressive behavior

Several meta-analyses of clinical trials of cholesterol-lowering interventions found that although mortality from coronary heart disease was reduced by such interventions, an increase in mortality from suicide and violence occurred (Frick et al., 1987; Muldoon et al., 1990, 1991; Strandberg et al., 1991). However, the WHO Multiple Risk Factor Intervention Trial Research Group study (1990) failed to confirm this finding. Initial low cholesterol levels were reported to predict death by suicide or injury in follow-up studies performed after six years (Lindberg et al., 1992), after 25 years (Pekkanen et al., 1989), and in working men (Persson and Johanssen, 1984). These findings have been supported by Neaton et al. (1992) but not by Chen et al. (1991), Jacobs et al. (1992), Smith et al. (1992), and Vartainen et al. (1994).

Low serum cholesterol levels also appear to correlate with personality factors that have relevance to adolescent suicide, such as violent responses to alcohol (Virkkunen, 1983a), criminality and anti-social personality (Virkkunen, 1979), and to attention problems and conduct disorder (Virkkunen and Pentinnen, 1984). High serum cholesterol levels are associated with adherence to social norms, dependency, high morality, and self-criticism (Jenkins et al., 1969). Low cholesterol diets also may increase aggression and hostility in animals (Kaplan et al., 1991), although one study found that such a diet decreased aggression and depression in humans (Weidner et al., 1992).

Several studies of psychiatric patients found a relationship between low serum cholesterol and suicide in depressed patients (Modai et al., 1994; Sullivan et al., 1994), in males who had made serious suicide attempts (Gollier et al., 1995), and in children with adjustment disorder and depression (Glueck et al., 1994). The latter study found that children with these disorders showed more suicidal tendencies than child inpatients with other disorders.

In a study by Apter et al. (1997) of 152 adolescent inpatients, the correlation between serum cholesterol levels, suicidal behavior, and psychopathological traits and symptoms, such as aggression, impulsivity, depression, and anxiety, were examined. Compared to the nonsuicidal adolescents, the suicidal adolescents showed significantly **higher** levels of serum cholesterol. This difference was not accounted for by gender. In the suicidal group of adolescents, however, there was an **inverse** relationship between serum cholesterol levels and severity of suicidal behavior. There does not seem to be any relationship between the low serum cholesterol levels found in suicidal patients and indices of serotonin function (Sarchiapone et al., 2001).

## Gamma-aminobutyric acid/benzodiazepine system in aggressive and suicidal behavior

Animal studies have provided increasing evidence that the gamma-aminobutyric acid (GABA)/benzodiazepine system may function as a modulator of aggressive behavior. Increasing central GABAergic activity appears to decrease some types of aggressive behavior in rats and mice, while GABA antagonists appear to induce aggressive behavior (Simler et al., 1983; Skolnick et al., 1985). Aggressive mice may also have lower regional GABA concentrations than their nonaggressive counterparts (Simler et al., 1982).

In addition, Potegal et al. (1983) showed that intracranial administration of GABA-modulating agents produces differing effects upon muricide, depending upon the specific neuroanatomical region affected. They suggested that, since

GABA is an inhibitory neurotransmitter, GABAergic activation in a nuclear region excitatory to aggression will be inhibitory, while GABAergic activation in a nuclear region inhibitory to aggression will be disinhibitory, which seems to occur in some areas of the septum and the caudal ventral tegmental area.

Benzodiazepines, drugs which stimulate the GABA/benzodiazepine receptor and, therefore, increase central GABAergic function, have been shown to reduce aggressive behavior in humans and in a wide variety of animals. However, there is also evidence that chronic low dosage administration of these drugs can cause increased aggressive behavior in humans and animals.

The peripheral benzodiazepine receptor (PBR) is involved in cholesterol translocation from the outer mitochondrial membrane to the inner membrane and hormonal changes and steroidogenesis influence its activity. Acute stress produces up-regulation, while down-regulation occurs in chronic stress (Drugan et al., 1988), and in conditions such as posttraumatic stress disorder and general anxiety disorder (Weizman et al., 1995). Apter et al. (1997) examined the PBR in a group of adolescent inpatients. The PBR density in the suicidal patients was significantly lower than in the nonsuicidal group. In addition, there was a significant inverse correlation between the severity of the suicidal behavior (as measured by the Suicide Risk Scale) and PBR density. This finding probably reflects the influence of stress on suicidal behavior, but may also be related to the association between cholesterol and suicidal behavior described above.

## The catecholamine systems

A few animal models have been developed for studying the catecholamine system and aggression. Pucilowski et al. (1982) have reported that 6-hydroxydopamine-induced lesions of the ventral mesencephalic tegmental area produce decreased foot-shock-induced fighting but fail to influence muricidal behavior in rats.

While a variety of studies investigating the relationship between the catecholamine system and human aggressive behavior have been undertaken, results have often been contradictory (Valzelli, 1981). Woodman et al. (1978) reported on a group of prisoners with hyperactivity of the sympathetic system who excreted more NE and less epinephrine in their urine than did the control prisoners and patients. These individuals showed similar differences in plasma catecholamines. Interestingly, these prisoners had also committed the most violent set of crimes compared to the control group of prisoners. Brown et al. (1979) found a significant positive correlation between CSF MHPG and aggressive behavior in military men, while Sandler et al. (1978) reported that prisoners with histories of violent crimes had higher levels of urinary phenylacetic acid than prisoners with histories of nonviolent crimes. In 1983, Davis et al. repeated this result.

Beta-adrenergic antagonists, such as propranolol, have been utilized to some effect in a subset of individuals (generally with some type of organic brain injury or mental retardation) who exhibit ongoing aggressive behaviors.

Data are sparse regarding the role of the catecholamine system in the link between aggression and suicidality. Brown et al. (1979) reported increased levels of MHPG in patients with personality disorders and life histories of aggressive and suicidal behavior, suggesting the involvement of the NE system in aggression regulation. However, this finding has not been replicated.

Ostroff et al. (1982) studied the 24-hour urinary norepinephrine/epinephrine (NE/E) ratio in psychiatric patients and reported interesting data on the peripheral NE system and aggression. Their work was based on an expanded model proposed by Woodman et al. (1978) indicating differences in psychophysiological responses (e.g., galvanic skin response) in subjects who reported anger against others, in contrast to subjects who reported anger against themselves during stressful situations. They hypothesized that "anger out" was associated with NE-like substances and "anger in" was associated with epinephrine-like substances. Three patients who made violent suicide attempts were shown to have a significantly lower NE/E ratio than other patients, thus appearing to confirm this hypothesis. Studies with prison inmates, however, have shown a positive correlation between low NE/E ratios and assaultiveness (Woodman et al., 1978).

## Hormones

Persky et al. (1971) demonstrated a high correlation between the production of testosterone and measures of aggression in young human male volunteers, with a significant positive correlation between age and testosterone production, but no correlation with aggression measures in male volunteers over 30 years of age. Scaramella and Brown (1978) found a trend toward positive correlations between plasma testosterone and aggressive behavior in male hockey players, with significant correlations in only one out of seven aggressiveness items.

Matthews (1979) found no difference in testosterone levels between male prisoners who had committed violent crimes and those who had committed nonviolent crimes. It is interesting to note that Virkkunen (1983b) reported on enhanced insulin secretion during a glucose tolerance test in boys and young men with antisocial personality disorder and unsocialized aggressive conduct disorder, while Virkkunen and Pentinnen (1984) also demonstrated low serum cholesterol levels correlated with violent behavior in boys and young men with antisocial personality disorder and aggressive conduct disorder.

In animals, castration reduces fighting behavior, as does the administration of anti-androgenic substances or estrogens. Irritative aggression has been shown to be androgen-dependent, so that male rats respond more aggressively to foot-shock than do female rats. Castration causes a decrease in this behavior, while exogenous testosterone reverses the effect of castration. There is accumulating evidence that competitive aggression may also be associated with the metabolism of androgens. This is based on the greater prostate and preputial gland weights of dominant mice, compared to subordinate mice and higher blood titers of testosterone in dominant, compared to submissive, macaque monkeys. In addition, both maternal protective aggression and sex-related aggression have clearly been shown to be hormonally controlled (Valzelli, 1981).

Searcy and Wingfield (1980) reported that androgen levels are positively correlated with the level of social dominance in male red-winged blackbirds due to influences on aggression, while there are similar findings for rats and vervet monkeys.

Attempts have also been made to link hormones to autoaggression, primarily focusing on cortisol secretion and the dexamethasone suppression test, although the data from such studies have been unconvincing (van Praag, 1986a,b,c). Other studies found that a blunted TSH response to TRH may characterize violent suicide attempters (Linkowski et al., 1983, 1984; van Praag, 1986a,b,c). Testosterone levels have been examined in correlation with outwardly directed aggression in animal and human studies (see above).

## Hormones and suicide

The influence of hormonal factors on suicidal behavior has not been well studied (see reviews by van Praag (1986c) and by Roy and Linnoila (1988)). A number of investigators have reported a positive correlation between urinary 17-hydroxycorticosteroid measures and suicide, but others have not found any such correlation (reviewed by van Praag (1986c) and by Roy and Linnoila (1988)). Dysregulation of the hypothalamic-pituitary-adrenal axis (HPA) has also been studied. Traskman-Bendz et al. (1984) reported that depressed patients with hypercortisolemia were more likely to show suicidal behavior than depressed patients with normal cortisol levels. When compared to patients with a history of violent suicide attempts, patients with such a history were characterized by higher urinary cortisol levels and reduced MHPG plasma levels (van Heeringen et al., 2000).

The hypothalamic-pituitary-thyroid axis (HPT) has also been the focus of study. Roy et al. (1987) reported blunted thyroid stimulating hormone (TSH) responses to thyroid releasing hormone (TRH) stimulation among depressed suicide attempters, although this finding may relate more to aggression than to suicide itself. This area of research is promising, as there may be a relationship between 5-HT metabolism and HPT function (Roy and Linnoila, 1988).

## Carbohydrate (CHO) metabolism

There has been a great deal of interest in the relationship between carbohydrate (CHO) metabolism, 5-HT systems and aggression. Some of this interest stems from the work of Yamamoto et al. (1985), who have shown that lesions of the suprachiasmatic nucleus produce rats that are vulnerable to mild hypoglycemia. These rats show hyperinsulinemic and hypoglucagonemic responses to glucose and desoxyglucose challenges, respectively. The suprachiasmatic nucleus is thought to play a role in feeding and satiety, as well as in control of the circadian regulation of glucose metabolism. The suprachiasmatic nucleus receives 5-HT input from the brainstem raphe nuclei and, thus, there may be an anatomical, as well as a functional, linkage between glucose metabolism and the 5-HT system.

Clinical evidence for such a relationship comes from a case report of a 13-year-old girl whose antisocial behavior comprised largely of stealing sweets. She also had a low level of CSF 5-HIAA (Kruesi et al., 1985).

Virkkunen (1983b) showed that violent offenders often become hypoglycemic and hyperinsulinemic after an oral glucose load. Patients with explosive personality disorder show more rapid onset and recovery of the hypoglycemia than did patients with antisocial personality disorder. Virkkunen (1983b) also showed a relationship between hypoglycemic and hyperinsulinemic responses and a lifetime history of aggressive, violent, and antisocial behaviors. Moreover, they are also more likely to have fathers with histories of antisocial and criminal behaviors.

Virkkunen (1983b) also found that 11 out of 20 arsonists became hypoglycemic in the oral glucose tolerance test (OGTT). These individuals also had low CSF 5-HIAA, but the correlation between these two measures was not significant. In a larger sample of 57 arsonists, Virkkunen found mild hypoglycemia during the OGTT.

## The electroencephalogram

Altered electroencephalographic (EEG) activity has been associated with various psychiatric disorders and behaviors, including depression, suicide, and aggression. Graae et al. (1996) examined quantitative resting EEG activity in adolescent female suicide attempters. Normal adolescents had greater alpha (less activation) over the right than left hemisphere, whereas suicidal adolescents had significant asymmetry in the opposite direction. Alpha asymmetry over the posterior regions was related to ratings of suicidal intent. Thus, reduced posterior activation may be related to suicidal and/or aggressive behavior.

## Conclusion

The development of operational criteria for nosological diagnosis (i.e., the DSM and ICD systems) have enabled biological researchers to focus on more clearly defined disorders in their search for biological markers. Nonetheless, it has become increasingly apparent that there are some basic psychopathological dimensions which cut across nosological boundaries and which appear to be related to specific biological mechanisms. As can be seen from the above review, aggression dysregulation, encompassing both autoaggression (such as suicide) and outwardly directed aggression, is one such dimension that deserves further study.

Both in animals and humans, the biological marker that correlates most strongly with aggression dysregulation seems to be low CSF 5-HIAA (van Praag, 1986a; Valzelli, 1985). However, to date, most studies in this area have not controlled for other psychometric variables, such as anxiety / distress and impulsivity, which may also be related to 5-HT dysregulation, and which very often accompany aggression dysregulation. The interrelationships between these 5-HT-related psychometric variables and their correlation with different measures of 5-HT metabolism would appear to be important areas for further research.

While little research to date has been done on the role of other catecholamines, such as DA and NE, in aggression regulation, they may also be involved, either by themselves or more likely in combination with 5-HT and other neurotransmitters (such as GABA) that have not been widely studied with respect to suicide and human aggression. Brown et al. (1982b) have strongly advocated further research into such combined neurotransmitter systems.

Finally, while hormonal studies of autoaggression have not been conclusive and have not controlled for related psychopathological dimensions, such as anxiety / distress and impulsivity, early data are quite intriguing and a number of leads remain to be followed-up. The HPA and HPT axes have yet to be studied in outwardly directed aggression. Testosterone and the hypothalamic-pituitary-gonadal axis (HPG) have not yet been examined in suicide. Similarly, glucose and fat metabolism seem to have become promising areas regarding violence research but not, as yet, with respect to suicide, and this may prove to be another important avenue of study.

## REFERENCES

Abbar, M., Courted, P., Amadeo, S., Caer, Y., Mallet, J., Baldy-Moulinier, M., Castlenau D., and Malefosse, A. (1995). Suicidal behaviors and the tryptophan hydroxylase gene. *Archives of General Psychiatry*, **52**, 846–849.

Agren, H. (1980). Symptom patterns in unipolar and bipolar depression correlating with monoamine metabolites in the cerebrospinal fluid: l. General patterns. *Psychological Research*, **3**, 211–223.

Agren, H. (1983). Life at risk: markers of suicidality in depression. *Psychiatry Development*, **1**(1), 87–103.

Almeida-Montes, L. G., Valles-Sanchez, V., Moreno-Aguilar, J., Chavez-Balderas, R. A., Garcia-Marin, J. A., Cortes-Sotres, J. F., and Heinze-Martin, G. (2000). Relation of serum cholesterol, lipid, serotonin and tryptophan levels to severity of depression and to suicide attempts. *Journal of Psychiatry and Neuroscience*, **25**(4), 371–377.

Anderson, G. M., Segman, R. H., and King, R. A. (1995). Serotonin and suicidality: II. Acute neurobiological effects. *Israel Journal of Psychiatry and Related Science*, **32**(1), 44–50.

Apter, H. M., van Praag, S., Sevy, M., Korn, M., and Brown, S. (1990). Interrelationships among anxiety, aggression, impulsiveness and mood: a serotonergically linked cluster? *Psychological Research*, **32**, 191–199.

Apter, A., Kotler, M., Sevy, S., Plutchik, R., Brown, S., Foster, H., Hillbrand, M., Korn, M., and van Praag, H. (1991). Correlates of risk of suicide in violent and nonviolent psychiatric patients. *American Journal of Psychiatry*, **148**(7), 883–887.

Apter, A., Plutchik, R., and van Praag, H. M. (1993). Anxiety, impulsivity and depressed mood in relation to suicide and violent behavior. *Acta Psychiatrica Scandinavica*, **87**(1), 1–5.

Apter, A., Gothelf, D., Orbach, I., Har-Even, D., Weizman, R., and Tyano, S. (1995). Correlation of suicidal and violent behavior in different diagnostic categories in hospitalized adolescent patients. *Journal of the American Academy of Child and Adolescent Psychiatry*, **34**(7), 912–918.

Apter, A., Soreni, N., Don-Tufeled, O., Weizman, A., Karp, L., and Gavish, M. (1997). Decreased peripheral-type benzodiazepine receptor in suicidal adolescent in-patients. Paper presented at the WPA Regional Conference, Jerusalem. World Psychiatric Association, June 1997.

Arango, V., Ernsberger, P., Sved, A. F., and Mann, J. J. (1993). Quantitative autoradiography of alpha 1 and alpha 2-adrenergic receptors in the cerebral cortex of controls and suicide victims. *Brain Research*, **630**(1–2), 271–282.

Arango, V., Underwood, M. D., Gubbi, A. V., and Mann, J. J. (1995). Localized alterations in pre- and postsynaptic serotonin binding sites in the ventrolateral prefrontal cortex of suicide victims. *Brain Research*, **688**(1–2), 121–133.

Arango, V., Underwood, M. D., Pauler, D. K., Kass, R. E., and Mann, J. J. (1996). Differential age related loss of pigmented locus coerelus neurones in suicides, alcoholics and alcoholic suicides. *Alcoholism, Clinical and Experimental Research*, **20**(7), 1141–1147.

Arora, R. C., and Melzer, H. Y. (1993). Serotonin 2 receptor binding in blood platelets of schizophrenic patients. *Psychological Research*, **47**(2), 111–119.

Arranz, B., Blennow, K., Eriksson, A., Mansson, J. E., and Marcusson, J. (1997). Serotonergic, noradrenergic and dopaminergic measures in suicide brains. *Biological Psychiatry*, **41**(10), 1000–1009.

Asberg, M., Traskman, L., and Thoren, P. (1976). 5-HIAA in the cerebrospinal fluid: a biochemical suicide predictor? *Archives of General Psychiatry*, **33**, 1193–1197.

Audenaert, K., Van-Laere, K., Dumont, F., Slegers, G., Mertens, J., van-Heeringen, C., and Dierckx, R. A. (2001). Decreased frontal serotonin 5-HT2a receptor binding index in deliberate self-harm patients. *European Journal of Nuclear Medicine*, **28**(2), 175–182.

Banki, C. M., and Arato, M. (1983). Amine metabolites, neuroendocrine findings and personality dimensions as correlates of suicidal behavior. *Psychological Research*, **10**, 253–261.

Bellivier, F., Leboyer, M., Courtet, P., Buresi, C., Beaufils, B., Samolyk, D., and Allilaire, J. F. (1998). Association between the tryptophan hydroxylase gene and manic-depressive illness. *Archives of General Psychiatry*, **55**, 33–37.

Biegon, A., and Fieldlust, S. (1992). Reduced tyrosine hydroxylase immunoreactivity in the locus coeruleus of suicide victims. *Synapse*, **10**, 79–82.

Bioulac, B., Benezech, M., Renaud, B., Noel, B., and Roche, D. (1980). Serotonergic functions in the 47, XYY syndrome. *Biological Psychiatry*, **15**, 917–923.

Bondy, B., Erfuth, A., Jonge, S., Krüger, M., and Meyer, H. (2000). Possible association of the short allele of the serotonin transporter promoter gene polymorphism (5-HTTLPR) with violent suicide. *Molecular Psychiatry*, **5**, 193–195.

Botchin, M. B., Kaplan, J. R., Manuck, S. B., and Mann, J. J. (1993). Low versus high prolactin responders to fenfluramine challenge: marker of behavioral differences in adult cynomolgus macaques. *Neuropsychopharmacology*, **9**(2), 93–99.

Brent, D. A. (1989). The psychological autopsy: methodological considerations for the study of adolescent suicide and life threatening behavior. *Suicide and Life-Threatening Behavior*, **19**, 43–47.

Brent, D. A. (1997). Genetics of suicide [unpublished lecture]. WHO suicide meeting, Bern, Switzerland.

Brent, D. A., Perper, J. A., Moritz, G., Allma, C., Friend, A., Roth, D., Schweers, J., Balach, L., and Baugher, M. (1993). Psychiatric risk factors for adolescent suicide: a case control study. *Journal of the American Academy of Child and Adolescent Psychiatry*, **32**, 521–529.

Brent, D. A., Perper, J. A., Moritz, G., Allma, C., Friend, A., Roth, D., Schweers, J., Balach, L., and Baugher, M. (1994). Psychiatric risk factors for adolescent suicide: a case control study. *Acta Psychiatrica Scandinavica*, **89**, 52–58.

Brown, G. L., Goodwin, F. K., Ballenger, J. C., Goyer, P. F., and Major, L. F. (1979). Aggression in humans correlates with cerebrospinal fluid amine metabolites. *Psychiatry Research*, **1**, 131–139.

Brown, G. L., Ebert, M. H., Goyer, P. F., Jimerson, D. C., Klein, W. J., Bunney, W. E., and Goodwin, F. K. (1982a). Aggression, suicide and serotonin: relationships to CSF amine metabolites. *American Journal of Psychiatry*, **139**, 741–746.

Brown, G. I., Goodwin, F. K., and Bunney, W. E. Jr. (1982b). Human aggression and suicide: their relationship to neuropsychiatric diagnoses and serotonin metabolism. *Advances in Biochemistry and Psychopharmacology*, **34**, 287–307.

Buchsbaum, M. S., Coursey, R. D., and Murphy, D. L. (1976). The biochemical high risk paradigm: behavioral and familial correlates of low platelet monoamine oxidase activity. *Science*, **194**, 339–341.

Buresi, C., Courtet, P., Leboyer, M., Feingold, J., and Malafosse, A. (1997). Association between suicide attempt and the tryptophan hydroxylase gene. *American Journal of Human Genetics*, **61** (Suppl), 270.

Chen, Z., Petto, R., Collins, R., McMahon, S., Lu, J., and Li, W. (1991). Serum cholesterol concentration and coronary heart disease in population with low cholesterol concentrations. *British Medical Journal*, **303**, 276–282.

Coccaro, E. F. (1989). Central serotonin and impulsive aggression. *British Journal of Psychiatry*, **155** (Suppl), 52–62.

Coccaro, E. F., Silverman, J. M., Klar, H. M., Horvath, T. B., and Siever, L. J. (1994). Familial correlates of reduced central serotonergic system function in patients with personality disorders. *Archives of General Psychiatry*, **51**(4), 318–324.

Coccaro, E. F., Siever, L., Howard, M., Klar, H., Maurer, G., Cochrane, K., Cooper, T., Mohs, R. C., and Davis, K. (1989). Serotonergic studies in patients with affective and personality disorders. *Archives of General Psychiatry*, **46**, 587–599.

Cook, E. H., Lindgren, V., Leventhal, B. L., Courchesne, R., Lincoln, A., Shulman, C., and Courchesne, C. (1997). Autism or atypical autism in maternally but not paternally derived proximal 15q duplication. *American Journal of Human Genetics*, **60**, 928–934.

Correa, H., Duval, F., Mokrani, M., Bailey, P., Tremeau, F., Staner, L., Diep, T. S., Hode, Y., Crocq, M. A., and Macher, J. P. (2000). Prolactin response to D-fenfluramine and suicidal behavior in depressed patients. *Psychiatry Research*, **93**(3), 189–199.

Davis, B. A., Yu, P. H., Boulton, A. A., Wormith, J. S., and Addington, D. (1983). Correlative relationship between biochemical activity and aggressive behaviour. *Progress in Neuropsychopharmacology and Biological Psychiatry*, **7**(4–6), 529–535.

de Parmentier, F., Mauger, J. M., Lowther, S., Crompton, M. R., Katona, C. L., and Horton, R. W. (1997). Brain alpha adreno receptors in depressed suicide. *Brain Research*, **757**(1), 60–68.

Di Bella, D., Catalano, M., Balling, U., Smeraldi, E., and Lesch, K. P. (1996). Systematic screening for mutations in the coding region of the human serotonin transporter (5-HTT) gene using PCR and DGGE. *American Journal of Medical Genetics*, **67**, 541–545.

Drugan, R. C., Basile, A. S., Crawly, J. N., Paul, S. M., and Skolnick, P. (1988). Characterization of stress-induced alteration in $^3$H Ro 5-4864 binding to peripheral benzodiazepine receptors in rat heart and kidney. *Pharmacology, Biochemistry and Behavior*, **30**, 1015–1020.

Du, L., Faludi, G., Palkovitz, M., Demeter, E., Bakish Dlapierre, Y. D., Lapierre, Y. D., Sotonyi, P., and Hrdina, P. D. (1999). Frequency of long allele in serotonin transporter gene is increased in depressed suicide victims. *Biological Psychiatry*, **46**, 196–201.

Frick, M. H., Elo, O., and Haapa, K. (1987). Helsinki heart study primary prevention trial with gernfibrozil in middle aged men with dyslipedemia. *New England Journal of Medicine*, **317**, 1237–1245.

Furlong, R. A., Ho, L., Walsh, C., Rubinsztein, J. S., Jain, S., Paykel, E. S., and Rubinsztein, D. C. (1998a). Analysis and meta-analysis of two serotonin transporter gene polymorphisms in bipolar and unipolar affective disorders. *American Journal of Medical Genetics*, **81**, 58–63.

Furlong, R. A., Ho, L., Rubinsztein, J. S., Walsh, C., Paykel, E. S., and Rubinsztein, D. C. (1998b). No association of the tryptophan hydroxylase gene with bipolar affective disorder, unipolar affective disorder, or suicidal behavior in major affective disorder. *American Journal of Medical Genetics*, **81**, 245–247.

Garrison, C. Z., Jackson, K. L., Addy, C. L., McKeowan, R. E., and Waller, M. L. (1991). Suicidal behaviors in young adolescents. *American Journal of Epidemiology*, **133**, 1005–1014.

Geijer, T., Frisch, A., Persson, M. L., Wasserman, D., Rockah, R., Michaelovsky, E., Apter, A., Jonsson, E., Nothen, M. M., and Weizman, A. (2000). Search for association between suicide attempt and serotonergic polymorphisms. *Psychiatry and Genetics*, **10**, 19–26.

Gelernter, J., Pakstis, A. J., and Kidd, K. K. (1997). Linkage mapping of serotonin transporter protein gene SLC6A4 on chromosome 17. *Human Genetics*, **95**, 677–680.

Glueck, C. J., Kutler, F. E., Hammer, T., Rodriguez, R., Sosa, F., Sieve-Smith, L., and Morrison, J. A. (1994). Hypocholesterolemia, hyperglyceridemia, suicide and suicide ideation in children hospitalized for psychiatric diseases. *Pediatric Research*, **35**, 602–610.

Gollier, J. A., Marzuk, P. M., Leon, A. C., Weiner, C., and Tardiff, K. (1995). Low serum cholesterol levels and attempted suicide. *American Journal of Psychiatry*, **152**, 419–423.

Gould, M. S., Shaffer, D., and Fisher, P. (1992). The clinical prediction of adolescent suicide. In Maris, R. W. (ed.) *Assessment and Prediction of Suicide*. New York, NY: Guilford Publications.

Graae, F., Tenke, C., Bruder, G., Rotheram, M. J., Piacentini, J., Castro-Blanco, D., Leite, P., and Towey, J. (1996). Abnormality of EEG alpha asymmetry in female adolescent suicide attempters. *Biological Psychiatry*, **40**(8), 706–713.

Hallikainen, T., Saito, T., Lachman, H. M., Volavka, J., Pohjalainen, T., Ryynanen, O. P., Kauhanen, J., Syvalahti, E., Hietala, J., and Tiihonen, J. (1999). Association between low activity serotonin transporter genotype and early onset alcoholism with habitual impulsive violent behavior. *Molecular Psychiatry*, **4**, 385–388.

Halperin, J. M., Newcorn, J. H., Schwarz, S. T., Sharma, V., Siever, L. J., Koda, V. H., and Gabriel, S. (1997). Age related changes in the association between serotonergic function and aggression in boys with ADHD. *Biological Psychiatry*, **41**(6), 682–689.

Heilis, A., Teufel, A., Petri, S., Stober, G., Riederer, P., Bengel, D., and Lesch, K. P. (1996). Allelic variation of human serotonin transporter gene expression. *Journal of Neurochemistry*, **66**, 2621–2624.

Heilis, A., Mossner, R., and Lesch, K. P. (1997). The human serotonin transporter gene polymorphism – basic research and clinical implications. *Journal of Neural Transmission*, **104**, 1005–1014.

Jacobs, D., Blackburn, H., Higgins, M., Reed, D., Iso, H., McMillan, G., Neaton, J., Nelson, J., Potter, J., Rivkind, B., Rossuow, J., Shekelle, R., and Yousuf, S. (1992). Report of the conference on low blood cholesterol mortality associations. *Circulation*, **86**, 1046–1060.

Jenkins, C. D., Holmes, C. J., Zizanski, S. G., Rosenman, R. H., and Friedman, M. (1969). Psychological traits and serum lipids I. Findings from the California Psychological Inventory. *Psychosomatic Medicine*, **31**, 115–128.

Kaplan, J., Manuck, S., and Shively, C. (1991). The effect of fat and cholesterol on social behavior in monkeys. *Psychosomatic Medicine*, **53**, 634–642.

Kruesi, M. J., Linnoila, M., Rapoport, J. L., Brown, G. L., and Petersen, R. (1985). Carbohydrate craving, conduct disorder, and low 5HIAA. *Psychiatry Research*, **16**(1), 83–86.

Kruesi, M. J. P., Rapoport, J. L., Hamburger, S., Hibbs, E., Potter, W. Z., Lenane, M., and Brown, G. L., (1990). Cerebrospinal fluid monoamine metabolites, aggression and impulsivity in disruptive behavior disorders of children and adolescents. *Archives of General Psychiatry*, **47**, 419–426.

Kruesi, M. J. P., Hibbs, E. D., Zahn, T. P., Keysor, C. S., Hanburger, S. D., Bartko, J. J., and Rapoport, J. L. (1992). A 2-year prospective follow up of children and adolescents with disruptive behavior disorders. Prediction by CSF 5-HIAA, HVA and autonomic measures? *Archives of General Psychiatry*, **49**, 429–435.

Kunugi, H., Ishida, S., Kato, T., Tatsumi, M., Hirose, T., and Nank, S. (1999). No evidence for association of polymorphisms of the tryptophan hydroxylase gene with affective disorders or attempted suicide among Japanese patients. *American Journal of Psychiatry*, **156**, 774–776.

Kyes, R. C., Botchin, M. B., Kaplan, J. R., Manuck, S. B., and Mann, J. J. (1995). Aggression and brain serotonergic responsivity: response to slides in male macaques. *Physiology and Behavior*, **57**(2), 205–208.

Lesch, K. P., and Mossner, R. (1998). Genetically driven variation in serotonin uptake: is there a link to affective spectrum, neurodevelopmental and neurodegenerative disorders? *Biological Psychiatry*, **44**, 179–192.

Lesch, K. P., Wolozin, B. L., Estler, H. C., Murphy, D. L., and Riederer, P. (1993). Isolation of a cDNA encoding the human brain serotonin transporter. *Journal of Neural Transmission* [Gen Sect], **91**, 67–72.

Lesch, K. P., Balling, U., Gross, J., Strauss, K., Wolozin, B. L., Murphy, D. L., and Riederes, P. (1994). Organization of the human serotonin transporter gene. *Journal of Neural Transmission* [Gen Sect], **95**, 157–162.

Lesch, K. P., Gross, J., Franzek, E., Wolozin, B. L., Riederer, P., and Murphy, D. L. (1995). Primary structure of the serotonin transporter in unipolar depression and bipolar disorder. *Biological Psychiatry*, **37**, 215–223.

Li, T., Xu, K., Deng, H., Cai, G., Liu, G., Liu, X., Wang, R., Xiang, X., Zhao, J., Murray, R. M., Sham, P. C., and Collier, D. A. (1997). Association analysis of the dopamine D4 gene exon III VNTR and heroin abuse in Chinese subjects. *Molecular Psychiatry*, **2**, 413–416.

Lidberg, L., Asberg, M., and Sundquist-Stensman, U. B. (1984). 5-Hydroxyindoleacetic acid in attempted suicides who have killed their children. *Lancet*, **ii**, 928.

Lidberg, L., Tuck, J. R., Asberg, M., Scalia-Tomba, G. P., and Bertilsson, L. (1985). Homicide, suicide and CSF 5-HIAA. *Acta Psychiatrica Scandinavica*, **71**, 230–236.

Lindberg, G., Rastam, L., Gullberg, G., and Ecklund, G. A. (1992). Low serum cholesterol concentration and short time mortality from injuries in men and women. *British Medical Journal*, **305**, 277–297.

Linkowski, P., Van Wettere, J. P., Kerkhofs, M., Brauman, H., and Mendlewicz, J. (1983). Thyrotrophin response to thyreostimulin in affectively ill women relationship to suicidal behaviour. *British Journal of Psychiatry*, **143**, 401–405.

Linkowski, P., Van Wettere, J. P., Kerkhofs, M., Gregoire, F., Brauman, H., and Mendlewicz, J. (1984). Violent suicidal behavior and the thyrotropin-releasing hormone-thyroid-stimulating hormone test: a clinical outcome study. *Neuropsychobiology*, **12**(1), 19–22.

Linnoila, M., Virkkunen, M., Scheinin, M., Nuutila, A., Rimon, R., and Goodwin, F. K. (1983). Low cerebrospinal fluid 5-hydroxyindoleacetic acid concentration differentiates impulsive from non-impulsive violent behavior. *Life Science*, **33**, 2609–2614.

Little, K. Y., Clark, T. B., Ranc, J., and Duncan, G. E. (1995). Beta-adrenergic receptor binding in frontal cortex from suicide victims. *Biological Psychiatry*, **34**, 596–605.

Lowther, S., De Paermentier, F., Cheetham, S. C., Crompton, M. R., Katona, C. L., and Horton, R. W. (1997). 5-HT1A receptor binding sites in post mortem brain samples from depressed suicides and controls. *Journal of Affective Disorders*, **42**(2–3), 199–207.

Malone, K. M., Haas, J. M., Sweeney, J., and Mann, J. J. (1995). Major depression and the risk of attempted suicide. *Journal of Affective Disorders*, **34**, 173–175.

Malone, K. M., Corbitt, E. M., Li, S., and Mann, J. J. (1996). Prolactin response and suicide attempt lethality in major depression. *British Journal of Psychiatry*, **168**(3), 324–329.

Mann, J. J., and Arango, V. (1992). Integration of neurobiology and psychopathology in a unified model of suicidal behavior. *Journal of Clinical Psychopharmacology*, **12**, 2–7.

Mann, J. J., and Malone, K. M. (1997). Cerebrospinal fluid amines and higher – lethality suicide attempts in depressed inpatients. *Biological Psychiatry*, **41**(2), 162–171.

Mann, J. J., McBride, P. A., Brown, R. P., Linnoila, M., Leon, A., De Meo, M., Mieczkowski, T., Myers, J., and Stanley, M. (1992). Relationship between central and peripheral serotonin indexes in depressed and suicidal psychiatric inpatients. *Archives of General Psychiatry*, **49**, 442–446.

Mann, J. J., McBride, P. A., Malone, K. M., and DeMeo, M. (1995). Blunted serotonergic responsivity in depressed inpatients. *Neuropsychopharmacology*, **13**, 53–64.

Mann, J. J., Henteleff, R. A., Lagattuta, T. F., Perper, J. A., Li, S., and Arango, V. (1996a). Lower [3]H-paroxetine binding in cerebral cortex of suicide victims is partly due to fewer high affinity, non-transporter sites. *Journal of Neural Transmission*, **103**(11), 1337–1350.

Mann, J. J., Malone, K. M., Psych, M. R., Sweeney, J. A., Brown, R. P., Linnoila, M., Stanley, B., and Stanley, M. (1996b). Attempted suicide characteristics and cerebrospinal fluid amine metabolites in depressed patients. *Neuropsychopharmacology*, **16**(6), 576–586.

Mann, J. J., Malone, K. M., Nielsen, D. A., Goldman, D., Erdos, J., and Gelernter, J. (1997). Possible association of a polymorphism of the tryptophan hydroxylase gene with suicidal behavior in depressed patients. *American Journal of Psychiatry*, **154**, 1451–1453.

Mann, J. J., Oquendo, M., Underwood, M. D., and Arango, V. (1999). The neurobiology of suicide risk: a review for the clinician. *Journal of Clinical Psychiatry*, **60** (Suppl 27–11), 113–116.

Mann, J. J., Huang, Y. Y., Underwood, M. D., Kassir, S. A., Oppenheim, S., Kelly, T. M., Dwork, A. J., and Arango, V. (2000). A serotonin transporter gene promoter polymorphism (5-HHTTLPR) and prefrontal cortical binding in major depression and suicide. *Archives of General Psychiatry*, **57**(8), 729–738.

Manuck, S. B., Flory, J. D., Ferrell, R. E., Dent, K. M., Mann, J. J., and Muldoon, M. F. (1999). Aggression and anger-related traits associated with a polymorphism of the tryptophan hydroxylase gene. *Biological Psychiatry*, **45**, 603–614.

Marazzati, D., Presta, S., Silvestri, S., Battistini, A., Mosti, L., Balestri, C., Palego, L., and Conti, L. (1995). Platelet markers in suicide attempters. *Progress in Neuro-Psychopharmacology and Biological Psychiatry*, **19**(3), 375–383.

McBride, P. A., Brown, R. P., DeMeo, M., Keilip, J., Mieczowski, T., and Mann, J. J. (1994). The relationship of platelet 5 HT2 receptor indices to major depressive disorder, personality traits and suicidal behavior. *Biological Psychiatry*, **35**(5), 295–308.

McCay, K., Halperin, R., Grayson, S., Hall, N., and Newcorn, J. H. (1993). The children's aggression scale. Parent and teacher version. Scientific Proceedings of the Annual Meeting of the American Academy of Child and Adolescent Psychiatry 9 [abstract].

Modai, I., Walevski, A., Dror, S., and Weizman, A. (1994). Serum cholesterol levels and suicidal tendencies in psychiatric inpatients. *Journal of Clinical Psychiatry*, **55**, 252–254.

Muldoon, M. F., Manuck, S. B., and Mathews, K. A. (1990). Lowering cholesterol concentrations and mortality: a quantitative review of primary prevention trials. *British Medical Journal*, **301**, 309–314.

Muldoon, M. F., Manuck, S. B., and Mathews, K. A. (1991). Does cholesterol lowering increase non-illness related mortality? *Archives of Internal Medicine*, **151**, 1453–1459.

Neaton, J. D., Blackburn, H., Jacobs, D., and the Multiple Risk Factor Intervention Research Group (1992). Serum cholesterol levels and mortality findings for men screened in the Multiple Risk Intervention Trial. *Archives of Internal Medicine*, **152**, 1490–1500.

New, A. S., Trestman, R. L., Mitropoulo, V., Coccaro, E., Silverman, J., and Siever, L. J. (1997). Serotenergic function and self injurious behavior in personality disorder patients. *Psychiatry Research*, **69**(1), 17–26.

Nielsen, D. A. (1996). TPH replication study. Not! *Archives of General Psychiatry*, **53**, 964–965.

Nielsen, D. A., Dean, M., and Goldman, D. (1992). Genetic mapping of the human tryptophan hydroxylase gene on chromosome 11, using an intronic conformational polymorphism. *American Journal of Human Genetics*, **51**, 1366–1371.

Nielsen, D. A., Goldman, D., Virkkunnen, M., Tokola, R., Rawlings, R., and Linnoila, M. (1994). Suicidality and 5-HIAA concentration associated with a tryptophan hydroxylase polymorphism. *Archives of General Psychiatry*, **51**, 34–40.

Nielsen, D. A., Jenkins, G. L., Stefasko, K. M., Jefferson, K. K., and Goldman, D. (1997). Sequence, splice site and population frequency distribution analyses of the tryptophan hydroxylase intron 7. *Molecular Brain Research*, **45**, 145–148.

Nielsen, D. A., Virkkunen, M., Lappalainen, J., Eggert, M., Brown, G. L., Long, J. C., Goldman, D., and Linnoila, M. (1998). Tryptophan hydroxylase gene marker for suicidality and alcoholism. *Archives of General Psychiatry*, **55**, 593–602.

Ninan, P. T., van Kammen, D. P., Scheinin, M., Linnoila, M., Bunney, W. E., and Goodwin, F. K. (1984). CSF 5-hydroxyindoleacetic acid levels in suicidal schizophrenic patients. *American Journal of Psychiatry*, **141**(4), 566–569.

Nolan, K. A., Volavka, J., Lachman, H. M., and Saito, T. (2000). An association between a polymorphism of the tryptophan hydroxylase gene and aggression in schizophrenia and schizoaffective disorder. *Psychiatry and Genetics*, **10**, 109–115.

Nordstrom, P., Samuelsson, M., Asberg, M., Traskman-Bendz, L., Aberg-Widstedt, A., Nordin, C., and Bertilsson, L. (1994). CSF5-HIAA predicts suicide risk after attempted suicide. *Suicide and Life Threatening Behavior*, **24**(1), 1–9.

O'Neil, M., Page, N., Adkins, W. N., and Eicelman, B. (1986). Tryptophan-trazodone treatment of aggressive behavior. *Lancet*, **11**, 859–860.

Oquendo, M. A., and Mann, J. J. (2000). The biology of impulsivity and suicidality. *Psychiatric Clinics of North America*, **23**(1), 11–25.

Ordway, G. A., Smith, K. S., and Haycock, J. W. (1994). Elevated tyrosine hydroxylase in the locus coerulus of suicide victims. *Journal of Neurochemistry*, **58**, 494–502.

Oreland, L., Wiberg, A., Asberg, M., Traskman, L., Sjostrand, L., Thoren, P., Bertilsson, L., and Tybring, G. (1981). Platelet MAO activity and monoamine metabolites in cerebrospinal fluid in depressed and suicidal patients and in healthy controls. *Psychiatry Research*, **4**, 21–29.

Ostroff, R., Giller, E., Bonese, K., Ebersole, E., Harkness, L., and Mason., J. (1982). Neuroendocrine risk factors of suicidal behavior. *American Journal of Psychiatry*, **139**, 1323–1325.

Pacheco, M. A., Stockmeir, C., Meltzer, H. Y., Overholzer, J. C., Dilley, G. E., and Jope, R. S. (1966). Alterations in phosphoinositide signaling and G-protein levels in depressed suicide brain. *Brain Research*, **713**(1–2), 37–45.

Pandey, G. N., Pandey, S. C., Dwivedi, Y., Sharma, R. P., Janicak, P. G., and Davis, J. M. (1995). Platelet serotonin-2A receptors: a potential marker for suicidal behavior. *American Journal of Psychiatry*, **152**(6), 850–855.

Pandey, G. N., Dwivedi, Y., Pandey, S. C., Conley, R. R., Roberts, R. C., and Taminga, C. A. (1997). Protein kinase C in the postmortem brain of teenage suicide victims. *Neuroscience Letters*, **228**(2), 111–114.

Pekkanen, J., Nissinen, A., Punsar, S., and Karonen, M. J. (1989). Serum cholesterol and risk of accidental death in a 25 year follow up: the Finnish cohort of the Seven Countries Study. *Archives of Internal Medicine*, **149**, 1589–1591.

Persson, B., and Johanssen, B. W. (1984). The Kockum study: 22 year follow up. *Acta Medica Scandinavica*, **216**, 85–493.

Persson, M. L., Wasserman, D., Geijer, T., Jonsson, E, and Terenius, L. (1997). Tyrosine hydroxylase allelic distribution in suicide attempters. *Psychiatry Research*, **72**, 73–80.

Pfeffer, C. R., Normandin, L., and Tatsyuki, K. (1994). Suicidal children grow up: suicidal behavior and psychiatric disorders among relatives. *Journal of the American Academy of Child and Adolescent Psychiatry*, **33**, 1087–1097.

Pichot, W., Ansseau, M., Gonzalez-Moreno, A., Wauthy, J., Hansenne, M., and von Frenckell, R. (1995). Relationship between alpha 2-adrenergic function and suicidal behavior in depressed patients. *Biological Psychiatry*, **38**, 201–203.

Pickar, D., Roy, A., Breier, A., Doran, A., Wolkowitz, O., Colison, J., and Agren, H. (1986). Suicide and aggression in schizophrenia. In Mann, J. J., and Stanley, M. (eds.) Psychobiology of Suicidal Behavior. Special issue of *Annals of the New York Academy of Sciences*, pp. 189–196.

Pliszka, S. R. (1987). Tricyclic antidepressants in the treatment of children with attention deficit disorder. *Journal of the American Academy of Child and Adolescent Psychiatry*, **26**(2), 127–132.

Plutchik, R., and van Praag, H. M. (1986). The measurement of suicidality, aggressivity and impulsivity. *Clinical Neuropharmacology*, **9** (Suppl.), 380–382.

Plutchik, R., and van Praag, H. M. (1990). A self-report measure of violence risk, II. *Comprehensive Psychiatry*, **31**, 450–456.

Potegal, M., Yoburn, B., and Glusman, M. (1983). Disinhibition of muricide and irritability by intraseptal muscimol. *Pharmacology, Biochemistry and Behavior*, **19**, 663–669.

Pucilowski, O., Kostowski, W., Bidzinski, A., and Hauptmann, M. (1982). Effect of 6-hydroxydopamine–induced lesions of A-10 dopaminergic neurons on aggressive behavior in rats. *Pharmacology, Biochemistry and Behavior*, **16**, 547–551.

Ramamoorthy, S., Bauman, A., Moore, K., Han, H., Yang-Feng, T., Chang, A., Ganapathy, V., and Blakely, R. D. (1993). Antidepressant- and cocaine-sensitive human serotonin transporter: molecular cloning, expression, and chromosomal localization. *Proceedings of the National Academy of Science of the USA*, **90**, 2542–2546.

Reissner, I. R., Mann, J. J., Stanley, M., Huang, Y. Y., and Houpt, K. A. (1966). Comparison of cerebrospinal fluid monoamine metabolites levels in dominant aggressive and non-aggressive dogs. *Brain Research*, **714**(1–2), 57–64.

Roy, A., and Linnoila, M. (1988). Suicidal behavior, impulsiveness and serotonin. *Acta Psychiatrica Scandinavica*, **78**(5), 529–535.

Roy, A., Pickar, D., Linnoila, M., Doran, A. R., Ninan, P., and Paul, S. M. (1985). Cerebrospinal fluid monoamine and monoamine metabolite concentrations in melancholia. *Psychiatry Research*, **15**(4), 281–292.

Roy, A., Agren, H., Pickar, D., Linnoila, M., Doran, A., Cultler, N., and Paul, S. (1986). Reduced concentrations of HVA and 5HT ratios in depressed patients: relationship to suicidal behavior and dexamethazone nonsuppression. *American Journal of Psychiatry*, **143**, 1539–1545.

Roy, A., Everett, D., Pickar, D., and Paul, S. M. (1987). Platelet tritiated imipramine binding and serotonin uptake in depressed patients and controls. Relationship to plasma cortisol levels before and after dexamethasone administration. *Archives of General Psychiatry*, **44**(4), 320–327.

Roy, A., De Jong, J., and Linnoila, M. (1989). Cerebrospinal fluid monoamine metabolites and suicidal behavior in depressed patients. *Archives of General Psychiatry*, **4**, 609–612.

Russ, M. J., Lachman, H. M., Kashdan, T., Saito, T., and Bajmakovic-Kacila, S. (2000). Analysis of catechol-*O*-methyltransferase and 5-hydroxytryptamine transporter polymorphisms in patients at risk for suicide. *Psychiatry Research*, **93**, 73–78.

Ryan, N. D., Birmaher, B., Perel, J. M., Dahl, R. E., Meyer, V., al-Shabbout, M., Iyengar, S., and Puig-Antich, J. (1992). Neuroendocrine response to L-5-hydroxytryptophan challenge in prepubertal major depression. Depressed vs normal children. *Archives of General Psychiatry*, **49**(11), 843–851.

Rydin, E., Schalling, D., and Asberg, M. (1982). Rorschach ratings in depressed and suicidal patients with low levels of 5-hydroxyindoleacetic acid in cerebrospinal fluid. *Psychiatry Research*, **7**, 229–243.

Sanders-Bush, E., and Mayer, S. E. (1996). 5-Hydroxytryptamine (serotonin) receptor agonists and antagonists. In: Hardman, Limbird, Molinoff, Ruddon, Gilman, (eds.) *Goodman and Gilman's The Pharmacological Basis of Therapeutics* (9th edition). McGraw-Hill companies, pp. 249–256.

Sandler, M., Ruthven, C. R., Goodwin, G. L., Field, H., and Matthews, R. (1978). Phenylethylamine overproduction in aggressive psychopaths. *Lancet*, **2**, 1269–1270.

Sarchiapone, M., Camardese, G., Roy, A., Della-Casa, S., Satta, M. A., Gonzalez, B., Berman, J., and De-Risio, S. (2001). Cholesterol and serotonin indices in depressed and suicidal patients. *Journal of Affective Disorders*, **63**(3), 217–219.

Scaramella, T. J., and Brown, W. A. (1978). Serum testosterone and aggressiveness in hockey players. *Psychosomotor Medicine*, **40**(3), 262–265.

Searcy, W. A., and Wingfield, J. C. (1980). The effects of androgen and antiandrogen on dominance and aggressiveness in male red-winged blackbirds. *Hormones and Behavior*, **14**(2), 126–135.

Sedvall, G., Fyro, B., Gullberg, B., Nyback, H., Wiesel, F.-A., and Wode-Helgodt, B. (1980). Relationships in healthy volunteers between concentration of monoamine metabolites in cerebrospinal fluid and family history of psychiatric morbidity. *British Journal of Psychiatry*, **136**, 366–374.

Sheard, M. H., Marini, J. L., Bridges, C. I., and Wagner, E. (1976). The effect of lithium on impulsive aggressive behavior in man. *American Journal of Psychiatry*, **133**(12), 1409–1413.

Shimon, H., Agam, C., Belmaker, R. M., Hyde, T. M., and Kleinman, J. E. (1997). Reduced frontal cortex inositol levels in postmortem brain of suicide victims and patients with bipolar disorder. *American Journal of Psychiatry*, **154**(8), 1148–1150.

Simler, S., Puglisi-Allegra, S., and Mandel, P. (1982). Gamma-aminobutyric acid in brain areas of isolated aggressive or non-aggressive inbred strains of mice. *Pharmacology, Biochemistry and Behavior*, **16**(1), 57–61.

Simler, S., Puglisi-Allegra, S., and Mandel, P. (1983). Effects of n-di-propylacetate on aggressive behavior and brain GABA level in isolated mice. *Pharmacology, Biochemistry and Behavior*, **18**(5), 717–720.

Skolnick, P., Reed, G. F., and Paul, S. M. (1985). Benzodiazepine-receptor mediated inhibition of isolation-induced aggression in mice. *Pharmacology, Biochemistry and Behavior*, **23**(1), 17–20.

Smith, G. D., Shipley, M., Marmot, M. G., and Rose, G. (1992). Plasma cholesterol concentration and mortality. The Whitehall Study. *Journal of the American Medical Association*, **267**, 70–76.

Spreux-Varoquax, O., Alvarez, J. C., Berlin, I., Batista, G., Despierre, P. G., Gilton, A., and Cremniter, D. (2001). Differential abnormalities in plasma 5-HIAA and platelet serotonin concentrations in violent suicide attempters: relationships with impulsivity and depression. *Life Sciences*, **69**(6), 647–657.

Stanley, B., Molcho, A., Stanley, M., Winchel, R., Gameroff, M. J., Parsons, B., and Mann, J. J. (2000). Association of aggressive behavior with altered serotonergic function in patients who are not suicidal. *American Journal of Psychiatry*, **157**(4), 609–614.

Strandberg, T. E., Salomaa, W., Naukkanin, V. A., Vanhanen, H. T., Sarna, S. J., and Miettinen, T. A. (1991). Long term mortality after five year multifactorial primary prevention of cardiovascular diseases in middle aged males. *Journal of the American Medical Association*, **266**, 1225–1229.

Sullivan, P. F., Joyce, P. R., Bilih, C. N., Muhler, R. T., and Oackley-Browne, M. (1994). Total cholesterol and suicidality in depression. *Biological Psychiatry*, **36**, 472–477.

Traskman, L., Asberg, M., Bertilsson, L., and Sjostrand, L. (1981). Monoamine metabolites in CSF and suicidal behavior. *Archives of General Psychiatry*, **38**(6), 631–636.

Traskman-Bendz, L., and Asberg, M. (1986). Serotonergic function and suicidal behavior in personality disorders. In Mann, J. J., and Stanley, M. (eds.) Psychobiology of Suicidal Behavior. Special issue of *Annals of the New York Academy of Sciences*, pp. 168–1774.

Traskman-Bendz, L., Asberg, M., Bertilsson, L., and Thoren, P. (1984). CSF monoamine metabolites of depressed patients during illness and after recovery. *Acta Psychiatrica Scandinavica*, **69**, 333–342.

Tripodianakis, J., Markianos, M., Sarantidis, D., and Leotsakou, C. (2000). Neurochemical variables in subjects with adjustment disorder after suicide attempts. *European Psychiatry*, **15**(3), 190–195.

Tsuang, M. T. (1983). Risk of suicide in the relatives of schizophrenics, manics, depressives and controls. *Journal of Clinical Psychiatry*, **44**, 396–400.

Turker, T., Sodmann, R., Goebel, U., Jatzke, S., Knapp, M., Lesch, K. P., Schuster, R., Schutz, H., Weiler, G., and Stober, G. (1998). High ethanol tolerance in young adults is associated with the low-activity variant of the promoter of the human serotonin transporter gene. *Neuroscience Letters*, **248**, 147–150.

Valzelli, L. (1981). *Psychobiology of Aggression and Violence*. New York, NY: Raven Press.

Valzelli, L. (1984). Reflections on experimental and human pathology of aggression [review]. *Progress in Neuropsychopharmacology and Biological Psychiatry*, **8**(3), 311–325.

Valzelli, L. (1985). Animal Models of behavioral pathology and violent aggression. *Methods and Findings of Experimental and Clinical Pharmacology*, **7**(4), 189–193.

van Heeringen, K., Audenaert, K., Van-de-Wielde, E., and Verstraete, A. (2000). Cortisol in violent suicidal behaviour. Association with personality and monoaminergic activity. *Journal of Affective Disorders*, **60**(3), 181–189.

van Praag, H. M. (1982a). Biochemical and psychopathological predictors of suicidality. *Bibliotheca-psychiatrica*, **162**, 42–60.

van Praag, H. M. (1982b). Depression, suicide and the metabolism of serotonin in the brain. *Journal of Affective Disorders*, **4**, 275–290.

van Praag, H. M. (1983). CSF 5-HIAA and suicide in non-depressed schizophrenics. *Lancet*, **II**, 977–978.

van Praag, H. M. (1986a). (Auto)Aggression and CSF 5-HIAA in depression and schizophrenia. *Psychopharmacology Bulletins*, **22**(3), 669–673.

van Praag, H. M. (1986b). Biological suicide research: outcome and limitations. *Biological Psychiatry*, **21**, 1305–1323.

van Praag, H. M. (1986c). Monoamines and depression: the present state of the art. In Plutchik, R. (ed.) *Emotion: Theory, Research and Experience*. New York, NY: Academic Press.

van Praag, H. M. (1996). Serotonin-related, anxiety / aggression-driven, stressor related depression. A psychobiological hypothesis. *European Journal of Psychiatry*, **11**, 57–67.

van Praag, H. M. (2000). Serotonin disturbances and suicide risk: is aggression or anxiety the interadjacent link? *Crisis*, **21**(4), 160–162.

Vartainen, E., Pouska, P., Pekkanen, J., Tuomilehto, J., Lonquist, J., and Ehnholm, C. (1994). Serum cholesterol and accidental or other violent death. *British Medical Journal*, **309**, 445–447.

Vestergaard, P., Sorensen, T., Hoppe, E., Rafaelsen, O. J., Yates, C. M., and Nicolaou, N. (1978). Biogenic amine metabolites in cerebrospinal fluid of patients with affective disorders. *Acta Psychiatrica, Scandinavica*, **58**, 88–96.

Virkkunen, M. (1979). Serum cholesterol in antisocial personality. *Neuropsychobiolology*, **5**, 27–30.

Virkkunen, M. (1983a). Serum cholesterol levels in homicidal offenders. *Neuropsychobiology*, **10**, 65–69.

Virkkunen, M. (1983b). Insulin secretion during the glucose tolerance test in antisocial personality. *British Journal of Psychiatry*, **142**, 598–604.

Virkkunen, M., and Pentinnen, H. (1984). Serum cholesterol in aggressive conduct disorder. *Biological Psychiatry*, **19**, 435–439.

Virkkunen, M., Goldman, D., Nielsen, D. A., and Linnoila, M. (1995). Low brain serotonin turnover rate (low CSF-5-HIAA) and impulsive violence. *Journal of Psychiatry and Neuroscience*, **20**(4), 271–275.

Weidner, G., Connor, S. L., Hollis, J. F., and Connor, W. E. (1992). Improvements in hostility and depression in relation to dietary change and cholesterol lowering. The Family Heart Study. *Annals of Internal Medicine*, **117**, 820–823.

Weizman, A., Burgin, R., Harel, Y., and Gavish, M. (1995). Platelet peripheral type benzodiazepine receptor in major depression. *Journal of Affective Disorders*, **33**(4), 257–261.

WHO Multiple Risk Factor Intervention Trial Research Group. (1990). Mortality rates after 10.5 years for participants in the Multiple Risk Factor Intervention Trial. Findings related to a priori hypotheses of the trial. *Journal of the American Medical Association*, **263**(13), 1795–1801.

Woodman, D. D., Hinton, J. W., and O'Neill, M. T. (1978). Plasma catecholamines, stress and aggression in maximum security patients. *Biological Psychology*, **6**(2), 147–154.

Yamamoto, H., Nagai, K., and Nakagawa, H. (1984). Additional evidence that the suprachiasmatic nucleus is the center for regulation of insulin secretion and glucose homeostasis. *Brain Research*, **304**(2), 237–241.

Yamamoto, H., Nagai, K., and Nakagawa, H. (1985). Lesions involving the suprachiasmatic nucleus eliminate the glucagon response to intracranial injection of 2-deoxy-D-glucose. *Endocrinology*, **117**(2), 468–473.

Zalsman, G., Frisch, A., Bromberg, M., Gelernter, J., Michaelovsky, E., Campino, A., Erlich, Z., Tyano, S., Apter, A., and Weizman, A. (2001a). Family-based association study of serotonin transporter promoter in suicidal adolescents: possible role in violence traits. *American Journal of Medical Genetics*, **105**, 239–245.

Zalsman, G., Frisch, A., King, R. A., Pauls, D. L., Grice, D. E., Gelernter, J., Alsobrook, J., Michaelovsky, E., Apter, A., Tyano, S., Weizman, A., and Leckman, J. F. (2001b). Case–control and family-based association studies of tryptophan hydroxylase A218C polymorphism and suicidality in adolescents. *American Journal of Medical Genetics*, **105**, 451–457.

# 6

# Psychodynamic approaches to youth suicide

Robert A. King

## Introduction

The psychodynamic perspective seeks to understand the meaning of suicidal behavior in terms of feelings, motives, and their conflicts, in the context of past and present interpersonal relationships. For example, in looking at the immediate experiential antecedents of suicidal action, we may ask, what are the intolerable affects from which suicide is a perceived means of escape? What kinds of internal or external events serve to trigger suicidal feelings and behavior and what is their significance in the broader context of the suicidal youngster's life? The psychodynamic approach is also a developmental one that attempts to understand the origins of the vulnerability to suicide and depression in the related developmental vicissitudes of the capacity for self-care and comfort; the ability to develop, sustain and make use of protective affiliations; and the regulation of self-esteem (King and Apter, 1996). Finally, the psychodynamic perspective seeks clues as to how the challenges of a given developmental epoch, such as adolescence, may confer a particular vulnerability to suicidal behavior. The psychodynamic approach to suicide is thus intended not to supplant but to complement the biological, sociological, and nosological approaches to suicide.

The earliest psychoanalytic attempts to understand suicide came early in the twentieth century against the background of a perceived epidemic of youth suicide in Germany and Austria (Neubauer, 1992). Much as in our own day, lay writers sought to blame the schools and the decline of family and social values, while medical writers looked for hormonal defects or "hereditary taints." In 1910, the Vienna Psychoanalytic Society held a symposium "On Suicide with Particular Reference to Suicide among Young Students" (Friedman, 1967) to examine the problem from a psychoanalytic perspective. No comprehensive theory emerged, but several vivid insights emphasized the distinctive themes of guilt, aggression turned against the self, and thwarted love which were to characterize much of later psychoanalytic thinking on suicide. For example, Stekel emphasized the aggressive and self-punitive aspects of the talion principle: "No one kills himself who has never wanted to kill another, or at least wished the death of another" (Friedman, 1967, p. 87). In contrast, Sadger emphasized the libidinal element: "[T]he only person who puts an end to his life is one who has been compelled to give up all hope of love" (Friedman, 1967, p. 76).

In his own later writings on suicide, Freud attempted to move beyond motives such as a refusal to accept loss of libidinal gratification or guilt over death wishes towards others. In trying to understand how the self became the target of its own hatred and destructiveness, Freud (1917) concluded "The analysis of melancholia now shows that the ego can kill itself only if, . . . it can treat itself as an object – if it is able to direct against itself the hostility which relates to an object and which represents the ego's original reaction to objects in the external world" (p. 252). As Freud (1923) put it later, ". . . [T]he ego gives itself up because it feels itself hated and persecuted by the super-ego, instead of loved. To the ego, therefore, living means the same as being loved – loved by the superego, which . . . fulfills the same function of protecting and saving that was fulfilled in earlier days by the father and later by Providence or Destiny" (p. 58). Freud's formulation thus combined both the aggressive and libidinal strands in the notion that the attack on the self is prompted by the experienced or threatened loss of an intensely needed, but ambivalently loved, object whose own attitude towards the subject is felt to be potentially hateful, critical, or rejecting.

Freud's evocative insights about suicide have proven fertile for theory building and clinical practice (King and Apter, 1996). The challenge for contemporary psychodynamic research, however, is to relate our understanding of suicide to the broader context of developmental psychopathology. To do so, it is essential to operationalize psychodynamic constructs in such a way as to permit their empirical study and to move beyond the consulting room to the study of larger clinical and community populations. The purpose of this paper is to present some of the recent advances in meeting this challenge.

## Escape from unbearable affects

Most commonly, suicidal behavior occurs as a desperate attempt to escape from an intolerable affect, such as rage, intense isolation, or self-loathing (Hendin, 1991; Shneidman, 1989). Less frequently in adolescence, unbearable anxiety, a sense of inner deadness, or fear of fragmentation may also play a role. Self-awareness becomes unbearable and self-destruction beckons as means of sur-cease (Baumeister, 1990; Dean and Range, 1999; Dean et al., 1996).

In a study of adolescent self-poisoners, Hawton and colleagues (1982) found, using a card sort procedure, that the commonest reported affective state prior to the ingestions were "angry with someone" (54%), "lonely or unwanted" (54%), and "worried about the future" (40%). Only 54% of these adolescents, however, reported that they clearly wanted to die at the time of their ingestion. Among the other reasons given for their ingestions were: "to get relief from a terrible state of mind" (42%) or "to escape for a while from an impossible situation" (42%).

Negron et al. (1997) found that two-thirds of adolescent suicide ideators or attempters seen in the emergency room reported intense anger, hopelessness, depression, or crying while contemplating suicide.

Kienhorst et al. (1995) studied the reasons endorsed by adolescent suicide attempters and found the most frequently endorsed factor consisted of items related to stopping of consciousness, specifically "I wanted to get relief from a terrible state of mind," "I wanted to stop feeling pain," and "I wanted to die" (endorsed respectively by 58%, 75%, and 73% of attempters).

Although the card sort procedure used by Hawton and others forces the choice of a specific response, in clinical practice it is striking how many adolescents are unable to give a reason for their impulsive suicide attempts or parasuicidal gestures; responses such as "I don't know why I did it; I just felt like it" or "I was upset" are common. Indeed, White (1974) found over half of adolescent self-poisoners unwilling or unable to provide an explanation or motive for their act and Beautrais et al. (1997) found that one-third of adolescents making serious suicide attempts were unable to describe any precipitating factor. In the study of Kienhorst et al. (1995), 39% of subjects endorsed "I seemed to lose my self-control and I don't know why I did it then." Further research is warranted to evaluate to what extent this inability represents an acute cognitive disorganization in the face of sudden upset or, alternatively, a more enduring alexithymic cognitive-affectual style that, linked to a paucity of emotional problem-solving skills, renders youngsters vulnerable to feeling unable to cope. Along these lines, Rourke et al. (1989) speculate that nonverbal learning disabilities, which they believe to be associated with impaired social perception, judgment, and skills, constitute an important risk factor for social isolation, depression, and suicidality.

Understanding the meaning and intensity of the unbearable affects which trigger self-destructive acts requires examining not only their immediate precipitants, but also their longer-standing origins from a developmental, interpersonal context.

Although completed suicides and suicide attempts are sometimes precipitated by extraordinary stresses, such as assault or abuse, in most cases the identifiable precipitants are the commonplace travails of adolescence such as a disciplinary crisis, argument with a parent or romantic partner, teasing, or some form of perceived failure (Apter et al., 1993; Beautrais, 2001; Shaffer et al., 1988). The catastrophic reverberation these events evoke in the suicidal adolescent can be viewed from several perspectives. Emphasizing the *reactive* element, we might ask what special significance these events hold for the vulnerable youngster. Alternatively, emphasizing *personality* and *temperamental* factors, we may ask, what are the impairments in the youngster's capacity for self-comfort, affect regulation, or problem-solving skills (including the ability to elicit support or comfort from others) that render him or her vulnerable to feeling so desperately overwhelmed? Often, the interpersonal upset that serves as the proximate trigger of a suicidal episode stands against the background of a life-long propensity to form insecure or ambivalent relationships.

Clinicians sometimes infer an underlying interpersonal motive for suicide attempts, such as retaliation against an ambivalently regarded other, an attempt to restore a tie to a vital attachment figure, or an effort to coerce change in what is perceived as an intolerable interpersonal or family situation (e.g., Cohen-Sandler et al., 1982a,b; Orbach, 1988; Orbach et al., 1999). It is interesting to note, however, that adolescent suicide attempters are less likely than their clinicians to perceive an instrumental interpersonal motive in their attempts (Hawton et al., 1982). In Kienhorst et al. (1995)'s study, only 18% to 27% of adolescent attempters endorsed a revenge motive ("to frighten," "get back," or "to make people sorry") and less than half endorsed an appeal motive ("to show how much I loved someone" (23%), "to get help from someone" (27%), "to find out whether someone really loved me" (30%), or "to make people understand how desperate I was feeling" (46%)). Only 11% endorsed "I wanted to try and get someone to change their mind," but a full 80% endorsed "the situation was so unbearable that I had to do something and I didn't know what else to do."

## The role of loss and interpersonal vulnerability

Loss plays a particularly important role, both as an immediate precipitant of adolescent suicide and as a potential antecedent to the vulnerability to depression and suicide (Adams, 1990). As noted, the breakup or disruption of a significant relationship is among the commonest precipitants of attempted or completed adolescent suicides (Adams, 1990; Apter et al., 1993; Shaffer et al., 1988). Although an acute loss may serve as an important proximate precipitant, cumulative losses also appear to confer particular vulnerability. For example, in a sample of preadolescent psychiatric inpatients, we found that, compared to nonsuicidal depressed subjects and other psychiatric subjects, suicidal subjects had significantly higher levels of stressful life events, especially losses, both in the year preceding admission and over their entire life-span (Cohen-Sandler et al., 1982 a,b). (The other distinguishing feature of these suicidal youngsters was their high level of aggression directed both towards self and others.)

The term "loss" has been used to cover a variety of disparate stresses, ranging from death or permanent separation from an important other (e.g., by parental divorce) through estrangement or loss of the other's emotional availability or positive regard. Such losses often co-occur and may accompany other forms of family disruption and pathology (which may reflect partially heritable factors); in the untidiness of real life, disentangling the impact of these different elements can be difficult (see Chapters 1 and 4).

Following the loss of one parent, the remaining parent's or surrogate's parenting style and degree of affectionate involvement with the child appear to affect the extent of the child's vulnerability to later depression (Adams, 1990; Brown et al., 1986; Tennant, 1988). Weller et al. (1991) found that 37% of recently bereaved prepubertal children met criteria for major depression; 37% were self-deprecating; and 61% had morbid or suicidal ideation. Those with a prior psychiatric history and a family history of depression were most troubled.

## The role of attachment

Drawing on studies of experimental and naturally occurring separations and losses, the work of Bowlby (1973, 1980) and colleagues (Ainsworth et al., 1978; Carlson and Sroufe, 1995) provides clues as to the mechanisms by which early, ongoing losses or deprivations may confer vulnerability. Further, they also provide a possible empirical paradigm for classifying individuals' characteristic styles of response to interpersonal loss or frustration and the corresponding risk for depression or suicide these styles may convey.

Bowlby (1973, 1980) proposed that the young child's actual experience of the caretaker's physical and emotional availability shaped the child's development of persisting expectations ("working models of attachment") concerning the availability of significant others. Reflecting these working models of attachment, the child also developed enduring styles of interaction or response to disruptions (Carlson and Sroufe, 1995).

As empirically operationalized for infants by Ainsworth et al. (1978), these attachment styles can be classified as: (a) *secure* – characterized by the ability to accept comfort and re-establish positive relations after separation; (b) *insecure-ambivalent* – characterized by helplessness and, despite open expression of distress, trouble being comforted; and (c) *insecure-avoidant* – characterized by failure to initiate interaction and unresponsiveness to and avoidance of the caretaker following reunion.

Although the relative role of experience vs. constitutional factors remains unclear, these attachment styles appear to persist into later childhood, adolescence, and even adulthood, and exert an ongoing influence on the quality of perceived reciprocity, support, and closeness with others (Priel et al., 1998).

For example, empirical studies find that *secure* attachment persists as a strong but flexible emphasis on relationships. Children with a history of secure attachment as infants are able to express distress directly, to use the caretaker for reassurance when threatened or upset, and to remain confident in the availability of the other and their own ability to effectively elicit care (see review by Carlson and Sroufe, 1995). Such children report having at least one good friend whom they consider reliable and more often report relationship-oriented solutions to stressful situations. As adults, studied using the Adult Attachment Interview (Main and Goldwyn, 1989), they value relationships and, while able to describe freely difficult early relationships, do so from a realistic and flexible perspective. In contrast, *insecure-ambivalent* attachment endures as an overvaluation of dependent relationships, colored by persistent and intense struggles with attachment figures. Children with such histories are often easily frustrated, overtly anxious, socially inept, and dependently helpless. As adults, they recall earlier dependency issues easily, but remain preoccupied with difficulties with parents and unable to resolve attachment-related issues (Main and Goldwyn, 1989). *Insecure-avoidant* attachment perpetuates itself in discounting and avoidance of relationships; children with such histories fail to initiate interaction or to seek contact in response to perceived threats. Their fantasy play and problem solving are impoverished and lack interpersonal themes. As adults, they are dismissive of attachments and have difficulty recalling attachment-related events (Main and Goldwyn, 1989). Idealized views of parents may persist unintegrated with anecdotes of rejecting or unempathic caretaking (Carlson and Sroufe, 1995).

In addition to the Adult Attachment Interview, a variety of scales, such as Revised Adult Attachment Scale and the Inventory of Parent and Peer Attachment, are suitable for assessing the attachment style or cognitions of adolescents. In longitudinal studies of adolescents, secure attachment style predicts higher levels of perceived and enacted social support (Herzberg et al., 1999). When followed into college, female high-school seniors with secure attachment style experienced less chronic strain and fewer stressful events, with less performance anxiety and greater school satisfaction than peers with insecure attachment styles (Burge et al., 1997a,b).

These studies and others utilizing attachment style and related concepts suggest that the life stresses associated with depression or externalizing disorders are, at least in part, often self-generated and that individuals' interpersonal expectations actively shape their social experiences (Daley et al., 1997; Hammen, 2000; Priel et al., 1998; Rudolph et al., 2000).

This schema of attachment styles suggests a typology which may also be useful in understanding distinctive forms of vulnerability to depression and even suicidality in reaction to frustration. Individuals differ in the forms of self-blame and self-reproach to which they are prone at different ages (A. Freud, 1965). Bibring (1953) proposed further that individuals also differ from each other in their vital aspirations which, when frustrated, lead to depression – a condition which he defined as a state of real or imagined helplessness to preserve cherished aspects of the self or to maintain crucial relationships. For different individuals, Bibring suggested, the vital aspirations, without which life felt unbearable, might be: (a) the wish to be appreciated or lovable, not unworthy; (b) the wish to be strong, superior, and secure, not weak; or (c) the wish to be good and loving, not hateful or destructive. One important research goal is to understand better how developmental, family, and cultural factors determine which aspirations become most problematic for a given youngster, render him or her most vulnerable to depression, and color the affective tone that self-reproach takes.

Drawing on these perspectives, two subtypes of vulnerability to depression have been proposed – the *dependent* and the *self-critical* – each having its own distinctive antecedents, characteristic preoccupation, and specific type of dysphoria (Arieti and Bemporad, 1980; Beck, 1983; Blatt, 1995). As summarized by Blatt (1995; Blatt et al., 1992, 1993; Blatt and Homann, 1992), individuals of the *dependent* subtype have a pattern of insecure-ambivalent attachment. As described above, they are characterized by an overvaluation of dependent relationships and a propensity for intense struggles with attachment figures; they are correspondingly preoccupied with dependency and the threat of abandonment and feel helpless in the face of perceived loss. In contrast, individuals of the *self-critical* type are characterized by compulsive self-reliance (Bowlby, 1980) and dismiss the importance of intimate relationships; instead, they are anxiously preoccupied with issues of self-worth and autonomy, with perceived failure triggering humiliating feelings of unworthiness, guilt, and loss of control.

These authors further speculate that these contrasting vulnerability profiles stem in part from distinctive early developmental experiences, with anxiously insecure attachment reflecting neglectful or overindulgent parenting and avoidantly insecure attachment resulting from excessively controlling, rejecting, judgmental, or punitive rearing (Ainsworth et al., 1978; Blatt, 1995; Blatt and Homann, 1992; Carlson and Sroufe, 1995).

This typology of depressive vulnerabilities has been operationalized in an assessment instrument, the Depressive Experiences Questionnaire (DEQ) (and a corresponding Depressive Experiences Questionnaire for Adolescents (DEQ-A)), which characterizes subjects' self-perceptions in a psychometrically reliable fashion along the dimensions of dependency (concerns about rejection or interpersonal loss); self criticism (feeling guilty, self-critical, or falling short of standards); and efficacy (feelings of personal goal-oriented accomplishment) (Blatt et al., 1992). The instrument has proven useful in studying the relationship of these depressive traits to a variety of adolescent problem behaviors (Blatt et al., 1993; Kuperminc et al., 1997; Leadbeater et al., 1995; Luthar and Blatt, 1995).

Hewitt and Flett (1991, 1993; Hewitt et al., 1992, 1994, 1997) have developed a Multidimensional Perfectionism Scale to assess self-oriented, other-oriented, and socially-prescribed forms of perfectionism and have studied the empirical relationship of these measures to suicidality. They found both socially prescribed and self-oriented perfectionism associated with suicidal ideation, with life stress playing a role in the association with self-oriented perfectionism (Hewitt et al., 1994).

Among our adolescent psychiatric inpatients, levels of self-critical or dependent concerns (as measured on the DEQ-A) correlated strongly with the presence of suicidal ideation and attempts (King et al., unpublished data). Other studies using this typology find that dependent individuals are prone to impulsive, manipulative, nonlethal suicide attempts, while self-critical individuals are prone to more planful and serious suicide attempts (Blatt, 1995; Faazia, 2001).

These empirically measurable subtypes may also predict the types of stress likely to precipitate depression or suicidality in different individuals. Studies show that, in dependent individuals, distress or depression is more likely to be precipitated by negative interpersonal events (e.g., rejections or losses) (e.g., Priel and Shahar, 2000). In contrast, self-critical individuals are more likely to become depressed in response to perceived failures in achievement (Brown et al., 1995; Hammen et al., 1989; Hewitt and Flett, 1991, 1993).

This body of research and other studies drawn from Action Theory (Shahar, 2001) examine how individuals create the conditions that contribute to their depression and distress by generating contextual risk factors (such as negative life events) and fail to generate contextual protective factors (such as supportive social relations and positive life events) (Shahar, 2002, poster presentation). For example, adolescents high on the self-critical scale of the DEQ-A were less likely to initiate behavior that is intrinsically rewarding (autonomous motivation) and were more likely to initiate behavior to appease, impress or influence people (controlled motivation). As a result, self-critical youngsters experienced more negative achievement-related and interpersonal-related life events and fewer interpersonal- or achievement-related positive events (Shahar and Priel, 2003; Shahar et al., 2003).

(These personality traits may also have implications for response to treatment (Blatt et al., 1998). Depressed self-critical individuals may also have difficulty using psychotherapy (including Interpersonal Therapy and Cognitive-Behavioral Therapy), because of their difficulty forming a therapeutic alliance and deriving satisfaction with social relations (Shahar et al., 2002; Zuroff et al., 2000).)

## Self-criticism and suicide

For some highly self-critical youngsters, the proximate cause of suicide may be a narcissistic blow or disappointment, such as a perceived or threatened humiliation or failure to meet an impossibly high, self-imposed standard of achievement. For other, more dependent, youngsters a romantic disappointment or other interpersonal upset may be more likely to precipitate suicidal action.

The perfectionistic or self-critical type of suicide has a special tragic salience for certain high-performing, self-demanding youngsters. A systematic postmortem study of Israeli adolescent suicides occurring in the context of compulsory military service found a substantial proportion of recruits, many serving in prestigious front-line units, who committed suicide despite having received, at the time of their rigorous preinduction screening, outstanding ratings of psychological, intellectual, and physical fitness for combat duty (Apter et al., 1993; King and Apter, 1996). The immediate precipitants of these unanticipated suicides were frequently seemingly unremarkable frustrations. Only as viewed with the clarity of hindsight through the psychological autopsy did it become clear that these young men's high self-expectations, often combined with isolative traits, magnified their distress and left them unable to cope when they encountered external setbacks which they perceived as failures. In some cases, a recent, reactive, and undetected depression appeared to have exacerbated this lethal downward spiral, but help was not sought, apparently out of feelings of intense privacy or shame. In other cases, even on extensive postmortem inquiry, no evidence of depression could be found; however, these young suicides' need to maintain a self-presentation of high achievement and to suppress acknowledgement of personal limitations or dysphoric feelings make this absence of reported symptoms hard to assess.

In contrast to young suicides in the U.S. and Western Europe, substance abuse was absent and antisocial personality rare among Israeli late-adolescent suicides at the time of our original report, while seemingly high-functioning youngsters with high combat fitness scores appeared over-represented (Apter et al., 1993). This pattern may be changing over time, however, as reflected in a progressive decline in the proportion of suicides by recruits with high preinduction fitness scores (Dycian, 1995).

In many respects, these late-adolescent Israeli suicides resemble those of elite students (Thernstrom, 1996), young athletes (Berkow, 1995), and military officers (Lewis, 1996) reported over the past few years in the U.S. press, as well as those of academics and politicians described by Blatt (1995) and Trillin (1993). Similarly, in a review of completed suicides at Oxford over a period of 15 years, Hawton et al. (1995) noted that two-thirds were worried about their academic work. "[S]ome students, often despite considerable achievements in various spheres of university life, were tormented by low self-esteem . . . [that] appeared to lead some to set themselves impossibly high standards" (p. 49). In his pioneering postmortem study of child and early adolescent suicides, Shaffer (1974) noted a subgroup of anxiously perfectionistic subjects.

Although these case studies are intriguing, the need for controlled studies is underlined by the finding of Shaffer et al. (1996) in their large New York area postmortem study that perfectionism (as defined by items drawn from the symptom interview) was equally common in adolescent suicides and controls. Similarly, in their analysis of the Methods for the Epidemiology of Child and Adolescent Mental Disorders (MECA) Study data, Gould et al. (1998) examined the influence of perfectionism, as defined by four items from the Anxiety Disorders module of the structured diagnostic interview: worrying about schoolwork/job performance; worrying about athletic performance; worrying about making a mistake; or worrying about "making a fool of themselves." Once psychiatric diagnoses were adjusted for, perfectionism was not a significant risk factor of suicidality. (These items related primarily to Hewitt and Flett (1991)'s construct of self-oriented perfectionism, whereas it is socially prescribed perfectionism that Hewitt et al. (1997) found to have the strongest association with suicide.)

The interactive dangers of perfectionism combined with social isolation are tragically illustrated by the widely publicized story of Sinedu Tadesse, an Ethiopian student at Harvard who, with much premeditation, hanged herself after murdering her roommate, against whom she turned when the latter announced her intention not to room together again the next semester. As profiled in contemporary newspaper accounts and by Thernstrom (1996), Sinedu was from childhood an academically driven, but deeply isolated young woman, for whom achievement became not only a promised escape ticket from her war-ravaged country, but a substitute for social intimacy. Acknowledging her lack of social skills, she exhorted herself to study social conversation as though it were a required academic course. Caught in a downward spiral of depression, further withdrawal, and deteriorating academic performance, she received word that she was unlikely to be accepted at the elite medical school on which she had set her sights. Far from home, she also withdrew from relatives living nearby. Viewed in retrospect, her diary records a profound inability to use or experience others, past or present, as sustaining presences. As quoted by Thernstrom (1996), Sinedu wrote,

I don't understand what people mean by the warmth of a family, the love of their mother and the security of their home. I grew up feeling lonely & cold amidst two parents & four siblings . . . it took me all my life to figure out what [others] had & what I did not have . . . . My parents did not beat me or abuse me. They fed me, bought me clothes, sent me to good schools and wished the best for me. As a result I was unable to point at any tangible cause . . . . (p. 70)

Returning our attention to the Israeli context, suicide also took a high toll among the early, intensely idealistic, young Zionist pioneers (*chalutzim*) of the second and third aliyah (1904–1923), who had to struggle against harsh and debilitating physical conditions, hunger, illness, military hostilities, and radical cultural dislocation, which included often permanent separation from their families of origin and intense dependence on the group (Lieblich, 1981; Tzur, 1974, 1979). Faced with the near-impossible demands of their ideals, many young men and women appear to have killed themselves when confronted with the void opened by their inability to sustain these ideals or to expose their perceived shortcomings to the collective's anticipated disapproving scrutiny. By one estimate (Tzur, 1974), suicides accounted for over 10% of the obituaries in the labor movement's newspapers of the period. So common were these demoralized and demoralizing young suicides that some observers echoed the discouraged reports of the spies sent by Moses into Canaan (Numbers, XIII, 32): "The land devours its inhabitants" (Tzur, 1979).

## Pathological narcissism

As these many cases illustrate, certain types of perfectionism confer a malignant vulnerability for suicide (Blatt, 1995; Hamachek, 1978). Perfectionism is adaptive for individuals who have high but attainable goals, derive pleasure from their efforts, and acknowledge reasonable personal limitations. In contrast, neurotically or maladaptively perfectionistic individuals draw little pleasure from their achievements, which they are prone to denigrate, and dread each new task with anxious preoccupation lest they fail (Hamachek, 1978).

Much remains to be learned about the development of these various styles of self-evaluation and self-esteem regulation including the impact of parental style and cultural influences. For example, Shahar (2001) suggests that youth with elevated perfectionism may be especially permeable to contemporary society's emphasis on achievement and individuality.

Although the formulations discussed earlier contrast dependent and self-critical depressive traits, both strands may co-exist in anxiously perfectionistic individuals who perceive their parents' (and others') approval and love as conditional on meeting high standards of achievement. These individuals' often life-long, intensely self-critical attitudes and anxious pursuit of perfection seem to represent a desperate, but unending attempt to win approval and a sense of worth (Koestner et al., 1991).

## Adolescent suicide and the development of self-care

Closely related to the development of attachment and maintenance of self-esteem are other important self-regulatory capacities, such as the capacity for bodily self-care, self-protection, and self-soothing. The child's gradual internalization of the parents' attentiveness to the child's bodily care is an important component of the child's ability to see their body and self as worth protecting and caring for (A. Freud, 1965; Khantzian and Mack, 1983; King and Apter, 1996; Orbach et al., 1996a,b, 1997, 2001). When this process goes well, the child is able to transform early experiences of parents' empathic care into a sense of his or her body as being cherished and pleasurable. In addition, the securely attached child is able to evoke a sustaining image of the caring, comforting, or approving other, even when physically absent (Winnicott, 1958). When this process goes awry – as it may for a variety of reasons including chronic illness; temperamental unsoothability; or parental ambivalence, neglect, or abuse – the child may come to feel alienated from or hostile towards his or her body, which is perceived as the source of troubling, problematic feelings (Ritvo, 1984). This hostility or alienation from the body may constitute a risk factor for suicidality (King and Apter, 1996). Children with a history of physical abuse show elevated rates of self-mutilation and suicidal ideation and attempts (Green, 1978; Wagner, 1997), although a parental propensity for domestic violence and child abuse may also imply genetically transmissible vulnerabilities (e.g., impulsivity, aggressiveness) that influence the child in addition to the early experiential factors (cf. Chapter 4).

As part of a larger study of adolescent self-destructiveness and the capacity for self-care, we developed a questionnaire assessing adolescents' perceptions of parental attitudes towards their bodily care during childhood. In a sample of adolescent psychiatric inpatients, self-reported life-time history of suicide attempts, as well as the lethality and severity of intent of current (past-month) suicide attempts correlated significantly with perceived lack of empathic parental attentiveness to the child's physical care and perceived paternal physical punitiveness (King, Quinlan, Gammon, unpublished data).

Orbach and colleagues (1996a,b, 1997, 2001) employed a psychophysiological paradigm to assess suicidal adolescents' alienation from their bodies. Compared to psychiatric and normal controls or accident victims, suicidal adolescents had significantly elevated pain thresholds and increased tolerance for experimentally inflicted pain (Orbach et al., 1996b). In another study, Orbach and colleagues (1995) found that, compared to nonsuicidal depressed and normal adolescents, suicidal adolescents had more negative feelings towards their body (including greater perceived discrepancy between ideal and actual body features), and greater dissociative tendencies, with the magnitude of these measures correlating with the degree of suicidal tendencies. The authors speculated that these potential risk factors for suicidal behavior reflected early trauma and sadomasochistic relationships (Orbach, 1994). In this connection it is interesting to note that anorexics, who suppress pangs of hunger or discomfort and feel alienated from and wary of the body's needs, also have high rates of suicidal feelings and attempts (Apter et al., 1995).

## Adolescence as a developmental period of risk for suicide

Although the rate of completed suicide rises gradually with age throughout the life span for females in the U.S., in males it takes a large jump in adolescence and rises even higher in old age (Conwell, 2001; see also Chapter 1). If there are developmental vulnerabilities to depression and suicide, why do depression or suicidal behavior become manifest at one point in an individual's life rather than another?

Certain developmental epochs appear more vulnerable to the hazards of object or narcissistic loss. In elderly males, infirmity, such as the loss of a spouse, is a major trigger for suicide (Osgood and Thielman, 1990). In the case of illness or infirmity, the objective degree of physical impairment appears to be a less important predictor of suicide than its narcissistic impact on the individual. Based on the "disparity between aspiration and accomplishment," Shneidman (1971) was able to identify correctly four of the five suicides in his blind study of the data from the Terman long-term prospective study of gifted students; these suicides, however, did not occur before the fifth decade of life. Certain narcissistically organized individuals may decompensate in middle age, when they are unable to maintain the same level of accomplishment or attractiveness, when cumulative interpersonal difficulties catch up with them, or when it becomes clear that the fantasied rewards of success will not bring satisfaction (Kernberg, 1975).

As discussed elsewhere in this volume (Chapters 1 and 4), the increased rates of depression seen in adolescence are certainly one factor in the increased levels of suicidality seen in this developmental epoch. Risk factors such as a developmental propensity for recklessness, impulsivity, aggression, or problem behaviors (Clark et al., 1990; Jessor, 1991; Shaffer et al., 1988, 1996), with all of their potentially deleterious consequences, undoubtedly also play a role in the adolescent vulnerability to self-destructive behavior, including suicide (Chapter 2). In addition to these risk factors, however, adolescence also appears to be a period of particular vulnerability to object loss or narcissistic disappointment. The process of separating and individuating from parents leaves adolescents particularly sensitive to loss (King, 1990, 2002; Tabachnik, 1981). Friendships and romantic attachments take on a special intensity as a means of establishing independence from the family (A. Freud, 1958). Adolescents who are ambivalently attached to their families may have a propensity to turn to friends and romantic partners with particular intensity in order to find a substitute for the parental tie, but unfortunately frequently re-create the same stormy patterns in these new relationships. Since these friendships are frequently highly charged, but unstable, such youngsters are particularly vulnerable to suffer frequent and intense upsets around their disruption. Similarly, the need to prove one's worth through achievement takes on a new importance in adolescence as a means of establishing an identity; perceived failures, although appearing minor to others, may produce despair in the vulnerable adolescent.

## Conclusion

The psychodynamic perspective on youth suicide helps to supplement other biological, sociological, phenomenological, and nosological approaches. The challenge ahead is to develop better means of empirically studying these psychodynamic constructs and to harness them in the service of identifying more effective means of treatment and prevention.

### REFERENCES

Adams, K. S. (1990). Environmental, psychosocial, and psychoanalytic aspects of suicidal behavior. In Blumenthal, S. J., and Kupfer, D. J. (eds.) *Suicide over the Life Cycle: Risk Factors, Assessment, and Treatment of Suicidal Patients* (pp. 39–96). Washington DC: American Psychiatric Press.

Ainsworth, M. D. S., Blehar, M. C., Waters, E., and Wall, S. (1978). *Patterns of Attachment: A Psychological Study of the Strange Situation*. Hillsdale, NJ: Erlbaum.

Apter, A., Bleich, A., King, R. A., Kron, S., Fluch, A., Kotler, M., and Cohen, D. J. (1993). Death without warning? A clinical postmortem study of suicide in 43 Israeli adolescent males. *Archives of General Psychiatry*, **50**, 138–142.

Apter, A., Gothelf, D., Orbach, I., Weizman, R., Ratzoni, G., Har-Even, D., and Tyano, S. (1995). Correlation of suicidal and violent behavior in different diagnostic categories in hospitalized adolescent patients. *Journal of the American Academy of Child and Adolescent Psychiatry*, **34**, 912–918.

Arieti, S., and Bemporad, J. R. (1980). The psychological organization of depression. *American Journal of Psychiatry*, **137**, 1360–1365.

Baumeister, R. F. (1990). Suicide as escape from Self. *Psychological Review*, **97**, 90–113.

Beautrais, A. L. (2001). Child and young adolescent suicide in New Zealand. *Australian and New Zealand Journal of Psychiatry*, **35**(5), 647–653.

Beautrais, A. L., Joyce, P. R., and Mulder, R. T. (1997). Precipitating factors and life events in serious suicide attempts among youths aged 13 through 24 years. *Journal of the American Academy of Child and Adolescent Psychiatry*, **36**(11), 1543–1551.

Beck, A. T. (1983). Cognitive therapy of depression: new perspectives. In Clayton, P. J. and Barrett, J. E. (eds.) *Treatment of Depression: Old Controversies and New Approaches*. New York, NY: Raven Press.

Berkow, I. (1995). An athlete is dead at 17 and no one can say why. *The New York Times*. October 1, 1995, Sports section, pp. 1 and 7.

Bibring, E. (1953). The mechanism of depression. In Greenacre, P. (ed.) *Affective Disorders* (pp. 13–48). New York, NY: International University Press.

Blatt, S. J. (1995). The destructiveness of perfectionism: implications for the treatment of depression. *American Psychologist*, **50**, 1003–1020.

Blatt, S. J., and Homann, E. (1992). Parent–child interaction in the etiology of dependent and self-critical depression. *Clinical Psychology Review*, **12**, 47–91.

Blatt, S. J., Schaffer, C. E., Bers, S. A., and Quinlan, D. M. (1992). Psychometric properties of the Depressive Experiences Questionnaire for Adolescents. *Journal of Personality Assessment*, **59**, 82–98.

Blatt, S. J., Hart, B., Quinlan, D. M., Leadbeater, B., and Auerbach, J. (1993). Interpersonal and self-critical dysphoria and behavioral problems in adolescents. *Journal of Youth and Adolescence*, **22**, 253–269.

Blatt, S. J., Zuroff, D. C., Bondi, C. M., Sanislow, C. A. III, and Pilkonis, P. A. (1998). When and how perfectionism impedes the brief treatment of depression: further analyses of the National Institute of Mental Health Treatment of Depression Collaborative Research Program. *Journal of Consulting and Clinical Psychology*, **66**(2), 423–428.

Bowlby, J. (1973). *Attachment and Loss*, vol. II, *Separation*. New York, NY: Basic Books.

Bowlby, J. (1980). *Attachment and Loss*, vol. III, *Loss, Sadness and Depression*. New York, NY: Basic Books.

Brown, G. P., Hammen, C. L., Craske, M. G., and Wickens, T. D. (1995). Dimensions of dysfunctional attitudes as vulnerabilities to depressive symptoms. *Journal of Abnormal Psychology*, **104**(3), 431–435.

Brown, G. W., Harris, T. O., and Bifulco, A. (1986). Long-term effects of early loss of parent. In Rutter, M., Izard, C. E., and Read, S. B. (eds.) *Depression in Young People: Developmental and Clinical Perspectives* (pp. 251–296). New York, NY: Guilford.

Burge, D., Hammen, C., Davila, J., and Daley, S. E. (1997a). The relationship between attachment cognitions and psychological adjustment in late adolescent women. *Development and Psychopathology*, **9**(1), 151–167.

Burge, D., Hammen, C., Davila, J., Daley, S. E., et al. (1997b). Attachment cognitions and college and work functioning two years later in late adolescent women. *Journal of Youth and Adolescence*, **26**, 285–301.

Carlson, E. A., and Sroufe, L. A. (1995). Contributions of attachment theory to developmental psychopathology. In Cicchetti, D., and Cohen, D. J., (eds.) *Developmental Psychopathology*, vol. 1, *Theory and Methods* (pp. 581–617). New York, NY: John Wiley and Sons.

Clark, D. C., Sommerfeldt, L., and Schwarz, M., et al. (1990). Physical recklessness in adolescence: trait or byproduct of depressive/suicidal states? *The Journal of Nervous and Mental Disease*, **178**, 423–433.

Cohen-Sandler, R., Berman, A. L., and King, R. A. (1982a). A Follow-up Study of Hospitalized Suicidal Children. *Journal of the American Academy of Child Psychiatry*, **21**, 389–403.

Cohen-Sandler, R., Berman, A. L., and King, R. A. (1982b). Life stress and symptomatology: determinants of suicidal behavior in children. *Journal of the American Academy of Child Psychiatry*, **21**, 178–186.

Conwell, Y. (2001). Suicide in later life: a review and recommendations for prevention. *Suicide and Life-Threatening Behavior*, **31**(Suppl.), 32–47.

Daley, S. E., Hammen, C., Burge, D., Davila, J. et al. (1997). Predictors of the generation of episodic stress: a longitudinal study of late adolescent women. *Journal of Abnormal Psychology*, **106**(2), 251–259.

Dean, P. J., and Range, L. M. (1999). Testing the escape theory of suicide in an outpatient clinical population. *Cognitive Therapy and Research*, **23**(6), 561–572.

Dean, P. J., Range, L. M., and Goggin, W. C. (1996). The escape theory of suicide in college students: testing a model that includes perfectionism. *Suicide and Life-Threatening Behavior*, **26**(2), 181–186.

Dycian, A. (1995). Suicide in the Israeli Military – trends and changes [Abstract]. Paper presented at the International Conference on Understanding Youth Suicide, Tel Aviv, August 30, 1995.

Faazia, N. (2001). Dependency, self-criticism and suicidal behavior. Unpublished Master's Thesis, University of Windsor, Windsor, Ontario.

Freud, A. (1958). Adolescence. *Psychoanalytic Study of the Child*, **13**, 255–278.

Freud, A. (1965). *Normality and Pathology in Childhood: Assessments of Development*. New York, NY: International University Press.

Freud, S. (1917). Mourning and Melancholia. *The Standard Edition of the Complete Psychological Works of Sigmund Freud*, **14**, 289–300.

Freud, S. (1923). The Ego and the Id. *The Standard Edition of the Complete Psychological Works of Sigmund Freud*, **19**, 12–59.

Friedman, P. (ed.) (1967). *On Suicide: With Particular Reference to Suicide Among Young Students. Discussions of the Vienna Psychoanalytic Society – 1910*. New York, NY: International University Press.

Gould, M. S., King, R., Greenwald, S., Fisher, P., Schwab-Stone, M., Kramer, R., Flisher, A. J., Goodman, S., Canino, G., and Shaffer, D. (1998). Psychopathology associated with suicidal ideation and attempts among children and adolescents. *Journal of the American Academy of Child and Adolescent Psychiatry*, **37**, 915–923.

Green, A. H. (1978). Self-destructive behavior in battered children. *American Journal of Psychiatry*, **135**, 579–582.

Hamachek, D. E. (1978). Psychodynamics of normal and neurotic perfectionism. *Psychology*, **15**, 27–33.

Hammen, C. (2000). Interpersonal factors in an emerging developmental model of depression. In Johnson, S. L., Hayes, A. M., et al. (eds.) *Stress, Coping, and Depression* (pp. 71–88). Mahwah, NJ: Lawrence Erlbaum Associates.

Hammen, C., Ellicott A., Gitlin, M., and Jamison, K. R. (1989). Sociotrophy / autonomy and vulnerability to specific life events in patients with unipolar and bipolar disorder. *Journal of Abnormal Psychology*, **98**, 154–160.

Hawton, K., Cole, D., O'Grady, J., and Osborn, M. (1982). Motivational aspects of deliberate self-poisoning in adolescents. *British Journal of Psychiatry*, **141**, 286–291.

Hawton, K., Simkin, S., Fagg, J., and Hawkins, M. (1995). Suicide in Oxford University Students, 1976–1990. *British Journal of Psychiatry*, **166**, 44–50.

Hendin, H. (1991). Psychodynamics of suicide, with particular reference to the young. *American Journal of Psychiatry*, **148**, 1150–1158.

Herzberg, D. S., Hammen, C., Burge, D., Daley, S. E., Davila, J., and Lindberg, N. (1999). Attachment cognitions predict perceived and enacted social support during late adolescence. *Journal of Adolescent Research*, **14**(4), 387–404.

Hewitt, P. L., and Flett, G. L. (1991). Perfectionism in the self and social contexts: conceptualization, assessment, and association with psychopathology. *Journal of Personality and Social Psychology*, **60**, 456–470.

Hewitt, P. L., and Flett, G. L. (1993). Dimensions of perfectionism, daily stress, and depression: a test of the specific vulnerability hypothesis. *Journal of Abnormal Psychology*, **102**, 58–65.

Hewitt, P. L., Flett, G. L., and Turnbull-Donovan, W. (1992). Perfectionism and suicide potential. *British Journal of Clinical Psychology*, **31**(2), 181–190.

Hewitt, P. L., Flett, G. L., and Weber, C. (1994). Dimensions of perfectionism and suicide ideation. *Cognitive Therapy and Research*, **18**, 439–460.

Hewitt, P. L., Newton, J., Flett, G. L., and Callender, L. (1997). Perfectionism and suicide ideation in adolescent psychiatric patients. *Journal of Abnormal Child Psychology*, **25**, 95–101.

Jessor, R. (1991). Risk behavior in adolescence: a psychosocial framework for understanding and action. *Journal of Adolescent Health*, **12**, 597–605.

Kernberg, O. F. (1975). *Borderline Conditions and Pathological Narcissism.* New York, NY: Jason Aronson.

Khantzian, E. J., and Mack, J. E. (1983). Self-preservation and the care of the Self. *Psychoanalytic Study of the Child,* **38,** 209–232.

Kienhorst, I. C. W. M., DeWilde, E. J., Diekstra, R. F. W., and Wolters, W. H. G. (1995). Adolescents' image of their suicide attempt. *Journal of the American Academy of Child and Adolescent Psychiatry,* **34,** 623–628.

King, R. A. (1990). Child and adolescent suicide. In Michels, R. (ed.) *Psychiatry,* vol. 2. Philadelphia, PA: Lippincott Co.

King, R. A. (2002). Adolescence. In Lewis, M. (ed.) *Comprehensive Textbook of Child and Adolescent Psychiatry,* 3rd edn. (pp. 332–342). Baltimore, MD: Lippincott Williams and Wilkins.

King, R. A., and Apter, A. (1996). Psychoanalytic perspectives on adolescent suicide. *Psychoanalytic Study of the Child,* **51,** 491–511.

Koestner, R., Zuroff, D. C., and Powers, T. A. (1991). Family origins of adolescent self-criticism and its continuity into adulthood. *Journal of Abnormal Psychology,* **100,** 191–197.

Kuperminc, G. P., Blatt, S. J., and Leadbeater, B. J. (1997). Relatedness, self-definition, and early adolescent adjustment. *Cognitive Therapy and Research,* **21**(3) 301–320.

Leadbeater, B. J., Blatt, S. J., and Quinlan, D. M. (1995). Gender-linked vulnerabilities to depressive symptoms, stress, and problem behaviors in adolescents. *Journal of Research on Adolescence,* **5**(1), 1–29.

Lewis, N. A. (1996). Military strives to reduce a relatively low suicide rate. *The New York Times,* May 19, p.18.

Lieblich, A. (1981). *Kibbutz Makom.* New York, NY: Pantheon Books.

Luthar, S., and Blatt, S. J. (1995). Differential vulnerability of dependency and self-criticism among disadvantaged teenagers. *Journal of Research on Adolescence,* **5**(4), 431–449.

Main, M., and Goldwyn, R. (1989). *Adult Attachment Rating and Classification System.* Unpublished scoring manual, Department of Psychology, University of California, Berkeley, CA.

Negron, R., Piacentini, J., Graae, F., Davies, M., and Shaffer, D. (1997). Microanalysis of adolescent suicide attempters and ideators during the acute suicidal episode. *Journal of the American Academy of Child and Adolescent Psychiatry,* **36**(11), 1512–1519.

Neubauer, J. (1992). *The Fin-de-Siecle Culture of Adolescence.* New Haven, CN: Yale University Press.

Orbach, I. (1988). *Children Who Don't Want to Live.* San Francisco, CA: Jossey-Bass.

Orbach, I. (1994). Dissociation, physical pain, and suicide: a hypothesis. *Suicide and Life-Threatening Behavior,* **24**(1), 68–79.

Orbach, I., Lotem-Peleg, M., and Kedem, P. (1995). Attitudes towards the body in suicidal, depressed, and normal adolescents. *Suicide and Life-Threatening Behavior,* **25,** 211–221.

Orbach, I., Palgi, Y., Stein, D., Har-Even, D., Lotem-Peleg, M., Asherov, J., and Elizur, A. (1996a). Tolerance for physical pain in suicidal subjects. *Death Studies,* **20**(4), 327–341.

Orbach, I., Stein, D., Palgi, Y., Asherov, J., Har-Even, D., and Elizur, A. (1996b). Perception of physical pain in accident and suicide attempt patients: self-preservation vs self-destruction. *Journal of Psychiatric Research,* **30**(4), 307–320.

Orbach, I., Mikulincer, M., King, R., Cohen, D., Stein, D., and Apter, A. (1997). Thresholds and tolerance of physical pain in suicidal and non-suicidal patients. *Journal of Consulting and Clinical Psychology*, **65**, 646–652.

Orbach, I., Mikulincer, M., Blumenson, R., Mester, R., and Stein, D. (1999). The subjective experience of problem irresolvability and suicidal behavior: dynamics and measurement. *Suicide and Life-Threatening Behavior*, **29**(2), 150–164.

Orbach, I., Stein, D., Shan-Sela, M., and Har-Even, D. (2001). Body attitudes and body experiences in suicidal adolescents. *Suicide and Life-Threatening Behavior*, **31**(3), 237–249.

Osgood, N. J., and Thielman, S. (1990). Geriatric suicidal behavior: assessment and treatment. In Blumenthal, S. J., and Kupfer, D. J. (eds.) *Suicide Over the Life Cycle: Risk Factors, Assessment, and Treatment of Suicidal Patients* (pp. 39–96). Washington DC: American Psychiatric Press.

Priel, B., and Shahar, G. (2000). Dependency, self-criticism, social context and distress: comparing moderating and mediating models. *Personality and Individual Differences*, **28**(3), 515–525.

Priel, B., Mitrany, D., and Shahar, G. (1998). Closeness, support and reciprocity: a study of attachment styles in adolescence. *Personality and Individual Differences*, **25**(6), 1183–1197.

Ritvo, S. (1984). The image and uses of the body in psychic conflict. *Psychoanalytic Study of the Child*, **39**, 449–469.

Rourke, B. P., Young, G. C., and Leenaars, A. A. (1989). A childhood learning disability that predisposes those afflicted to adolescent and adult depression and suicide risk. **22**, 169–174

Rudolph, K. D., Hammen, C., Burge, D., Lindberg, N., Herzberg, D., and Daley, S. E. (2000). Toward an interpersonal life-stress model of depression: the developmental context of stress generation. *Development and Psychopathology*, **12**(2), 215–234.

Shaffer, D. (1974). Suicide in childhood and early adolescence. *Journal of Child Psychology and Psychiatry*, **15**, 275–291.

Shaffer, D., Garland, A., Gould, M., Fisher, P., and Trautman, P. (1988). Preventing teen-age suicide: a critical review. *Journal of the American Academy of Child and Adolescent Psychiatry*, **27**, 675–687.

Shaffer, D., Gould, M. S., Fischer, P., Trautman, P., Moreau, D., Kleinman, M., and Flory, M. (1996). Psychiatric diagnosis in child and adolescent suicide. *Archives of General Psychiatry*, **53**, 339–348.

Shahar, G. (2001). Personality, shame, and the breakdown of social bonds: the voice of quantitative depression research. *Psychiatry: Interpersonal and Biological Processes*, **64**(3), 228–239.

Shahar, G., and Priel B. (2003). Active vulnerability, adolescent distress, and the mediating/suppressing role of life events. *Personality and Individual Differences* (in press).

Shahar, G., Blatt, S. J., Zuroff, D. C., Krupnick, J., and Sotsky, S. M. (2003). Perfectionism impiedes social relations and response to brief treatment of depression. *Journal of Social and Clinical Psychology* (in press).

Shneidman, E. S. (1971). Perturbation and lethality as precursors of suicide in a gifted group. *Suicide and Life-Threatening Behavior*, **1**.

Shneidman, E. S. (1989). Overview: a multidimensional approach to suicide. In Jacobs, D., and Brown, H. N. (eds.) *Suicide: Understanding and Responding* (pp. 1–30). Madison, CT: International Universities Press.

Tabachnik, N. (1981). The interlocking psychologies of suicide and adolescence. *Adolescent Psychi-atry*, **9**, 399–410.

Tennant, C. (1988). Parental loss in childhood: its effect in adult life. *Archives of General Psychiatry*, **45**, 1045–1050.

Thernstrom, M. (1996). Diary of a murder. *The New Yorker*, June 3, pp. 62–71.

Trillin, C. (1993). *Remembering Denny*. New York, NY: Farrar, Straus and Giroux.

Tzur, M. (1974). *Not in a Coat of Many Colors (Le lo Kutonet Pasim)*. Tel Aviv: Am Oved.

Tzur, M. (1979). That which is not yet will build that which is. (Ma she'od eynenu yivne et ma she'yesh). *Shdemot*, **71**, 72–76.

Wagner, B. M. (1997). Family risk factors for child and adolescent suicidal behavior. *Psychological Bulletin*. **121**, 246–298.

Weller, R. A., Weller, E. B., Fristad, M. A., and Bowes, J. M. (1991). Depression in recently bereaved prepubertal children. *American Journal of Psychiatry*, **148**, 1536–1540.

White, H. C. (1974). Self-poisoning in adolescents. *British Journal of Psychiatry*, **124**, 24–35.

Winnicott, D. W. (1958). The capacity to be alone. In *The Maturational Process and the Facilitating Environment*, (pp. 29–36). New York, NY: International Universities Press. 1965.

Zuroff, D. C., Blatt, S. J., Sotsky, S. M., Krupnick, J. L., Martin, D. J., Sanislow, C. A. III, and Simmens, S. (2000). Relation of therapeutic alliance and perfectionism to outcome in brief outpatient treatment of depression. *Journal of Consulting and Clinical Psychology*, **68**(1), 114–124.

# 7

# Cross-cultural variation in child and adolescent suicide

Michael J. Kelleher and Derek Chambers

## Introduction

This chapter endeavors to explore the relationship between cultural influences and child and adolescent suicide in several empirical ways. The World Health Organization (WHO) figures for suicides in young people worldwide are reviewed. In doing so, we will examine the influence of cultural factors, using the work of Ronald Inglehart (1990, 1997) to divide by "type" the countries for which youth suicide rates are available. Inglehart (1997) employs the World Values Surveys (World Values Study Group, 1994) to "explore the hypothesis that mass belief systems are changing in ways that have important economic, political, and social consequences." Finally, the suicide rates of children as well as younger and older adolescents will be examined in one country, the Republic of Ireland, that has recently experienced a considerable change in suicide rates, in order to examine the explanatory power of cultural interpretations.

## Cultural sources of international epidemiological differences

A cultural explanation may be sought for international differences in the rates of child and adolescent suicide, as returned to the WHO. Cultural factors may also explain further differences, including the ratio of male to female suicide rates and differences in the methods used. Analysis of international variation in adolescent suicide rates is confounded by inconsistent recording practices, but this inconsistency in itself reflects social and cultural influences. For example, a study of the member countries of The International Association for Suicide Prevention found that the countries with religious sanctions against suicide returned lower suicide rates to the WHO and, indeed, the countries with religious sanctions were more likely not to return any rates of suicide at all (Kelleher et al., 1998a).

Further differences, in relation to method, appear to be influenced by differential access to means of self-harm in different societies. For example, jumping from a height is more common in commercial and residential areas that are characterized by a high density of multi-storey buildings, while the use of firearms in suicide seems to be more prevalent in rural areas and in societies with a "gun culture," such as the larger American cities. The choice of method thus reflects the influence of a particular culture.

## Defining suicide and the concept of suicide in children and adolescents

The concept of culture has been variably defined from many different perspectives. From a socio-psychological point of view it has been defined as "the system of information that codes the manner in which the people in an organized group, society or nation interact with their social and physical environment" (Reber, 1985). This implies the learning of rules, regulations, values and modes of interacting within and without the social group. This learning of a culture, or socialization, includes the learning or development of culturally specific concepts of death, in general, and suicide in particular (Canetto and Silverman, 1998).

The definition of suicide as applied to children and adolescents may also be problematic. "To intentionally bring about one's own death" may suffice as a brief definition of suicide in adults. Children, however, may mature and individuate at different rates in different cultures. Hence the concept of intention may, itself, be the subject of cultural variation.

With regard to recording practices, child suicide in particular is subject to case-specific and cultural influences, as suicidal intent in children can be extremely difficult to establish postmortem "beyond reasonable doubt." Even if suicide is recorded in a particular jurisdiction on the basis of the "balance of probability," the issue of determining intention remains a significant factor that is difficult to assess.

Death may convey different meanings to children and adolescents around the world. Just as the goings and comings of attachment figures may not be seen as permanent, children may also not conceive death as permanent. Not only is the concept of intention influenced by cultural variation, but it is likely that the development of the concept of suicide also influences actual rates among children and adolescents.

This development is thought to be influenced by exposure to suicidal behavior or the completed suicide of siblings, parents, peers or neighbors (Shafii, 1989). Pillay (1995) speculates that, because of the influence of peers, significant others, and the media, children's perceptions of suicidal and self-destructive behavior may be a significant factor in the onset of such behavior and in its prediction and prevention. So while suicide under the age of 10 years is rare, it does occur.

Indeed, it has been reported that almost all children in Canada have a basic understanding of suicide by grade 5 (9–10 years old) (Ministry of National Health and Welfare Canada, 1994). Another likely cultural influence on child and adolescent suicide is variation in child-rearing practices that influence the nature of children's relationships with the world around them.

## Inaccurate assumptions and real differences

International variations in suicide rates from countries around the world reflect the different social conditions and changes in each country. While there are many widespread assumptions about suicide, research has shown vast international differences in age- and gender-specific rates worldwide that contradict these assumptions. For example, the idea that suicide is universally a predominantly male phenomenon is inaccurate. In fact, in a number of countries, WHO figures reveal rates of suicide among girls and young women that are higher than among young males. This is the case in both Brazil and Cuba (Barraclough, 1988) as well as in those regions of mainland China for which rates are returned (He and Lester, 1997; Yip, 2001). Regional studies also find that among the Maring people of Papua New Guinea, only females commit suicide (Healey, 1979), while in the Deganga region of India, women constitute more than two-thirds of all suicides (Banerjee et al., 1990).

Despite these exceptions, male suicide rates are, in general, higher than female rates. However, considerable variation exists in the ratio of male-to-female suicide rates. Between 1988 and 1992, the average ratio of male-to-female young suicides (aged 15–24 years) varied from 1.1:1 in Mauritius to 7.1:1 in the Republic of Ireland, with Tajikistan returning higher female rates than male rates in this age group.

Inaccurate preconceptions regarding perceived cultural differences distort perceptions of suicide in other cultures. For example, the media and popular culture often imply an acceptance of suicide in Japanese culture. Indeed, scholars from various disciplines have focused on the apparent difference in attitude to suicide and suicidal behavior in Japan as compared to western countries (Takahashi, 1997). Takahashi points out that overemphasis on culturally specific aspects of suicidal behaviour in Japan – such as World War II *kamikaze* pilots or *hara-kiri*– have encouraged a "myth" that suicide is relatively common in Japan. References to the presumed high academic stress on Japanese youth, such as the experience of "examination hell" (Reischauer and Jansen, 1995), imply that Japanese youth are a high-risk group due to a particularly competitive education system. Yet, as Takahashi points out, the suicide rate in Japan has been decreasing since the 1950s and the average rates there for 1988–1992 are relatively low in international terms. Indeed, the age-specific suicide rate for 15- to 24-year-old Japanese males is lower than those for all of the English-speaking or Northern European countries.

Marked differences also exist across countries in the epidemiology of youth suicide in terms of preferred choice of method (e.g., Bignall, 1993; Central Statistics Office Ireland, 1976–2001; Commonwealth Department of Health and Family Services Australia, 1997; Ho et al., 1995; Office for National Statistics, England and Wales, 1994; Shaffer et al., 1988). Availability or access to means appears to strongly influence the choice of method. For example, in Hong Kong, with its considerable density of high-rise buildings, jumping from a height is the commonest method of suicide and between 1990 and 1992 accounted for over two-thirds of the suicides in the under-30-year-old age group (Ho, 1996). In the U.S., where gun licensing laws are relatively unrestrictive, firearms account for more than half of all youth suicides (Lipschitz, 1995). Similarly, among the wealthiest nations, Finland reports both the highest youth suicide rate and the highest firearms-related youth suicide rate (Johnson et al., 2000). In the Kuopio region of Finland, 62% of all 15- to 24-year-old male suicides were committed by shooting and licensed guns were used in 74% of these acts (Hintikka et al., 1997). In contrast, in Ireland, where gun licensing laws are restrictive and tall buildings are scarce, hanging is the primary method among young males, while self-poisoning, drowning, and hanging are the prevalent methods among young females (Central Statistics Office Ireland, 1976–2001). Hanging is also the primary method of youth suicide (15- to 24-year olds) in Australia, accounting for 39% of suicides. Drowning would appear to be extremely rare in Australia, as no figures are reported for this method by the Commonwealth Department of Health and Family Services Australia (1997). Rates of paracetamol-(acetaminophen-) related suicide vary by nation depending on national policies limiting package size or requiring prescription (Gunnell et al., 2000). In many poor and agricultural areas (including Fiji, Sri Lanka, and Trinidad), paraquat, a widely available but highly lethal herbicide, is a very common means of suicide (Hutchinson et al., 1999).

Recognition of these differences is not to deny that suicide reflects universal elements of our very humanity, but rather to acknowledge the social and cultural influences on this most individual of acts. Therefore, while there are common characteristics of all acts of suicide, the physical and social environment influences both the aggregate rate and the means of committing suicide in a particular society.

## Social change

The current social trends towards large-scale globalization, increased economic security, and the shift towards postmodernist values provide the best perspective for understanding worldwide differences in youth suicide. Changes in the value system of any society reflect the values of its young population, as they are often the most sensitive to social change (Arnett, 1999; Schlegel, 2000). Inglehart (1997) observes that in countries that have experienced economic growth and increasing economic security, postmaterial values tend to be emphasized more heavily by the younger birth cohorts. (Postmaterial values reflect a more fragmented social structure where class or race are unimportant and the construction of individual identity is by personal choice and not by ascription.) Thus, existential security leads to a rise in postmodern values.

At the same time, the rise in youth suicide is unevenly distributed worldwide and may be associated with the shift towards postmodernism as experienced in the so-called developed countries. Indeed, it has been speculated that modern society, as it is developing, "fails to meet the most fundamental requirements of any culture, i.e., to provide a sense of purpose and belonging, and so a sense of meaning and self-worth, and a moral framework to guide our conduct" (Eckersley, 1993, p.16 abstract).

The conditions described by Eckersley imply an increase in *anomie*, the term employed by Durkheim to describe normlessness and moral deregulation, which he believed carried with it a greater susceptibility to suicide (Durkheim, 1897/1993). To this end, it is useful to consider the conditions in Hong Kong, where indicators of normlessness and deregulation such as crime rate, drug abuse rate, and unemployment have remained steady over the past 30 years, as has the overall suicide rate. In fact, the rate for young females has actually decreased in the time period 1963–1992 (Ho, 1996). The same trend has been found in other Asian countries that have also enjoyed low levels of anomie, in particular as indicated by stable levels of unemployment.

This stability stands in stark contrast to western countries where a consistent rise in youth suicide (Cantor, 2000; Johnson et al., 2000; Retterstøl, 1993) has coincided with a period of social deregulation, whereby the traditional social institutions such as the Church, the state, and the family become less influential (Giddens, 1983). In particular, there has been a disproportionate rise in young male suicides under the age of 35 throughout Western Europe (Pritchard, 1996).

## Comparative analysis of national youth suicide rates

### Methodology

*World Health Statistics Annuals* (WHO, 1989–1995) were used to calculate five-year averages for the time period bracketing the study period of the most recent World Values Survey (1991–1993) (World Values Study Group, 1994). (For the most recent statistics, see WHO, 2001 and Table 1.2.) The age-specific suicide statistics for young people reported in the *WHO Statistics Annuals* are unfortunately only available in 10-year age bands. From a developmental and social psychology perspective, more specific data on 10- to 14-year-old and 15- to 19-year-old age-specific suicide rates would be of greater scientific value.

The World Values Survey (1991–1993) (World Values Study Group, 1994) was then used to divide countries by type, following the work of Inglehart. Inglehart (1990, 1997) grouped countries as defined by their position in relation to postmodernism (as measured by the Values Surveys), as well as proximate geographical location, shared language, or common cultural background. For example, the English-speaking countries are bound by a common history within the British Empire. Although the groupings of countries in such a crude manner may be open to debate, the extensive research into values and attitudes of societies worldwide, in particular the World Values Survey, provides an important framework for international comparison.

However, not all of the countries that return suicide rates for young people are covered by Inglehart's scheme. Of the 46 countries for which comprehensive youth suicide figures for the years 1988–1992 were available, only 31 are covered in the World Values Surveys. In the case of the United Kingdom, rates were obtained for each separate jurisdiction as well as for the whole United Kingdom, while in the World Values Surveys the United Kingdom is treated as two separate jurisdictions, Britain and Northern Ireland.

For those countries not included in Inglehart's work, we have grouped them based on the WHO regional divisions. Classifying the nation states that have emerged in the wake of the redrawing of the political map of Eastern Europe was particularly problematic. For example, in the *United Nations Demographic Yearbook* (United Nations, 1995) the following former-Soviet Union countries are considered South Central Asian: Kazakstan, Kyrgyzstan, Tajikistan, Turkmenistan, and Uzbekistan, while Azerbaijan is considered to be Western Asian. All of these countries are in the European region of the WHO and, because of their geographical location in relation to the former Eastern Bloc, are considered Eastern European/former Soviet Union for the purpose of this study, despite the prominence of other cultural influences on them.

Two other anomalous countries that were excluded from the World Values Survey, Israel and Mauritius, are considered independently of other countries. Mauritius was the only African state that returned comprehensive mortality data over the period of the study. Not obviously associated with any specific part of

**Table 7.1.** Countries examined, by cultural "type"

| | |
|---|---|
| Eastern Europe/former Soviet Union: | Estonia, Russia, Kazakstan, Slovenia, Latvia, Lithuania, Hungary, Croatia, Poland, Czech Republic, Kyrgyzstan, Moldova, Turkmenistan, Bulgaria, Uzbekistan, Tajikistan, and Azerbaijan |
| Northern Europe: | Finland, Norway, Switzerland, Sweden, Germany, Denmark, and The Netherlands |
| English-speaking: | New Zealand, Australia, Canada, United States of America, Scotland, Republic of Ireland, Northern Ireland, United Kingdom and England & Wales |
| Catholic Europe: | Austria, France, Spain, Portugal, Italy, and Greece |
| Asian: | Singapore, Japan, and Hong Kong |
| Latin American: | Argentina and Mexico |
| Others: | Israel and Mauritius (Africa) |

Europe, Israel is included by WHO in the European region, while the United Nations Demographic Yearbook classifies it as Western Asian.

Although disproportionately western, the reporting countries represent diverse cultures including Eastern Europe, Catholic Europe, Latin America, Africa, and Asia. As well as examining the five-year average rates for young people in these countries, the gender ratio in youth suicide rates are calculated. The countries examined, listed by "type" are shown in Table 7.1.

Because the WHO does not report methods of suicide, a comparison is made between several countries, chosen from the available literature, for which the prevalence of given methods appear markedly different.

## Results

The figures, where available, reveal significant differences between countries in different geographical and cultural groupings. For example, Finland in Northern Europe has an average rate for 15- to 24-year-old males of 43.7 per 100 000 compared with Japan (9.7), Mexico (5.2), and Azerbaijan (3.4). Rates for 15- to 24-year-old females have an even wider range, from 0.8 per 100 000 in Greece to 17.3 per 100 000 in Mauritius.

Rates for 5- to 14-year-olds tell their own story. The numbers of suicide in this age group are low, with the male suicide rate varying from 0.1 (England & Wales) to 1.6 per 100 000 (Hungary) for the period 1988–1992. The age-specific suicide rate for 5- to 14-year-old females varies from none in England & Wales and Ireland to 0.4 per 100 000 in Hungary and Norway for the same five-year period.

In the sections that follow we will examine this diversity in suicide rates for each gender in more detail.

### Rates for young males

The reported age-specific rates of 15- to 24-year-old male suicides vary almost 12-fold from Azerbaijan (3.4 per 100 000) to Finland (43.7 per 100 000) (Figure 7.1). Of the traditionally Catholic European countries, only Austria (25.9 per 100 000) reports a higher rate than the international mean of 16.7. Similarly, the Asian states of Singapore, Japan, and Hong Kong all report rates lower than average. While these figures would appear to represent a pattern, there is also great variability even within groupings, with the rates for Northern European and Eastern European/former Soviet Union countries, as well as the English-speaking countries, showing greater diversity. Indeed the Eastern European/former Soviet Union countries vary greatly from the lowest reported figures in Tajikistan and Azerbaijan to some of the highest figures in Estonia, Russia, and Kazakstan. The Eastern European/former Soviet Union grouping, however, contains a tremendous diversity in terms of language, religion, economic and political situation, and culture. Indeed, with the exception of Kazakstan, it is those Eastern European/former Soviet Union countries that are closer to Asia, geographically and culturally, that have lower than average suicide rates for this age group.

It is remarkable that for the 5- to 14-year-old males (Figure 7.2), the 11 highest age-specific suicide rates are all from Eastern European/former Soviet Union countries. In contrast, the three East Asian countries examined return lower than average rates. All of the traditionally Catholic European countries report below-average rates for the 5- to 14-year-old males. As with the rates for 15- to 24-year-old males, English-speaking and Northern European Countries do not display a readily apparent pattern. Representing Latin America, Argentina and Mexico have lower rates than the mean for both age groups of young males.

### Rates for young females

Compared to young male suicide rates, there is even wider variance in the suicide rates of young women (aged 15–24 years) across the various country groupings. The most notable feature of Figure 7.3 is the high suicide rate for 15- to 24-year-old females in Mauritius (17.3 per 100 000), which is over three times greater than the international mean rate of 5.1 per 100 000. As with young male suicides, the rates of young female suicide for the Eastern European countries are generally quite high, with the exception of Azerbaijan. Paralleling the high rate of 15- to 24-year-old male suicides, Austria has the highest rate for young female suicides of all the Catholic European countries – 6.1 per 100 000. Young female suicide

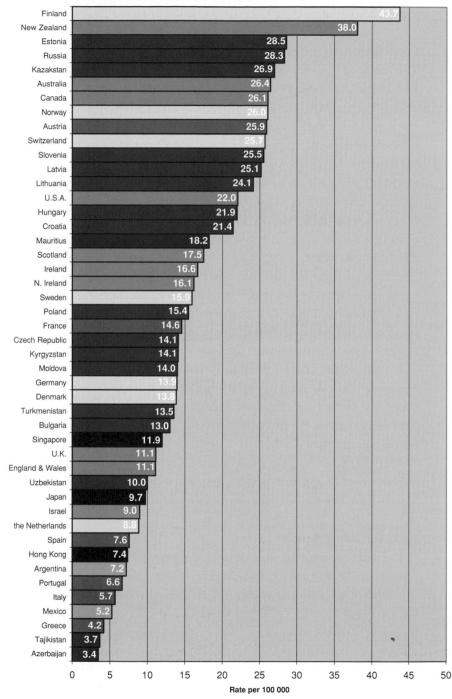

**Average male 15- to 24-year-old suicide, 1988–1992**

| Country | Rate |
|---|---|
| Finland | 43.7 |
| New Zealand | 38.0 |
| Estonia | 28.5 |
| Russia | 28.3 |
| Kazakstan | 26.9 |
| Australia | 26.4 |
| Canada | 26.1 |
| Norway | 26.0 |
| Austria | 25.9 |
| Switzerland | 25.7 |
| Slovenia | 25.5 |
| Latvia | 25.1 |
| Lithuania | 24.1 |
| U.S.A. | 22.0 |
| Hungary | 21.9 |
| Croatia | 21.4 |
| Mauritius | 18.2 |
| Scotland | 17.5 |
| Ireland | 16.6 |
| N. Ireland | 16.1 |
| Sweden | 15.9 |
| Poland | 15.4 |
| France | 14.6 |
| Czech Republic | 14.1 |
| Kyrgyzstan | 14.1 |
| Moldova | 14.0 |
| Germany | 13.9 |
| Denmark | 13.8 |
| Turkmenistan | 13.5 |
| Bulgaria | 13.0 |
| Singapore | 11.9 |
| U.K. | 11.1 |
| England & Wales | 11.1 |
| Uzbekistan | 10.0 |
| Japan | 9.7 |
| Israel | 9.0 |
| the Netherlands | 8.8 |
| Spain | 7.6 |
| Hong Kong | 7.4 |
| Argentina | 7.2 |
| Portugal | 6.6 |
| Italy | 5.7 |
| Mexico | 5.2 |
| Greece | 4.2 |
| Tajikistan | 3.7 |
| Azerbaijan | 3.4 |

Rate per 100 000

Figure 7.1  Average male 15–24 years suicide rate per 100 000, 1988–1992.

Current Check-Outs summary for Burkhardt
Thu Jan 12 14:24:13 PST 2012

BARCODE: 35369002738498
TITLE: Suicide in children and adolescen
DUE DATE: Feb 02 2012

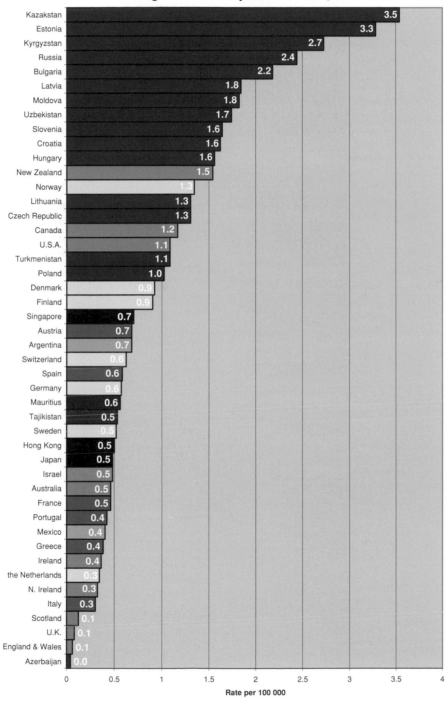

Figure 7.2  Average male 5–14 years suicide rate per 100 000, 1988–1992.

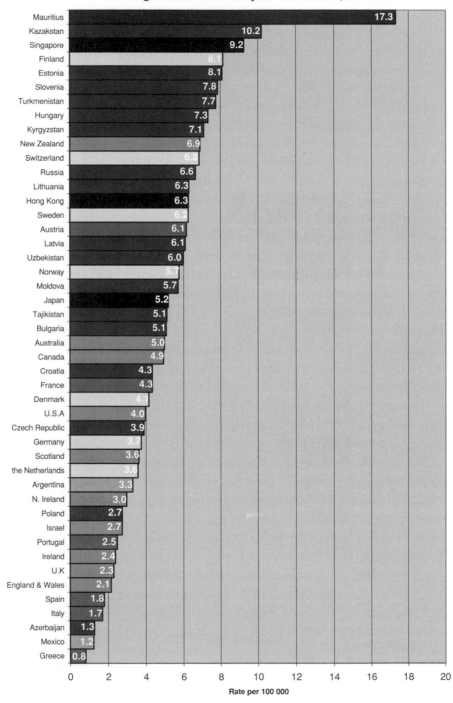

Figure 7.3  Average female 15–24 years suicide rate per 100 000, 1988–1992.

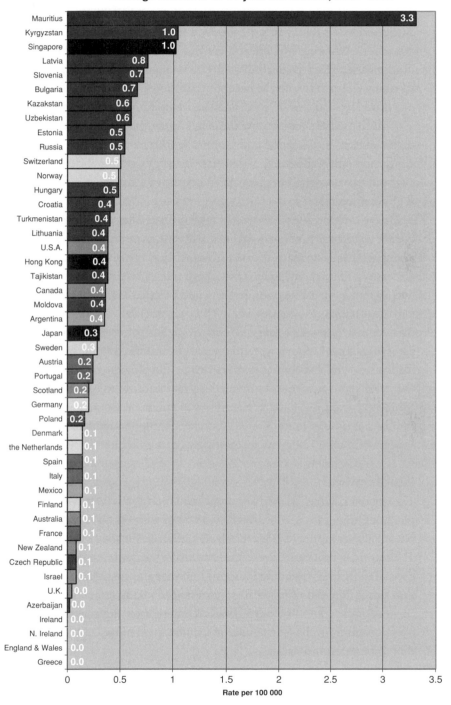

Figure 7.4  Average female 5–14 years suicide rate per 100 000, 1988–1992.

rates in the Northern European countries vary from the Netherlands to Finland, with rates of 3.6 and 8.1 per 100 000 respectively. Paralleling the pattern of young suicide rates across Western European countries, the northern Scandinavian countries – Norway, Sweden, and Finland – return higher rates than most of the other Western European countries. The young female suicide rates for English-speaking countries, with the exception of New Zealand, are all below the mean of 5.1 per 100 000, as are Israel and the Latin American countries of Argentina and Mexico. Cross-national patterns in suicide rates are not always similar for males and females (Canetto and Silverman, 1998). For example, Singapore, Hong Kong, and Japan all return higher than average age-specific rates for 15- to 24-year-old females whereas these Asian countries return lower than average rates for young males.

Due to the extremely low suicide rates returned for 5- to 14-year-old females, it is difficult to interpret cross-national patterns. Several countries report average age-specific suicide rates for this group of less than 0.1 per 100 000. It is also interesting that Finland, which has a high rate of suicide for young males overall and for females between the ages of 15 and 24, returns a below-average rate of 0.1 per 100 000 for 5- to 14-year-old girls. In contrast, the 3.3 per 100 000 age-specific suicide rate for 5- to 14-year-old females for Mauritius dramatically exceeds the rates for all other reporting nations and is over three times greater than the rates for the next highest countries, Kyrgyzstan and Singapore. In general, however, the pattern of suicide rates for 5- to 14-year-old females is similar to the pattern for 15- to 24-year-old females and for young males across Catholic Europe (low); Azerbaijan (lowest in the Eastern Europe/former Soviet Union grouping); and Singapore, Hong Kong and Japan (high).

**Gender ratios**

The gender ratio of young male-to-female suicides also varies widely by national grouping (Figure 7.5). For example, the below-average suicide rate for young Asian males and the above-average suicide rate for young Asian females yield a relatively very low gender ratio for youth suicide in Asia (see also Yip, 2001), considerably lower than the international mean of 3.6. It has been hypothesized that this is due to poorer social conditions for young females in these countries (Barraclough, 1988; Pritchard, 1996). Despite their high level of technological advance, many of these societies have maintained more traditional gender roles than have western societies.

In contrast, English-speaking countries all have a gender ratio for youth suicide that is considerably higher than the international mean of 3.6. Of these countries, the Republic of Ireland has the highest ratio (7.1:1) which might best be explained

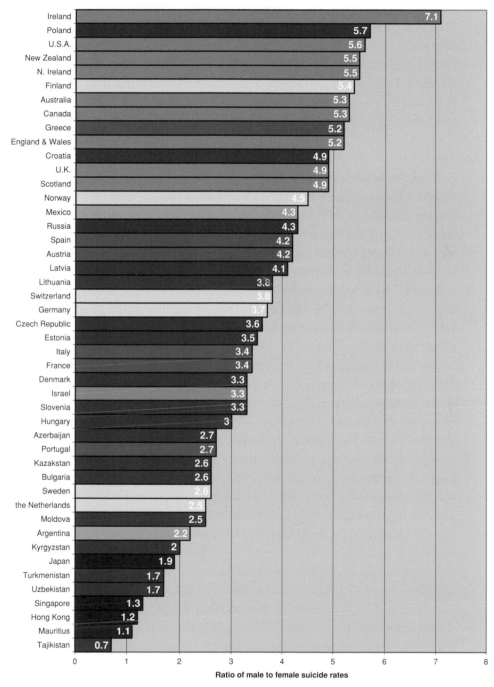

Figure 7.5  Gender ratio of 15- to 24-year-old suicides, 1988–1992.

by a combination of factors. First, the overall rise in the Irish suicide rate has occurred disproportionately in young rural males (Kelleher et al., 2002), while, in contrast, both the social conditions and expectations of young Irish females have risen considerably. For example, in 1995, for the first time in Irish national history, the number of female students in higher education outnumbered male students. Thus, an improvement in life-chances for young Irish women has coincided with a negative period for young Irish men in terms of uncertainty over changing gender roles in areas such as employment and family life.

## Discussion

### Culture and methods of suicide

As noted, the prevalence of different methods of suicide varies across societies, reflecting both ease of access and cultural influences. The impact of these differences on suicide rates is controversial. Two schools of thought dominate this area of suicidology, represented by the *availability hypothesis* and the *substitution hypothesis* (Marzuk et al., 1992).

Broadly speaking, the availability hypothesis suggests that differences in rates are directly influenced by the extent of the availability of lethal means of self-harm. In support of this thesis, Kreitman's (1976) celebrated study of the rates of suicide in England during the period of detoxification of domestic gas in the 1960s reported an overall decrease in suicide rates. However, other studies have suggested that restricting access to lethal means of self-harm only increases the use of more readily available means. For example, Marzuk et al. (1992) refer to a study in Ontario (Sloan et al., 1990) that concluded that when stricter gun control laws were passed in the late 1970s, the subsequent decline in the firearm suicide rate was accompanied by a rise in suicide by jumping from a height. A further study of Toronto and Quebec City (Rich et al., 1990) before and after the introduction of gun control legislation reported similar findings. In contrast, however, Lester and Leenaars (1993) and Carrington and Moyer (1994) observed reductions in firearm suicide rates without substitution of alternative methods.

Recent data from the U.S. (Birckmayer and Hemenway, 2001; Brent, 2001) underline the facilitating role of firearm availability with respect to impulsive suicide in youth. Community studies find that the association between suicide and firearms in the home is particularly high in the under-25-year-old age group. In adolescents under 16 years old, the risk for suicide attributable to home gun availability was greater than that due to psychopathology (Brent et al., 1999). A gun in the home confers a threefold elevation in risk for suicide in individuals with psychiatric disorder; however, for individuals without psychiatric disorder, a gun in the home conveys a 32- to 33-fold increased risk for suicide, illustrating the role firearms play in impulsive suicide even for individuals without diagnosable psychopathology (Brent, 2001; Brent et al., 1993a, 1993b; Kellerman et al., 1992).

How then can these opposing views on the effect of access to method be reconciled? Lester (1990) suggests that rates among those whose suicidal behavior may be deemed "impulsive" are most likely to be affected by ease of access to lethal means. Since impulsivity appears to play a significant role in youthful suicide and suicide attempts, the availability of various lethal methods of potential self-harm (such as firearms) may be particularly significant with regard to the epidemiology of suicide in young people.

The importance of availability or access to means of self-harm is further emphasized by trends in gender-specific suicidal behavior. While, in the western world at least, female suicides have traditionally been characterized by more passive means such as overdose, in Hong Kong the more violent method of jumping from a height accounted for the majority of young female suicides in 1986–1992 (Ho et al., 1995). Recently, however, the preferred method of choice by gender is changing in western countries (postmodern countries) perhaps reflecting the move away from traditionally defined gender roles in society (Brent et al., 1991; De Leo et al., 1995; Fischer et al., 1993; Pritchard, 1996).

Gender-specific choice of method of suicide in turn influences the ratio of male and female suicide rates. For example, jumping from a height, the preferred method for both genders in Hong Kong, is particularly lethal with minimal likelihood of surviving an impulsive attempt. In contrast, in Ireland, the prevalent method of self-harm among females is self-poisoning, which is generally less lethal. As a result, Hong Kong and Ireland lie at two extremes of the chart representing gender ratios for 15- to 24-year-old suicides (Ireland has a ratio male:female of 7.1:1 compared with 1.2:1 in Hong Kong) – see Figure 7.5.

It is not surprising then to note the considerable differences between diverse societies in the prevalence of various methods of suicide. In Hong Kong, as already mentioned, the preferred method for young males is jumping from a height. Between 1986 and 1992 jumping accounted for 93.8% of suicides for 10- to 14-year-olds, 71.9% for 15- to 19-year-olds and 66.3% for 20- to 24-year-olds. The remainder of suicides was mainly by hanging with a few in the older age groups overdosing. In the case of young females in Hong Kong, jumping accounted for 88.9%, 89.3%, and 67.2% of the three age groups respectively i.e. 10–14, 15–19 and 20–24 years (Ho et al., 1995). In Ireland, young male suicide is also dominated by a single, but different, method – hanging. In the three five-year age cohorts from 10 to 24 years of age, hanging accounts for 75%, 52%, and 44% of male suicides. Among young Irish females, poisoning, hanging, and drowning, in fairly even proportions, account for most suicides (Central Statistics Office Ireland, 1976–2001).

Ireland's neighbors, England and Wales, show an apparently different pattern of choice of suicide method. For both genders, between the ages of 10 and 24 years, only one suicide by drowning was recorded in all of 1994. This rarity is likely to be influenced by recording practices, as coroners in England and Wales must prove "beyond reasonable doubt" that a death from external causes was an actual suicide, with the most common alternative verdict being, of course, undetermined death. There are certain similarities, however; as amongst young males in England and Wales, as in Ireland, hanging is the commonest method, accounting for between 40% and 49% of suicides between 10 and 24 years of age. Self-poisoning, firearms, and jumping from a height are the most prevalent alternative methods of suicide. The overall number of young female suicides in 1994 in England and Wales was quite low, with only two suicides being recorded for those less than 15 years of age. Self-poisoning is the most common method of suicide for young women in England and Wales (67% of 15- to 19-year-olds, 42% of 20- to 24-year-olds), while hanging accounts for 26% of 20- to 24-year-old female suicide there.

In the U.S., firearms are the commonest choice of suicide method in under-19-year-olds males; firearms appear to account for almost all of the increase in youth suicide in the U.S. over the past 30 years (Bignall, 1993).

## Psychosocial correlates of suicide among young people

Given the international differences in youth suicide rates, method and gender ratios across different regions, it is important to consider the potential psychosocial factors that may contribute to these variations.

### Attachment relationships

Differences in child-rearing practices and the quality of child–parent attachments may be an important potential influential on cross-national variations in youth suicide rates. An enduring emotional tie between a child and a primary caretaker represents an attachment in developmental psychology. Attachment theory, as developed by John Bowlby (1969, 1973, 1980), gives an account of the formation and maintenance of the development of an enduring emotional tie between child and primary caretaker, a tie which Bowlby believed served the adaptive evolutionary function of promoting infant survival. In early childhood, attachment is commonly manifested in efforts to seek proximity and contact to the attachment figure, especially when the individual is under stress. Based on these experiences, the individual develops internal working models concerning the physical and emotional expectability and reliability of the caretaker, an emotional map that we all carry within us as a predictor of future relationships (Bowlby, 1987; Holmes, 1993).

Attachments have been seen as the prime initial transmitter of cultural "memes," which have been proposed as the environmental equivalents of genes (Dawkins, 1976). The "Strange Situation Test" (Ainsworth, 1969) provides an empirical means of assessing the quality of attachment styles, and cross-cultural meta-analysis of this test suggests possible international differences. The main classification schema has been between secure and insecure patterns of attachment, with a further subdivision into three insecure types in children (avoidant, ambivalent-resistant, and disorganized-disorientated) and two insecure types in adults (dismissive and enmeshed). For example, a high proportion (35%) of German children are classified as avoidant (Grossman et al., 1981). In cultures where parenting practices are characteristically highly protective, such as Japan and Israel, more children tend to manifest a resistant pattern of attachment (van Ijzendorn and Kroonenberg, 1988). Individuals' patterns of attachment (or "attachment dynamic" (Heard and Lake, 1986)) continue to influence the individual beyond childhood, even after emotional autonomy appears to have been achieved (Holmes, 1993).

The rise in suicide among the young in the West may possibly be explained in part by the hypothesis that societies with high levels of anomie tend to produce relationships that are characterized by separation and loss. Adam (1994) has developed a risk model for suicidal behavior based on attachment theory that argues that negative attachment experiences predispose to suicide. Divergent suicide rates worldwide may in part reflect cross-national differences in the quality of attachment relationships.

### Divorce

In keeping with the above, it is reasonable to assume that the quality of a child's relationship with the world is often dependent on the strength and closeness of the family unit. The stability of the social institution of the family in a given society may be measured to some extent by the level of divorce. Divorce is among the social factors shown to influence suicidal behavior in both case–control and epidemiological studies (Stack, 2000a,b) although its significance for youth suicide in the U.S. remains uncertain (Gould et al., 1998).

Using multiple regression to assess the association between social factors and suicide rates over the period 1951–1986 in Quebec, a significant association was found (Lester, 1995). A study of socio-demographic variables and suicide in the

U.S., which employed multiple regression analysis using aggregate data, found that suicide rates were significantly lower in States with low divorce rates (Lester, 1993).

In Norway, a similar type of study brought to light gender differences. Time-series analyses on differentiated data from 1911 to 1990 found that both alcohol consumption and divorce rates were independently and significantly associated with male suicide but not female suicide (Rossow, 1995). Also employing time-series analysis, Lester (1997) found that, in Israel, divorce rates were positively associated with male suicide but negatively with female suicide. This is consistent with the belief that marriage is protective of mental health in men but not in women. However, in Sweden, a country culturally similar to Norway, analyses of suicide and divorce between 1974 and 1986 did not reveal a gender difference (Hulten and Wasserman, 1992).

The influence of divorce as a social factor is not confined to the western world. Between 1975 and 1986, the divorce rate in Japan had a significantly high association with the suicide rate there for both sexes (Motohashi, 1991).

Further studies have shown that divorce not only affects the parents but also their offspring. Indeed, for children, parental divorce can have a devastating effect. While this effect varies in intensity and duration it is thought that the emotional effect is evidenced by "lowered self-esteem, declining sense of social competence, and a higher than usual propensity for substance abuse, depression and suicide" (Anable, 1991). A study of Kansan high-school students supports the notion that self-esteem is lower among children of divorced parents. The study also assessed levels of depression using the Beck Depression Inventory. Children of divorced parents scored higher on the depression scale while they also had consistently lower grade averages, which affect life-chances later in life (Brubeck and Beer, 1992).

A comparative analysis of psychiatric inpatients (aged 18–29) who had attempted suicide and two matching control groups (one consisting of nonsuicidal psychiatric patients and the other of "normal subjects") found that parental loss due to divorce had occurred significantly more often among suicide attempters than among either of the control groups (Benjaminsen et al., 1990).

In a comparative study of suicide among adolescents in the U.S. and Canada it was shown that in Canada, in particular, measures of domestic integration, especially divorce rates, predicted youth suicide rates more strongly than adult rates. The difference in the U.S. was less pronounced (Leenaars and Lester, 1995). An earlier study in Canada, however, showed the importance of temporal change on the effect of familial dissolution. The study covered the period from 1971 to 1981 and it was found that in 1981 there was a positive and significant association between family break-up through divorce and youth suicide for both young men and women whereas in 1971 this was not the case (Trovato, 1992).

In line with studies showing a positive relationship between youth suicide and divorce rates, a study in California found that as the divorce rate there declined, so too did the suicide rate (by 32%). The decline was pronounced among the young and coincided with an 88% decrease in teenage overdose and other poisoning deaths (Males, 1994).

Although a considerable body of work supports the positive association between parental divorce and youth suicide, the data are not conclusive. A recent study in the U.S. investigated factors that may modify the effect of parental divorce and separation on youth suicide (Gould et al., 1998). In a case–control psychological autopsy study, it was found that the impact of separation and divorce on youth suicide was small (especially once parental psychopathology is controlled for).

## Youth suicide trends in one culture: the case of the Republic of Ireland

The Republic of Ireland has traditionally had a very low reported rate of suicide (Daly and Kelleher 1987; Walsh et al., 1990). However, this has been consistently rising over the past 20 years from 5.7 per 100 000 in 1979 to 13.9 in 1998. This rise can be partly explained by improved methods of collecting statistics, as evidenced by the tenfold increase over the past 20 years in the ratio of suicide to undetermined death (from 2.2 to 28.6 for males and from 2.3 to 26.9 for females). However, the rise in youth suicide in Ireland is genuine. It has been estimated that the improved gathering of statistical information accounts for no more than 40% of the rise in male suicide since the late 1980s (Kelleher et al., 1996).

This rise in Irish suicide rates differs markedly by gender and these differences are increasing with time. Over the last 20 years, there has been a slight rise in the 20- to 24-year-old female suicide rate but, overall, the female suicide rate in Ireland has remained stable. The main increase in suicide rates is in 20- to 24-year-old males, with a less dramatic rise in 15- to 19-year-old males.

When the age-specific Irish male suicide rate is looked at for each one-year age cohort, a stepwise increase in the frequency of suicide with age is apparent, a pattern similar to that seen in the U.S. (e.g., Shaffer et al., 1988).

The causes of the secular increase in Irish young male suicides are unclear and have been the subject of considerable analyses in recent years (e.g., Kelleher, 1998). The various hypotheses parallel those advanced in other western developed countries, which share rising rates of young male suicide (Casey, 1997). The presence of cohort effects on rates of depression may provide one explanatory framework. Cultural factors may also influence the likelihood that a depressed young man today will more readily consider and act upon thoughts of suicide than a generation ago.

In this context, Ireland has experienced considerable social and cultural change over the past two or three decades. Although 94% of the population are nominally Roman Catholic (Central Statistics Office Ireland, 1991), rates of religious observance and doctrinal belief have greatly diminished (e.g., Breslin and Weafer, 1986; McGréil, 1991). Religious factors alone, however, do not provide a full explanation of the rise in suicide among Irish youth.

The greatest rise in youth suicide has occurred in the rural areas of Ireland, which have remained the most religiously observant, while the least rise has occurred in urban areas, which have experienced the greatest decline in the outward practice of religion (Kelleher et al., 1997).

A second major change in Irish society over the past 20 years, and, in particular, over the past decade, has been the increasing availability and use of illegal drugs, a factor which has been suggested as a major cause of the rise of youth suicide throughout the western world (Hawton et al., 1993; Neeleman and Farrell, 1997). However, in Ireland, the Dublin area, which has the highest prevalence of drug abuse, has the lowest suicide rate (Kelleher et al., 1998b).

Another major social change in Ireland relates to the growing proportion of young people continuing their education beyond the minimum school-leaving age of 15 years, with increasingly intense competition for school places.

The institution of the family in Ireland has also undergone considerable transformation. Although divorce was only legalized in 1996, the number of legal separations has been increasing over the years. Marriage rates have fallen steadily and the average age at marriage has increased. The average age of mothers is just over 30 and 30% of children are born outside of marriage, with the proportion even higher than this in some urban areas.

If secular changes in the nuclear family are important in contributing to a rise in suicide rates, then an explanation must be offered as to why it is that young males have shown this rise, but not young females. The overall trend seems to be towards the exclusion of males from the family unit. If there is a separation, it is usually the male parental figure that leaves the home. As a result, it may be speculated, male role models for adolescents may be perceived in a less permanent and more negative way today than they were in more traditional times.

There are many other changes in Irish society in recent years that have not yet been the subject of analysis. These include increasing urbanization, marked internal migration, and widespread industrialization, as well as a great increase in the gross national product. The economic life of the country is more competitive both internally and with respect to its European neighbors, with whom it is also increasingly better integrated. What potential role these factors play in the rise in Irish youth suicide rates is unclear. It should be emphasized, however, that the rise in young Irish male suicides parallels that in many Western societies and the relative role of factors specific to the Irish situation versus those shared with many other countries is also unclear.

## Conclusion

Reported rates of youth suicide from different countries are undoubtedly influenced by differing recording practices, but, as the variation in the gender ratio of youth suicide rates across countries suggests, there are also genuine underlying international differences in the rates of youth suicide. Differences in choice of lethal method are also wide and appear largely related to ease of access to lethal means, which in turn is subject to both environmental and cultural factors. For example, drowning is less common in areas where there is limited access to the sea, rivers, or lakes. In terms of cultural factors, societies with lenient gun-control policy have higher numbers of firearm suicide.

Culture also influences the timing, development, and shape of children's concept of death in general and suicide in particular. Culturally specific influences range from broad child-rearing practices through specific media coverage practices regarding suicide. In turn these largely cultural differences influence rates of suicide especially among preadolescents.

In the current climate of globalization, many of the convergent changes towards postmodernity are cross-national in their effects, blurring to some extent the influence of traditional cultural differences and carrying in their wake important implications for suicide patterns (Schlegel, 2000; Stack 2000a,b). Nonetheless, important differences persist, for example, between Europe and Asia or Africa. Some indicators of anomie and social instability are not apparent in Mauritius or any of the three East Asian countries in the study. The effects of the new social movements (such as environmentalism, feminism, and gay rights) associated with postmodernism are not felt as strongly in these countries as in Europe and the West. For example, feminism is not as strong, with the result that the gender ratio for suicide rates is lowest in these countries. Perhaps then, it is a positive thing that postmodernity has, as a core value, equality – not only equality of the genders but also equality for marginal groups such as homosexuals, minority religions, and racial minorities – as the risk associated with marginal groups may be reduced in time.

Children are brought up in different ways in different cultures and hence acquire different means of coping with both their human and physical environment. Because of the centrality of family relationships (especially the parent–child relationship) to children's psychological well being, it is likely that the demise of the traditional family unit in the postmodern era may have widespread detrimental effects on today's youth. The studies referred to above suggest potential links between the increases in youth suicide and divorce rates, but the data remain inconclusive.

In conclusion, it has not yet proven possible to identify the distinctive aspects of culture (including variations in method of suicide and differences in social institutions such as the family and religion) that offer a definitive explanation for national differences in child and adolescent suicidal behavior. Similarly, it is not yet clear which aspects of social change in the context of a small country like Ireland provide a reasonable explanation for the increase in youth suicide there. It does seem plausible that ease of access to lethal means of self-harm accounts for some of the cross-national variance in youth suicide rates. Overall, however, it seems that it is the shortcomings of increasingly modernized societies in failing to offer a meaning for existence that account for the rising youth suicide rates in advanced industrial or postmodern countries. As support of this notion, the highest rates of youth suicide are recorded in the modernized societies of Northern Europe and the English-speaking countries as well as those countries in Eastern Europe and the former Soviet Union that have been marked by political upheaval and social unrest. In light of these apparent trends, the impact of global change and the shift towards globalization provide an important focus for research on the epidemiological aspects of youth suicide.

## REFERENCES

Adam, K. S. (1994). Suicidal behaviour and attachment: a developmental model. In Sperling, M. B., and Berman, W. H. New York, NY: Guildford. (eds.) *Attachment in Adults: Theory Assessment and Treatment* (pp. 275–298).

Ainsworth, M. (1969). Object relations, dependency and attachment: a theoretical review of the mother-infant relationship. *Child Development*, **40**, 969–1025.

Anable, K. E. (1991). Children of divorce: ways to heal the wounds. *Clinical Nurse Specialist*, **5**(3), 133–137.

Arnett, J. (1999). Adolescent storm and stress, reconsidered. *American Psychologist*, **54**, 317–326.

Banerjee, G., Nandi, D., Nandi, S., Sarkar, S., Boral, G. C., and Ghosh, A. (1990). The vulnerability of Indian women to suicide: a field study. *Indian Journal of Psychiatry*, **32**, 305–308.

Barraclough, B. (1988). International variations in the suicide rate of 15–24 year olds. *Journal of Social Psychiatry and Epidemiological Psychiatry*, **23**, 75–84.

Benjaminsen, S., Krarup, G., and Lauritsen, R. (1990). Personality, parental rearing behaviour and parental loss in attempted suicide: a comparative study. *Acta Psychiatrica Scandinavica*, **82**(5), 389–397.

Bignall, J. (1993). Adolescents and guns [Letter]. *The Lancet*, **342**, 1169.

Birckmayer, J., and Hemenway, D. (2001). Suicide and firearm prevalence: are youth disproportionately affected? *Suicide and Life-Threatening Behavior*, **31**(3), 303–310.

Bowlby, J. (1969). *Attachment*. London: Penguin Books.

Bowlby, J. (1973). *Separation*. London: Penguin Books.

Bowlby, J. (1980). *Loss*. London: Penguin Books.

Bowlby, J. (1987). Attachment. In Gregory, R. (ed.) *The Oxford Companion to the Mind*. Oxford: Oxford University Press.

Brent, D. A. (2001). Firearms and suicide. *Annals of the New York Academy of Sciences*, **932**, 225–239 [discussion; 239–240].

Brent, D. A., Perper, J. A., and Allmain, C. J. (1991). The presence and accessibility of firearms in the homes of adolescent suicides. *Journal of the American Medical Association*, **21**, 2989–2995.

Brent, D. A., Perper, J., Moritz, G., Baugher, M., and Allman, C. (1993a). Suicide in adolescents with no apparent psychopathology. *Journal of the American Academy of Child and Adolescent Psychiatry*, **32**(3), 494–500.

Brent, D. A., Perper, J. A., Moritz, G., Baugher, M., Schweers, J., and Roth, C. (1993b). Firearms and adolescent suicide. A community case–control study. *American Journal of Diseases of Children*, **147**(10), 1066–1071.

Brent, D. A., Baugher, M., Bridge, J., Chen, T., and Chiappetta, L. (1999). Age- and sex-related risk factors for adolescent suicide. *Journal of the American Academy of Child and Adolescent Psychiatry*, **38**(12), 1497–1505.

Breslin, A., and Weafer, J. (1986). *Religious Beliefs, Practice and Moral Attitudes: A Comparison of Two Irish Surveys (1974–1984)*. Maynooth: St. Patrick's College Council for Research and Development.

Brubeck, D., and Beer, J. (1992). Depression, self-esteem, suicide ideation, death anxiety, and GPA in high-school students of divorced and non-divorced parents. *Psychological Report*, **71**(3.1), 755–763.

Canetto, S. S., and Silverman, M. M. (1998). Special Issue: Gender, culture and suicidal behavior. *Suicide and Life-Threatening Behavior*, **28**(1), 1–142 (entire volume).

Cantor, C. (2000) Suicide in the Western world. In Hawton, K., and van Heeringen, K. (eds.) *The International Handbook of Suicide and Attempted Suicide* (pp. 9–29). Chichester: Wiley.

Carrington, P. J., and Moyer, S. (1994). Gun control and suicide in Ontario. *American Journal of Psychiatry*, **151**, 606–608.

Casey, P. (1997). The psychiatric and social background to suicide – the problem of prevention [editorial]. *Irish Medical Journal*, **90**(1), 12.

Central Statistics Office Ireland (1976–2001). *Report on Vital Statistics*. Dublin: Government Stationery Office.

Central Statistics Office Ireland. (1991). *Census Report*, Volume I. Dublin: Government Stationery Office.

Commonwealth Department of Health and Family Services Australia (1997). *Youth Suicide in Australia: A Background Monograph*. Canberra: Australian Government Publishing Service.

Daly, M., and Kelleher, M. J. (1987). The increase in the suicide rate in Ireland. *Irish Medical Journal*, **80**(8), 233–234.

Dawkins, R. (1976). *The Selfish Gene*. Oxford: Oxford University Press.

De Leo, D. G., Carollo, M., and Mastinu, A. (1995). Epidemiology of suicide in the elderly population in Italy (1958–1988). *Archives of Suicide Research*, **1**, 3–18.

Durkheim, E. (1897/1993). *Suicide: a Study in Sociology* [Translated by J. A. Spaulding and G. Simpson.] London: Routledge.

Eckersley, R. (1993). Failing a generation: the impact of culture on the health and well-being of a nation. *Journal of Paediatrics and Child Health*, **29**(1), 16–19.

Fischer, E. P., Comstock, G. W., and Spencer, D. J. (1993). Characteristics of completed suicide. *Suicide and Life-Threatening Behaviour*, **23**, 91–100.

Giddens, A. (1983). Introduction. In Giddens, A. (ed.) *The Sociology of Suicide*. London: Frank Cass and Company Limited.

Gould, M. S., Shaffer, D., Fisher, P., and Garfinkel, R. (1998). Separation/divorce and child and adolescent completed suicide. *Journal of the American Academy of Child and Adolescent Psychiatry*, **37**(2), 155–162.

Grossman, K., Grossman, K. E., Huber, F., and Wartner, Y. (1981). German children's behaviour towards their mothers at 12 months and their fathers at 18 months in the Ainsworth Strange Situation. *International Journal of Behavioural Development*, **4**, 157–181.

Gunnell, D., Murray, V., and Hawton, K. (2000). Use of paracetamol (acetaminophen) for suicide and nonfatal poisoning: worldwide patterns of use and misuse. *Suicide and Life-Threatening Behavior*, **30**(4), 313–326.

Hawton, K., Fagg, J., Platt, S., and Hawkins, M. (1993). Factors associated with suicide after parasuicide in young people. *British Medical Journal*, **306**, 1641–1644.

He, Z. X., and Lester, D. (1997). The gender difference in Chinese suicide rates. *Archives of Suicide Research*, **3**(2), 81–89.

Healey, C. (1979). Women and suicide in New Guinea. *Journal of Social Analysis*, **2**, 89–107.

Heard, D., and Lake, B. (1986). The attachment dynamic in adult life. *British Journal of Psychiatry*, **149**, 430–438.

Hintikka, J., Lehtonen, J., and Viinamaki, H. (1997). Hunting guns in homes and suicides in 15–24 year old males in eastern Finland. *Australian and New Zealand Journal of Psychiatry*, **31**(6), 858–861.

Ho, T. P. (1996). Changing patterns of suicide in Hong Kong. *Social Psychiatry and Psychiatric Epidemiology*, **31**, 235–240.

Ho, T. P., Hung, S. F., Lee, C. C., Chung, K. F., and Chung, S. Y. (1995). Characteristics of youth suicide in Hong Kong. *Social Psychiatry and Psychiatric Epidemiology*, **30**, 107–112.

Holmes, J. (1993). Attachment Theory: a biological basis for psychotherapy? *British Journal of Psychiatry*, **163**, 430–438.

Hulten, A., and Wasserman, D. (1992). Suicide among young people aged 10–29 in Sweden. *Scandinavian Journal of Social Medicine*, **20**(2), 65–72.

Hutchinson, G., Daisley, H., Simeon, D., Simmonds, V., Shetty, M., and Lynn, D. (1999). High rates of paraquat-induced suicide in southern Trinidad. *Suicide and Life-Threatening Behavior*, **29**(2), 186–191.

Inglehart, R. (1990). *Culture Shift in Advanced Industrial Society*. New Jersey: Princeton University Press.

Inglehart, R. (1997). *Modernization and Postmodernization: Cultural, Economic and Political Change in 43 Societies*. New Jersey: Princeton University Press.

Johnson, G. R., Krug, E. G., and Potter, L. B. (2000). Suicide among adolescents and young adults: a cross-national comparison of 34 countries. *Suicide and Life-Threatening Behavior*, **30**(1), 74–82.

Kelleher, M. J. (1998). Youth suicide trends in the Republic of Ireland [editorial]. *British Journal of Psychiatry*, **173**, 196–197.

Kelleher, M. J., Corcoran, P., Keeley, H. S., Dennehy, J., and O'Donnell, I. (1996). Improving procedures for recording suicide statistics. *Irish Medical Journal*, **89**(1), 16–17.

Kelleher, M. J., Keeley, H. S., and Corcoran, P. (1997). The service implications of regional differences in suicide rates in the Republic of Ireland. *Irish Medical Journal*, **90**(7), 262–264.

Kelleher, M. J., Chambers, D., Corcoran, P., Williamson, E., and Keeley, H. S. (1998a). Religious sanctions and rates of suicide worldwide. *Crisis*, **19**(2), 78–86.

Kelleher, M. J., Corcoran, P., and Keeley, H. S. (1998b). Variation in suicide rates between Health Board areas. *Irish Medical Journal*, **91**, 53–56.

Kelleher, M. J., Corcoran, P., Keeley, H. S., Chambers, D., Williamson, E., Burke, U., and Byrne, S. (2002). Differences in Irish urban and rural suicide rates, (1976–1994). *Archives of Suicide Research*, **6**(2), 82–90.

Kellermann, A. L., Rivara, F. P., Somes, G., Reay, D. T., Francisco, J., Banton, J. G., Prodzinski, J., Fligner, C., and Hackman, B. B. (1992). Suicide in the home in relation to gun ownership. *New England Journal of Medicine*, **327**(7), 467–472.

Kreitman, N. (1976). The coal gas story: United Kingdom suicide rates, (1960–1971). *British Journal of Preventative and Social Medicine*, **30**, 86–93.

Leenaars, A., and Lester, D. (1995). The changing suicide pattern in Canadian adolescents and youth, compared to their American counterparts. *Adolescence*, **30**(119), 539–547.

Lester, D. (1990). The effects of detoxification of domestic gas on suicide in the United States. *American Journal of Public Health*, **80**, 80–81.

Lester, D. (1993). The effectiveness of suicide prevention centres. *Suicide and Life-Threatening Behaviour*, **23**(3), 263–267.

Lester, D. Suicide in Quebec, (1951–1986). (1995). *Psychological Reports*, **76**(1), 122.

Lester, D. (1997). Domestic social integration and suicide in Israel. *Israeli Journal of Psychiatry and Related Sciences*, **34**(2), 157–161.

Lester, D., and Leenaars, A. (1993). Suicide rates in Canada before and after tightening firearm control laws. *Psychological Reports*, **72**(3), 787–790.

Lipschitz, A. (1995). Suicide prevention in young adults. *Suicide and Life-Threatening Behaviour*, **25**(1), 155–170.

Males, M. (1994). California's suicide decline, (1970–1990). *Suicide and Life-Threatening Behaviour*, **24**(1), 24–37.

Marzuk, P. M., Leon, A. C., Tardiff, K., Morgan, E. B., Stajic, M., and Mann, J. (1992). The effect of access to lethal methods of injury on suicide rates. *Archives of General Psychiatry*, **49**, 451–458.

McGréil, M. (1991). *Religious Practice and Attitude in Ireland*. Maynooth: St. Patrick's College Survey and Research Unit.

Ministry of National Health and Welfare, Canada. (1994). *Suicide in Canada: Update of the Report of the Task Force on Suicide in Canada*.

Motohashi, Y. (1991). Effects of socio-economic factors on secular trends in Japan, (1953–1986). *Journal of Biosocial Science*, **23**(2), 221–227.

Neeleman, J., and Farrell, M. (1997). Suicide and substance misuse. *British Journal of Psychiatry*, **171**, 303–304.

Office for National Statistics, England and Wales (1994). *Mortality Statistics: Cause*. Series DH2(21). London: HMSO.

Pillay, B. J. (1995). Children's perceptions of suicide – a study at a primary school. In Schlebusch, L. (ed.) *Suicidal Behaviour, Proceedings of the Third South African Conference on Suicidology* (pp. 163–171). Durban: University of Natal.

Pritchard, C. (1996). New patterns of suicide by age and gender in the United Kingdom and the Western World (1974–1992); an indicator of social change? *Social Psychiatry and Psychiatric Epidemiology*, **31**, 227–234.

Reber, A. (1985). *Dictionary of Psychology*. London: Penguin Books.

Reischauer, E. O., and Jansen, M. B. (1995). *The Japanese Today: Change and Continuity*. Harvard: Harvard University Press.

Retterstøl, N. (1993). *Suicide: A European Perspective*. Cambridge: Cambridge University Press.

Rich, C. L., Young, J. G., Fowler, R. C., Wagner, J., and Black, N. A. (1990). Guns and suicide: possible effects of some specific legislation. *American Journal of Psychiatry*, **147**, 342–346.

Rossow, I. (1995). Suicide, alcohol and divorce; aspects of gender and family integration [comment]. *Addiction*, **90**(7), 985–988.

Schlegel, A. (2000). The global spread of adolescent culture. In Crockett, L. J., and Silbereisen, R. K. (eds.) *Negotiating Adolescence in a Time of Social Change*. Cambridge: Cambridge University Press.

Shaffer, D., Garland, A., Gould, M., Fisher, P., and Trautman, P. (1988). Preventing teenage suicide: a critical review. *Journal of the American Academy of Child and Adolescent Psychiatry*, **27**, 675–687.

Shafii, M. (1989). Completed suicide in children and adolescents: methods of psychological autopsy. In Pfeffer, C. R. (ed.) *Suicide Among Youth. Perspectives on Risk and Prevention*. Cambridge: Cambridge University Press.

Sloan, J. H., Rivara, F. P., Reay, D. T., Ferris, J. A., and Kellerman, A. L. (1990). Firearm regulations and rates of suicide: a comparison of two metropolitan areas. *New England Journal of Medicine*, **322**, 369–373.

Stack, S. (2000a). Suicide: a 15-year review of the sociological literature. Part I: cultural and economic factors. *Suicide and Life-Threatening Behavior*, **30**(2), 145–162.

Stack, S. (2000b). Suicide: a 15-year review of the sociological literature. Part II: modernization and social integration perspectives. *Suicide and Life-Threatening Behavior*, **30**(2), 163–176.

Takahashi, Y. (1997). Culture and suicide: from a Japanese psychiatrist's perspective. *Suicide and Life-Threatening Behaviour*, **27**(1), 137–145.

Trovato, F. (1992). A Durkheimian analysis of youth suicide: Canada, (1971) and (1981). *Suicide and Life-Threatening Behaviour*, **22**(4), 413–427.

United Nations (1995). *United Nations Demographic Yearbook*. New York: United Nations.

van Ijzendorn, M. H., and Kroonenberg, P. M. (1988). Cross-cultural patterns of attachment: a meta-analysis of the Strange Situation. *Child Development*, **59**, 147–156.

Walsh, D., Cullen, A., Cullivan, R., and O'Donnell, B. (1990). Do statistics lie: suicide in Kildare and Ireland. *Psychological Medicine*, **20**, 867–871.

World Health Organization. Suicide rates and absolute numbers of suicide by country (2001). Available at http://www 5. who.int./mental_health/main (accessed 3 September 2002).

*World Health Statistics Annual* (1989–1995). Geneva: World Health Organization.

World Values Study Group (1994). *World Values Survey, (1981–1984) and (1990–1993) (Computer file)*. ICPSR version. Ann Arbor, Michigan: Institute for Social Research (producer). Ann Arbor, Michigan: Inter-university Consortium for Political and Social Research (distributor).

Yip, P. S. (2001). An epidemiological profile of suicides in Beijing, China. *Suicide and Life-Threatening Behavior*, **31**(1), 62–70.

# 8

# An idiographic approach to understanding suicide in the young

Alan L. Berman

Harvard professor Edwin Boring, in his classic 1950 text, *A History of Experimental Psychology*, wrote that " . . . science begins in the evolutionary scale with the capacity to generalize in perceiving an object; . . . seeing in the observed object the uniformities of nature" (p. 5).

In the scientific study of suicide, our generalizations speak to epidemiologic trends. Aggregated sets of cases allow for temporal and subgroup comparisons (e.g., males vs. females, young vs. old, whites vs. nonwhites). Differences in the distribution of cases in different populations or at different times suggest general explanatory factors and theories that may, in turn, define risk variables. Once validated, these risk factors fuel our efforts at early detection of and intervention with defined "at-risk" youth, as well as larger scale preventive efforts.

Much has been learned from and much has been gained by this nomothetic approach. Recent epidemiological-, psychological-, sociological-, and biological-suicidological research permits us to paint reasonably well a profile of an adolescent at risk (for completion of suicide) as a mentally disordered, white male, who uses a gun (in the U.S.) or hangs himself (elsewhere in the world) "in the context of an acute disciplinary crisis or shortly after a rejection or humiliation" (Shaffer et al., 1988).

Yet, as valuable and important as these studies are, you might ask "Of what use are they?", and "How do I apply, clinically, this mass of aggregated data?". Typically these studies paint with such a broad brush that the caregiver, who is charged with translating the researchers' findings into clinical application, is potentially and inadvertently misled. For example:

- If diagnosed mental disorders are necessary conditions for suicidal behavior, and I work in a setting where all adolescents have diagnosed mental disorders, what then?
- If we have learned that 50% of suicidal females have made a prior suicide attempt, then 50% have not. Which of these is a risk factor?

- If substance abuse characterizes 37% of male completers over 17 years old, then no substance abuse characterizes a greater proportion of male completers. Even if the 37% who have abused is significantly greater than the proportion of substance abusers in the general population, it is dwarfed by populations of substance abusers (100% of whom abuse) who do not complete suicide.
- What of the young female sitting in your office, who presents with no family history of suicidal behavior, no recent exposure to suicide, and no exposure to family violence or abuse?
  Kristin is a good example. Kristin is:
- a 15-year-old, white female;
- from an intact family with no history of suicide, parental psychopathology, or substance abuse;
- not hopeless;
- attractive, likeable, seductive, and coquettish, in spite of being distrustful of adults, reactive to controls and authority, and therefore is noncompliant with treatment recommendations.
- difficult to form a therapeutic alliance with. She is diagnosed as having an Oppositional Disorder and has a history of learning disability.

Kristin made her first attempt at suicide at the age of 12 when her pet iguana died. For much of the past three subsequent years she has been sexually involved with a conduct-disordered, substance-abusing male. In addition to her sexual activity, mostly unprotected, she has run away from home, been arrested for breaking and entering and for stealing property. She carries with her a lethal supply of cyanide, which she says she will take if threatened with institutional control or incarceration.

Is Kristin typical of adolescents who attempt suicide? Does she reach some cut-off score on a static list of risk factors for suicide? Can you guess whether her story ends in a completed suicide; another attempt (near lethal or not); continued suicide threats; a life of continued acting out and trouble, but without suicidal behavior; or marriage and two kids by the time she's 30?

Kristin's case displays considerable risk, but no predictions. At the same time, she should remind us of how young a science suicidology is, and how much we remain in need of subgroup profiles; for example, research of risk factors specific to young females with early-onset sexual activity and object loss followed by suicidal behavior.

While the Holy Grail of science is discovering uniformities among observations, the heart of science is the observed object – the suicidal case. Kristin and I are here to remind you that the broad brush of the clinical epidemiologist paints a picture of the suicidal adolescent that is potentially and inadvertently misleading.

My role is to serve as a sort of transitional object. In the midst of excellent chapters on research findings and generalizations, I have the responsibility of reminding you of our roots and of the raw material of our science.

It is the intensive study of the individual that gives our science its richness and its texture. It, ultimately, is the unique and individual suicidal case, intensively studied, that provides the true understanding of suicidal behavior (Berman, 1991, 1992, 1997). As we search desperately for commonalities, it is only through the idiographic method that we can remind ourselves of the complexity of the suicidal character; that we can explore the myriad of exceptions to our established generalizations; that we can understand patterns, temporal dynamics, interactive effects between patients and caregivers, therapeutic issues of alliance, compliance, and countertransference, and how they apply once risk is detected; and particularly, the **meanings** of suicidal behaviors.

In this chapter, I hope merely to jog your mind and, perhaps, humble you before the idol of nomothetism. Obversely, I have but a simple point to make: the case study is a heuristic tool for understanding and teaching about suicide; a point we see less and less frequently in our literature as biological and epidemiological psychiatry have come to dominate our journals.

## Case studies provide explanatory hypotheses

As different as Kurt Cobain was from Marilyn Monroe, so were the apparent effects of their deaths on survivors. Our understanding of the Werther effect and the potential for copycat suicides when a celebrity suicide occurs is prophylactic; with awareness of the effect and its associated characteristics, increased observation and early detection of affected youth can be initiated. But the Werther effect is not universal and the idiographic understanding of case examples provides significant evidence for the efficacy of preventive actions.

According to David Phillips' (1974) research, Marilyn Monroe's suicide in August 1962 was followed by a rise in U.S. suicides of some 12% over expectation (and 9% in Great Britain). Phillips has argued that the effect is dose-specific, i.e., the more publicity devoted to a suicide story, the larger the rise in suicides thereafter. No doubt, Marilyn Monroe's suicide got considerable press.

Kurt Cobain's suicide in April 1994 was followed by an avalanche of publicity, yet it appears not to have had a Wertherian effect on his acolytes and admirers, many of whom we would expect to be among a high-risk subgroup of disaffected and troubled youth. While we await more national and international data, our

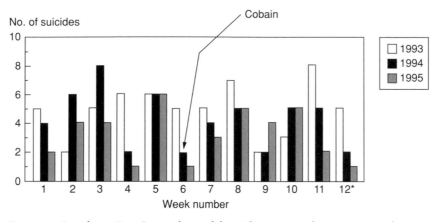

Figure 8.1  Suicides in King County, by week late February to mid-May over several years.
*Source:* Medical Examiner's Office, King County, Washington.
*Partial week.

preliminary case analysis presents a revealing look at this exception and possible reasons for it (Jobes et al., 1996). It is only through such intensive case study that exceptions can be better understood.

Cobain was a cultural icon, a symbol of and to the "lost generation." He pioneered an anti-fashion look, the grunge uniform of torn jeans; unwashed, chopped, and dyed hair; worn-out t-shirts, and unravelling sweaters. "Anti-fashion" soon became fashionable, Cobain attained extraordinary success with his group, Nirvana, and his depression and drug use ultimately killed him.

Figure 8.1 displays an interrupted time-series design for a seven-week surveillance period, with equivalent control periods in 1993 and 1995. In this seven-week period following Cobain's suicide, there were 24 suicides in King County, Washington; only one appeared linked to Cobain. Compared to both control years, there was no marked difference in the frequency of suicides in 1994.

Although anecdotal cases were reported in the States, Canada, and as far away as Slovenia (personal communication, Onja Grad, June, 1995), there was no statistically significant rise in the Seattle, Washington area, where Cobain lived and had a large local following.

What did we learn to explain the apparent absence of an imitation effect in Seattle? Here is what the intensive case study allows.

First, much was done right by the media. With few exceptions, the media did well in reporting on Cobain's suicide and life. There was a high degree of professionalism and responsibility exercised in both the print and visual media.

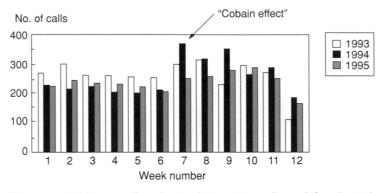

Figure 8.2  Suicide crisis calls to the Seattle Crisis Center, by week from late-February to mid-May, 1993–1995.

*Source:* Seattle Crisis Center.

*Partial week.

A concerted effort was made to distinguish Cobain the musician from Cobain the drug abuser and the suicide. The general message was, "Great artist . . . great music . . . stupid act . . . don't do it. Here's where to call for help."

Second, Cobain's use of a shotgun countered any romanticized visual image of a lonely misunderstood star drifting off into a sleepy overdose death à la Marilyn Monroe.

Third, and most importantly, a memorial service was held two days after his body was discovered. Over 7000 fans gathered in a downtown Seattle park. They listened to a tape-recorded message by Courtney Love, his widow, tearfully reading excerpts from Cobain's suicide note, interspersed with rageful cursing at him. This event was widely covered by the media. It turned out to be both tortured and healing. The grief-stricken cursing and wailing of Courtney Love made his death disturbing and real. Her honest and open grieving served to deromanticize Cobain's death and make it seem profoundly tragic, selfish, and ultimately wasteful.

Most importantly, the director of the Seattle Crisis Center made a concluding speech at the service. The Crisis Center's telephone number was widely publicized and made consistently available. The result, as evidenced in Figure 8.2, is that it was used.

In a similar vein, case studies are essential for exploring more thoroughly poorly understood or rare and complex phenomena. In North America, one identified high-risk suicide group is that of our Native Americans. Rates among native youth vary considerably from tribe to tribe, from one community to the next, and within any one tribe or community over time. For example, May and

Van Winkle (1994) have reported three-year average age-specific suicide rates over three decades for New Mexico Indian youth aged 15–19 years that ranged from a low of 5.54/100 000 to a high of 54.67/100 000. How does one explain such variability without resorting to more micro-oriented analyses? In my own work at one reservation on the border of Idaho and Nevada (Berman, 1979), where three-quarters of all deaths were nonnatural and the average age of the suicides was 23 years, several explanatory hypotheses emerged: high rates of alcoholism and depression; an extraordinary prevalence of gun ownership (an average of five guns per family); high unemployment (80% for most of the year); the destruction of traditional tribal cultures; community norms of tolerance and individualism; nonsupport for governance and achievement; a lack of help-seeking behavior and help-giving resources; and cultural sanctions against externalized expressions of rage. What a gold mine of interventive hypotheses! If there were an opportunity to accomplish a case–control study pairing this reservation with another, differentiating variables might further our understanding of protective factors, and also validate risk factors and potential targets for intervention.

## Case studies teach

As catalogued by Canada's Suicide Information and Education Center (SIEC), 12% of the over 1900 references appearing in the literature prior to 1970 included case illustrations (Tanney, personal communication, 1995). Since 1970, only 9% of the over 16 000 references published (and catalogued by SIEC) have included cases of suicidal individuals.

I fear the heartbeat of our science is growing faint.

As Case Consultation Editor of the American Association of Suicidology's journal, *Suicide and Life-Threatening Behavior*, between 1989 and 1995, I edited and presented a series of more than 20 cases. Each was discussed in print by two or more experts. I truly believe that these often quite lively presentations of contrasting views and interpretations had great pedagogic value.

Let me give but one brief example. One case (Berman, 1994) was that of a borderline, suicidal patient in long-term outpatient psychotherapy who, with great guilt and humiliation, had run up a balance of over $17 000 with an anticipated further debt estimated at $8000 per annum. This patient had made clear and significant gains in her treatment, leading her therapist to question whether he should continue her treatment pro bono or stop treating her and risk fulfilling her fears of abandonment, thereby increasing her risk for suicide. Four consultants responded to the question of management. One recommended a paradoxical intervention, a form of "therapeutic blackmail" by getting the patient to commit to therapeutic change in order to ward off the inevitable abandonment, i.e., "Either get better or I **will** abandon you." A second urged that the therapist articulate (i.e., interpret) the patient's debt as acting out a repetition compulsion, a reenactment of a fundamental sequence from childhood. A third urged the therapist to cut his losses and settle with the patient for what she could pay, perhaps $2000, then terminate therapy unless she could pay on a per-session, pay-as-you-go model. The fourth recommended an innovative compromise for the patient to work off the outstanding balance by contributing volunteer work in the community. Case studies of this sort offer unlimited opportunies for problem-oriented instruction.

Of course, the case study method is most profoundly illustrated by the psychological autopsy. Originally developed to assist medicolegal investigation of equivocal suicides (Litman et al., 1963), the psychological autopsy has increasingly been used in aggregated form and case–control analyses to provide in-depth, postdictive data regarding risk for and protection from suicide among youth. As a research tool, particularly in the hands of such accomplished researchers as David Brent and David Shaffer, who continue to refine procedures and methodology, the psychological autopsy yields both insights and validation to our hypotheses and theories.

The psychological autopsy, taken alone, has been used as a teaching tool since the first of two in-depth cases was presented and discussed in the *Bulletin of Suicidology*, the forerunner to *Suicide and Life-Threatening Behavior*, in the fall of 1970 (c.f., *Bulletin of Suicidology*, 1995). Case studies of suicidal individuals have been the central focus of at least two books (Berman, 1990; Niswander et al., 1973).

## Case studies illuminate

In Ed Shneidman's Festschrift, I (Berman, 1993) presented two psychological autopsies to illustrate and discuss what has, arguably, been called the most equivocal of all manners of death, asphyxiation by drowning. Unless witnessed, morphological criteria provide no evidence for determining how a body came to be in the water – an individual can slip, fall, jump, or be pushed. Although a popular form of suicide in Hollywood melodramas made during the 1920s, suicide by drowning is rare. The working hypothesis for medical examiners and coroners is that drownings are accidents, unless proven otherwise.

The case of Bobby Severn involved a 14-year-old boy who drowned near the end of a two-week wilderness adventure trip. Early one morning, his fellow campers and group leaders were awakened by the sound of a boy's voice yelling

59. While he was speaking to me I *butted in*

60. My mother always *yells.*

61. They didn't like him because *he was weird*

62. When they asked my opinion, *I didn't tell them*

63. Whenever he did poorly, he *tried to commit suicide*

64. He didn't study because *he knew he'd fail*

65. I lost out because *I didn't try*

66. In a group of people, I generally feel *fine*

Figure 8.3 Bobby Severn's sentence completions.

for help from somewhere in the lake by which they had camped. The fog prevented an immediate rescue and his body was not discovered until daybreak.

A strong swimmer, Bobby's presence in the water and inability to save himself suggested several hypotheses in explanation. If his death were a suicide, some evidence of intentionality had to be in evidence. If his death were an accident, sufficient evidence of some interference in or to his instinct toward self-preservation would be needed.

The psychological autopsy was rich in detail and included psychological testing some 18 months before his death. Included were his responses to sentence completions stems (see Figure 8.3; Item #63) and a projective drawing (Figure 8.4) depicting an underwater diver faced with an impending drowning. Note the shark approaching the oxygen line and the tombstone on the ocean floor.

I'll leave you in suspense about the final determination in this case (for which see Berman, 1993); I trust you see my point regarding this application of the intensive case study.

Psychological autopsy case studies of this sort are often called for in determining disputed insurance claims.

There are a variety of other applications of case study findings for teaching purposes. For example, the systematic analysis of suicide notes has been approached from a case–control method of inquiry, first posed to help differentiate genuine from simulated notes by Shneidman and Farberow (1961). Presentation of a note in the context of case information allows students to focus their interpretations of intent and evaluations of risk on the basis of actual communications from

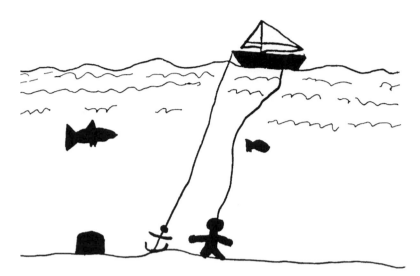

Figure 8.4  Bobby Severn's projective drawing.

the decedent or potential attempter. It also helps teach humility about what we do.

As one illustration, the communication illustrated in Figure 8.5 was presented to me by parents of an 18-year-old college freshman. He had been home recently on holiday and left a spiral notebook in which this was written. In consultation, his parents related that their son had always lived recklessly (e.g., he had five speeding tickets that past semester), had run away from home several times during his adolescence, and had more than a few physical altercations with his father. In addition, although they had discovered a bong in his bedroom, he denied he was using drugs and claimed he was "holding it for a friend." Test yourself here. What advice would you give these parents?

```
"MY SEARCH CONTINUES FOR A BLADE.
  A RAZOR'S EDGE TO SKIN THE FOX
TO DETERMINE THE ENTRAILS' CONFIGURATION
  TO ASCERTAIN THE COLOR OF HIS BLOOD."

"MY HAND JERKS DOWN AND IMMORTALITY
  RISES WITHIN MY SOUL, WITH FRIGHT
THE DIAL SWEEPS FROM LEFT TO RIGHT
  PROPELLING ME TOWARDS ECSTACY AGAIN."

"MY EYES SCRUTINIZE THE FRICTIONLESS SURFACE
  A METICULOUS SEARCH FOR THE FINAL OBSTACLE
THAT WILL JETTISON MY CORPOREAL BODY
  FROM REALITY TO HELL, VIA MUTILATION."

"BUT I WILL NOT HAVE EXISTED WITHOUT FEAR,
  A SURNAME FOR INSANITY, DELIGHT.
IN MY FINAL WILD RIDE, I CHANGE
  DIMENSIONS, ENTERING THROUGH A VIOLENT, SCARLET PORTHOLE."
```

Figure 8.5  A suicide note?

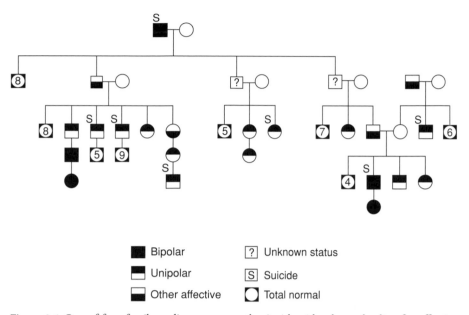

Figure 8.6 One of four family pedigrees among the Amish with a heavy loading for affective disorder and suicide. All seven suicides were found among individuals with a definite affective disorder. Squares denote males; circles, females. "Total Normal" means the total of normal offspring where no pathology was found. "Unipolar" means unipolar depression. From "Suicide and family loading for affective disorder" by J. Egeland and J. Sussex (1985) *Journal of the American Medical Association*, **254**, 915–918. Copyright 1985 by the American Medical Association. Reprinted by permission.

What little I have told you about this young man ought to give you much pause. Is this a suicidal message communicating impending death? Or is this the message of a thrill-seeker, an excessive risk-taker, a gambler who is likely to die through reckless misadventure?

Or, although only remotely likely, could it be that this is not the young man's poem at all, but one transcribed from some other source, e.g., as part of an academic course? As yet another possibility, were this a chapter on adolescent sexuality and my presentation on mastubartory fantasies, would you read this as a Rorschach and interpret it quite differently based on your mind-set?

I warned you that I might humble you!

Case studies also have value in teaching about biological bases to suicide. Egeland and Sussex (1985) presented fascinating evidence in a study of 26 suicides among the Amish of Pennsylvania over a 100-year period. Four families, in particular, had heavy loadings for affective disorder and suicide. For example, seven suicides occurred in this one family across four generations (see Figure 8.6) (see also Chapter 4).

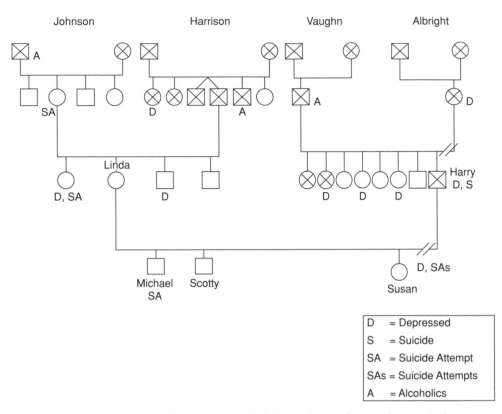

Figure 8.7  The Smith family genogram. A, alcoholic; D, depressed; S, suicide; SA, suicide attempt; SAs, suicide attempts. A cross indicates that the person is deceased.

You may have read of a widely publicized case in the U.S. involving a mother, named Susan Smith, who was convicted of murder for the deaths of her two young sons who drowned while strapped in her car. Her defense attorneys attempted to argue that she meant to go with them, i.e., that she was suicidal and had only at the last moment saved herself. Her family tree, also across four generations was presented to the court as part of this defense. Note the similarity between the family trees' loadings for depression and suicide attempt, and her father's suicide when she was six years old (see Figure 8.7).

## Case studies provide meaning and longitudinal perspective

Ed Shneidman, in speaking of the Inman Diaries (Shneidman, 1993), wrote, "They permit one to see the life in its longitudinal workings . . . glimpses over extended time into what William James called 'the recesses of feeling, the darker blinder strata of character.' We shall need to study these documents in greater detail to understand the psychological development of the suicidal drama."

What Shneidman understands and teaches us is that suicide is a dynamic process. Statistical studies of aggregated data provide static profiles of suicidal persons, statements of risk factors without the interplay of forces that give meaning and feel to the internal debate, the twists of ambivalent affects toward life and death, and the interactions between the person and environments, etc.

I believe the great value of the case study is to provide life to the deaths of individuals. It is in this belief that I respond with animation to the question of how I can study such a morbid subject. In this regard I refer you to the case of Kathy (Berman and Jobes, 1991) for an example of a case rich in texture and dynamics. The case study provides us the raw data for inductive reasoning. It humanizes our epidemiological and psychiatric statistics – statistics which too often fail us when we consider the tragedy of the suicidal adolescent.

In the end, as in the beginning, we have the individual case. The single case study design allows us to formulate treatment dynamics and plans and explore different theory-based formulations. It provides us the data for inductive reasoning. It humanizes our statistics. Although his intent at the time was quite tragically different, it is in this light that we might now read Joseph Stalin's oft-quoted, "When one man dies, it is a tragedy. When thousands die, it is statistics."

## REFERENCES

Berman, A. L. (1979). An analysis of suicidal and non-natural deaths among the Duck Valley Reservation Indians. Unpublished report to the McCormick Foundation, Chicago, IL.

Berman, A. L. (1990). *Suicide Prevention: Case Consultations.* [Springer Series on Death and Suicide.] New York: Springer-Verlag.

Berman, A. L. (1991). Child and adolescent suicide: from the nomothetic to the idiographic. In Leenaars, A. A. (ed.) *Life Span Perspectives of Suicide: Time-Lines in the Suicide Process* (pp. 109–120). New York, NY: Plenum Press.

Berman, A. L. (1992). Five potential suicide cases. In Maris, R. W., Berman, A. L. et al. (eds.) *Assessment and Prediction of Suicide* (pp. 235–254). New York, NY: The Guilford Press.

Berman, A. L. (1993). Forensic suicidology and the psychological autopsy. In Leenaars, A. A., Berman, A. L., Cantor, P., Litman, R. E., and Maris, R. W. (eds.) *Suicidology: essays in honor of Edwin S. Shneidman* (pp. 248–266). Northvale, NJ: Jason Aronson.

Berman, A. L. (ed.) (1994). Case consultation: a borderline dilemma. *Suicide and Life-Threatening Behavior,* **24**, 192–198.

Berman, A. L. (1997). The adolescent: the individual in cultural perspective. *Suicide and Life-Threatening Behavior,* **27**(1), 5–14.

Berman, A. L., and Jobes, D. A. (1991). *Adolescent Suicide: Assessment and Intervention.* Washington, DC: American Psychological Association.

Boring, E. (1950). *A History of Experimental Psychology.* New York, NY: Appleton-Century-Crofts.

*Bulletin of Suicidology* (1995). Washington, DC: American Association of Suicidology.

Egeland, J., and Sussex, J. (1985). Suicide and family loading for affective disorders. *Journal of the American Medical Association,* **254**, 915–918.

Jobes, D. A., Berman, A. L., O'Carroll, P. W., Eastgard, S., and Knickmeyer, S. (1996). The Kurt Cobain suicide crisis: perspectives from research, public health and the news media. *Suicide and Life-Threatening Behavior,* **26**(3), 260–271.

Litman, R. E., Curphey, T., Shneidman, E. S., Farberow, N. L., and Tabachnick, M. D. (1963). Investigations of equivocal suicides. *Journal of the American Medical Association,* **184**, 924–929.

May, P. A., and Van Winkle, N. (1994). Indian adolescent suicide: the epidemiologic picture in New Mexico. In Calling from the rim: suicidal behavior among American Indian and Alaska Native Adolescents. American and Alaska Native Mental Health Research. *The Journal of the National Center Monograph Series,* **4**, (pp. 1–34). Monograph, Denver, CO.

Niswander, G. D., Casey, T. M., and Humphreys, J. A. (1973). *A Panorama of Suicide.* Springfield, IL: Charles, C. Thomas.

Phillips, D. (1974). The influence of suggestion on suicide: substantive and theoretical implications of the Werther effect. *American Sociological Review,* **39**, 340–354.

Shaffer, D., Garland, A., Gould, M., Fisher, P., and Trautman, P. (1988). Preventing teenage suicide: a critical review. *Journal of the American Academy of Child and Adolescent Psychiatry,* **27**, 675–687.

Shneidman, E. S., and Farberow, N. L. (1961). Some comparisons between genuine and simulated suicide notes in terms of Mowrer's concepts of discomfort and relief. *Journal of General Psychology,* **56**, 251–256.

Shneidman, E. S. (1993). *Suicide as Psychache.* Northvale, NJ: Jason Aronson.

# 9

# Assessing suicidal behavior in children and adolescents

Cynthia R. Pfeffer

The assessment of suicidal behavior in children and adolescents presents several unique clinical issues, specifically related to developmental factors that make such assessment a dynamic task of arriving at a clinical judgment of how likely it is that a child or adolescent will behave in a suicidal manner. Extensive research of the epidemiology, clinical characteristics, and longitudinal course of suicidal behavior suggests that suicidal behavior occurs throughout the human life span with similarities that make it a clinical necessity to evaluate all individuals who come for medical or psychiatric attention for their level of suicidal risk. The importance of evaluating children and adolescents for suicidal behavior is supported by recent U.S. national epidemiological statistics indicating that in the last two decades the rates of suicide among children and young adolescents, age 5–14 years, have doubled and the rates of suicide among adolescents and young adults, age 15–24 years, are among the highest rates of all ages and they continue to increase (Singh et al., 1996). This chapter will discuss a systematic approach based on an understanding of developmental issues that are important for evaluating children and adolescents for suicidal behavior. It will focus also on evaluating the major issues that are associated with risk for such behavior (American Academy of Child and Adolescent Psychiatry, 2001; see also Pfeffer, 2001).

## The concept of suicidal behavior

Conceptualization of what constitutes suicidal behavior among children and adolescents is best considered within a schema of developmental psychopathology. Such a schema integrates "the interplay between normal and atypical development, an interest in diverse domains of functioning and an emphasis on the utilization of a developmental framework for understanding adaptation across the life course" (Cicchetti and Cohen, 1995, p. 3). Aspects of these issues will be discussed as they are specifically related to evaluating suicidal behavior among children and adolescents. Important to conceptualizing suicidal behavior among the young is the acknowledgement that "certain pathways signify adaptational failures in normal development that probabilistically forebode subsequent pathology" (Cicchetti and Cohen, 1995, p. 7). These adaptational failures may be considered risk or vulnerability factors that increase the likelihood of suicidal behavior. Also important in evaluating suicidal behavior among children and adolescents is the identification of "pathways to competent adaptation despite exposure to conditions of adversity" (Cicchetti and Cohen, 1995, p. 7). Identification of such protective factors can indicate how the likelihood for suicidal behavior is lessened. Furthermore, prospective and other types of longitudinal research have yielded information about the continuities and discontinuities that affect the profiles of suicidal states for individuals of varied ages or developmental levels.

A definition of suicidal behavior has two main features; that is, self-destructive behavior and the wish to kill oneself (Pfeffer, 1986). Suicidal behavior is defined as any self-destructive act in which a person *intends* to kill him or herself. Clinicians often ask if such self-destructive acts as self-cutting, reckless driving, or head banging are acts of suicidal behavior. In general, these behaviors can be considered to be suicidal behavior if a person intends to kill him or herself.

A clinical dilemma with regard to children and adolescents is that it is frequently difficult to identify intentionality or the wish to kill oneself because either children are so young that they are not able to verbalize their intent or they deny intentionality (Pfeffer, 1986). It is, therefore, often necessary to infer whether there is intent to kill oneself from the information obtained from other sources, such as parents, teachers, or others. It is also necessary to integrate all information about children's or adolescents' feelings, behaviors, and situations to infer whether there is intent to kill themselves. Regardless of whether intent to kill oneself is discerned, self-destructive behavior may cause serious damage to children or adolescents and techniques must be instituted to prevent such behavior.

Developmental schemas for cognitive capacities were described by Jean Piaget (1952). He stated that individuals construct a schema, which is "the internal representation . . . of some generalized class of situations, enabling the organism to act in a coordinated fashion over a whole range of analogous situations" (Gregory, 1987, p. 696). Piaget described the developmental levels of cognitive functioning of children and adolescents (Piaget, 1952) and these concepts are relevant in assessing suicidal behavior among children and adolescents (Pfeffer, 1986).

According to Piagetian concepts of cognitive development, children aged 2 to 5 or 7 years think at the level of preoperational concepts, in which the degree that their thinking is logical is limited. Such children often experience magical thinking and center their thinking on one dimension of an issue rather than integrating it with other concomitant features. Such children think in egocentric terms in which they understand things only from their own perceptions and experiences and do not appreciate another person's perception of a situation. Suicidal children, at this stage of cognitive development, may wish to die and think that if they overdose on a large quantity of sedating medication, it will make them die but their concept of death is to go to sleep. Such children equate death to sleep and do not understand the permanence of death.

Until recently, it was assumed that children should not be considered to be suicidal if they do not understand that death is final. This assumption has been shown to be wrong because direct observations of children's behavior indicate that self-destructive behavior has been observed as an outcome of children's intent to kill themselves (Pfeffer, 1986). It is critical to appreciate that children, even as young as three years old, have concepts of death. Such concepts may be immature but if a child wants to achieve the state they believe to be death, the child can carry out a self-destructive act to achieve this aim. Thus, intent to carry out suicidal behavior in children does not necessitate that the child has a mature concept of death (Pfeffer, 1986). This important notion makes it possible to understand the developmental nuances that are associated with suicidal states in children. In keeping with this, children can be considered to be suicidal because they have a concept of death, albeit immature, and they have an intent to die (Pfeffer, 1986). Appreciation of this developmental concept of death suggests that suicidal states can be defined in all stages of the life cycle.

By the approximate ages of 6–12 years, children have developed concrete cognitive concepts and, as a result, appreciate action in specific, logical ways that are limited in scope (Piaget, 1952). The thinking of such children is bound by logical rules that are predictable but based on present experiences. Children of this age make assumptions about their experiences that are based on limited information and do not change their concepts if new information is provided. Children at such cognitive developmental levels may think that if they jump out of a sixth floor window they will be hurt and taken to a doctor who will repair the damage. Their concepts of cause and effect may vary. For example, some children at this stage of cognitive development may believe that taking two aspirin tablets will be very dangerous and likely to kill someone, while other children will know that this action is not likely to kill someone.

Individuals from the age of 11 years through adulthood have developed operational concepts that enable them to think in abstract terms (Piaget, 1952). Their concepts about lethality should be similar to those of adults in appraising the dangerousness of a behavior (Gothelf et al., 1998). When evaluating adults for the degree of lethality of a self-destructive act, it is assumed that adults have achieved a relatively uniform level of cognitive development and, as a result, can comprehend whether a suicidal act will cause serious damage or death. Therefore, the concept of lethality can be measured by objective criteria with the assumption that most adults will consider the nature of a specific suicidal act in the same way. For example, jumping out of a sixth floor window will be uniformly considered a serious lethal act. In contrast, taking two tablets of aspirin will be considered by most adults to not be a serious lethal act. However, among young adolescents, there may be variability in their capacity to realistically know if a specific self-destructive act is lethal (Pfeffer, 1986). This is due to variation regarding when individuals achieve levels of abstract reasoning.

Considering these issues, the clinical assessment of suicidal behavior of children or adolescents must consider the developmental level of the cognitive capacity of a specific child or adolescent (Pfeffer, 1986). It is necessary to appraise what children or adolescents believe to be the outcome of self-destructive acts as well as to consider the objective outcome of carrying out a specific type of self-destructive act. For example, a seven-year-old child may believe that hanging oneself will cause someone to lose his or her breath but when taken out of the noose, the child will be able to breathe again. Such a child does not have an objective sense of the danger of hanging. Such a child believes the behavior not to be dangerous, but a clinician would rate such behavior as potentially lethal. A seven-year-old child may consider that taking two aspirins will kill them. However, objectively viewed this act is not very lethal. In such a case, should the clinician consider that the child's behavior is lethal? If a child believes that an objectively nonlethal act is lethal, such an act should be considered to be a serious suicidal act and appropriate interventions planned to prevent the likelihood of the child carrying out other dangerous behaviors.

## Interviewing about suicidal behavior

When interviewing children and adolescents about suicidal behavior, the context of the interview should be considered. In general, the assessment of suicidal behavior requires a sufficient amount of time to evaluate multiple factors that are associated with suicidal behavior. However, clinicians are frequently involved in emergency assessments of suicidal behavior of children or adolescents and little time is available to the assessment due to pressures of seeing other patients. In such circumstances, it is essential to ensure that a child or adolescent is comfortable with the interviewer and willing to talk. Such interviews are best conducted in a quiet area where there is little distraction. It is essential that the child or adolescent knows that the interviewer is able to help and that the purpose of the interview is to assist the child or adolescent. It is essential that the interviewer emphasizes that the child or adolescent will not be punished for ideas or behavior.

Interviewing about suicidal behavior involves direct discussion about the children's or adolescents' suicidal ideation or suicidal acts (Jacobsen et al., 1994; Pfeffer, 1986). The interviewer should begin with a hierarchical approach of addressing issues of suicidal tendencies. The purpose of this approach is to identify the degree of competence that children or adolescents have in discussing these issues as well as to establish an interview atmosphere that is nonthreatening for young patients. Thus, questions may begin as general concepts and progress to specific discussion about suicidal behavior.

An illustrative format for questions may be: Did you ever think that you wanted to hurt yourself? This general question enables the patient and interviewer to begin discussion of self-harmful ideation and behavior and focuses the interview process in the least threatening way for the patient. Other questions are: Did you ever try to hurt yourself? Tell me about what you did. When did you do this? This format of questions progresses from a discussion of thoughts to a discussion of behavior. It is essential that the interview process progresses to address questions about suicidal intent directly. Questions that can be asked are: Did you ever think about killing yourself? Did you ever plan to kill yourself? Did you ever try to kill yourself? When did you try to do this? Finally, it is important to discuss suicidal behavior directly. This should begin by asking children or adolescents if they know what suicide means. Often children and adolescents have concepts that suicide means to kill oneself.

If a patient does not know this, an interviewer may explain it to the patient. It is important to ask the following types of questions: Did you ever think about committing suicide? What did you think about? Do you have a plan to commit suicide? Did you ever try to commit suicide? When did you do this? Where were you when you tried to commit suicide? Not only is it important to ask about whether children or adolescents think about or have attempted suicide, but it is also important to identify the context in which this occurred. Important issues regarding the context involve the time, place, and triggering factors for suicidal behavior.

Some children or adolescents report auditory hallucinations about voices telling them to commit suicide or to kill themselves. These hallucinations should be considered suicidal ideation and it should be determined what the voices tell the child or adolescent to do and how the child or adolescent responds to these voices. If the child or adolescent cannot discern that these voices are his or her own thoughts and considers the voices as externally generated, the risk for responding actively to such hallucinatory commands may be high.

Suicidal plans and methods used should be determined. It is important to inquire about children's or adolescents' method for suicidal acts. Children and adolescents use the same self-destructive methods as adults to attempt or commit suicide (Pfeffer, 1986). In the U.S., guns and firearms are used to commit suicide in over 50% of all suicidal deaths regardless of the age, gender, or race/ethnicity of the suicidal person (Singh et al., 1996). Other methods used by suicidal children, adolescents, and adults are hanging, jumping from heights, overdosing, self-cutting, and running in front of an oncoming moving vehicle. In the assessment of planned or enacted suicidal methods, the interviewer should inquire if there is access to a gun or firearm in the home or in a place where the child or adolescent is able to use the weapon. Significant suicidal risk occurs whenever there is access to a gun or firearm, regardless of whether it is locked up, unloaded or dismantled (Brent et al., 1987).

Other issues regarding suicidal behavior should be discussed in relation to the context in which the suicidal act or idea occurs. This involves identifying whether the act would be, or was, carried out in close proximity to other people or whether a note or other communication of intent or plan was made. It should be explored whether there was a possibility that the child or adolescent could be rescued or took steps to seek help.

## Impact of other factors on identifying suicidal behavior

As noted above, the cognitive development of children and adolescents affects their understanding of the concept of suicidal behavior. Other factors, such as the current emotional state of children or adolescents, also affect the manner in which children and adolescents report their suicidal states. Specifically, the emotional condition of children and adolescents, such as presence of depression, anxiety, or anger, can affect the degree to which they report suicidal ideation or suicidal acts (Jacobsen et al., 1994). Intense affective states, such as anger or resentment, may cause children or adolescents to minimize, deny, or oppose discussion of their suicidal tendencies. It is as if the youngster is communicating "I'll show you what I will do for what you have done to me." This theme of revenge is a motivating factor for withholding important information about which children or adolescents are concerned. By withholding information about planned suicidal behavior, children or adolescents think that when they commit suicide, they will gain revenge by punishing people with their suicidal act.

Children or adolescents who are depressed may minimize their suicidal states because they are withdrawn, anhedonic, and not capable of interpersonal involvement, or because they want to keep secret their suicidal plan and state of hopelessness. Anxious children and adolescents may fear that talking about suicide may actually cause them to act out these preoccupations. The anxiety is a signal to retreat from direct communication regarding issues related to suicidal behavior.

In contrast, these affective states may lead to a heightened propensity to describe suicidal tendencies because such states are often present at the time of suicidal ideation or action. Depression, when severe, involves cognitive perceptions of self-blame, hopelessness, powerlessness, and guilt. The expression of these cognitive percepts may be acknowledgment that life is no longer tolerable, wishes to die, statements about ending one's life, planning methods to kill oneself, and overt verbalization of suicidal ideation. Intense anxiety may be associated with disorganized thinking, hyper-arousal, poor concentration, impulsive acts, and rapid conceptualization of ending one's life. The uncovering of suicidal impulses may be facilitated as a way of relieving these intolerable feelings. Anger may be so intense that children or adolescents fantasize about annihilating everyone, including themselves. They may express such impulses in the form of suicidal and homicidal ideation and acts (Pfeffer et al., 1983, 1989).

Emotional states may affect memory about past experiences. The concept of state-dependent recall is relevant in interviewing children and adolescents about their suicidal states (Jacobsen et al., 1994). This phenomenon suggests that the current emotional state may heighten or diminish recall of past conditions (Forgas et al., 1988). For example, children or adolescents who were severely depressed when they made a suicide attempt and who are presently not depressed may minimize the severity or the occurrence of the past suicide attempt. Their current emotional state affects recollection of the details of a past situation, especially if the emotional state in the past was different from that in the current situation. Thus, children or adolescents who have recovered from an episode of major depression may not recall the intensity or details of past suicidal ideation or a previous suicide attempt. Conversely, children or adolescents who continue to be in the emotional state in which they made a prior suicide attempt may describe that suicide attempt precisely as it had occurred. Therefore, when interviewing children and adolescents about their suicidal behavior, it is essential to evaluate the current affective state of the patient and to identify past affective conditions, especially those that may have been congruent with a past suicidal episode of ideation or behavior.

## Other procedures of identifying suicidal behavior

Assessing children and adolescents depends primarily on verbal methods to elicit details about suicidal behavior. Developmental cognitive and language limitations of children and adolescents may impede their ability to clarify the details about suicidal ideation or suicidal attempts. Younger children may not be as comfortable or confident in describing their suicidal states in verbal terms. In general, communication about past and current suicidal ideation or suicidal behavior may be very stressful for children and adolescents, and this may create a temporary loss of age-appropriate cognitive skills, thereby affecting the reliability and validity of their reports about suicidal states. Other approaches, such as play or drawing (Pfeffer and Richman, 1991; Zalsman et al., 2000), may be useful to augment the evaluation of suicidal states in children and adolescents.

Play is a universal behavior in all humans, and during childhood it has significant functions to enable children to master feelings related to stressful circumstances, to create fantasies helpful in solving problems, to imagine plans for future endeavors, and to communicate important concepts about their inner state of mind (Freud, 1963; Peller, 1954; Waelder, 1933; Winnicott, 1971).

Play is a natural method of identifying suicidal behavior in children and young adolescents. Specific characteristics of play have been described to be associated with suicidal states (Pfeffer, 1986). Children who have suicidal tendencies often play out intense destructive fantasies of killing others, killing themselves, and hopeless scenarios in which the only solution to problems is to die. Often such children misuse their play objects, causing them to be damaged, lost, or misplaced. Issues of loss and retrieval are common play themes of suicidal children. These can be observed in the representations of people, animals, or important objects that disappear and reappear. The reversibility of loss is a common fantasy associated with young children's immature concepts of the finality of death. Violent scenarios against the self and others abound in the play of suicidal children. The quality of such play is intense and it appears that the suicidal children are lost in their play and are unable to extract themselves from the play themes. Usually there is repetition of themes of violence, loss, death, abandonment, and despair. Such themes, however, are not pathognomonic of suicidal ideation or suicide attempts in children, but they are indicators to alert a clinician to inquire about suicidal states and other traumatic experiences.

Other techniques useful in identifying the presence and features of children's and adolescents' suicidal states involve interviewing other informants, who may be able to describe children's and adolescents' suicidal ideation and suicide attempts. Specifically, parents, teachers, and others who know the youngster may be reliable informants. However, multiple studies aimed to evaluate the degree of agreement between parental and child reports of psychiatric symptoms of the children or adolescents suggest that there is poor agreement for certain symptoms, especially those that are internalized and not obvious to an observer (Angold et al., 1987; Kazdin et al., 1983; Reich et al., 1982; Weissman et al., 1987). Such studies suggest that children are the most reliable informants regarding their suicidal states. Nevertheless, interviewing parents and others may assist a clinician in integrating the history and context of children's and adolescents' suicidal condition.

Other reasons for poor parent–child agreement may be that parents do not know of their child's or adolescent's suicidal behavior because they did not directly observe it. Some parents may deny or minimize their child's suicidal behavior because of its associated stigma. Parents may feel guilty that their child is suicidal and they consider such self-destructive behavior to be a reflection on their parenting style or skills.

Parental psychopathology may affect parents' reporting about their children's suicidal tendencies. Research suggests that parents who have mood disorders or who have a history of suicidal behavior may report more suicidal behavior among their children than parents who do not have a history of these psychiatric problems (Weissman et al., 1987). This trend may be related to state-dependent recall, to parents' identification of their own psychological states with their children's psychological states, or to their greater ability to identify subtle clues of problems that are similar to the ones that the parents themselves have experienced. It is essential for clinicians to consider these issues when interviewing parents as historians about their children's suicidal states.

## Suicide rating scales

A variety of self-administered suicide scales have been developed for screening normal, at-risk, and clinical populations for the vulnerability to, or presence of suicidal behavior or ideation (see AACAP, 2001; Goldston, 2000; Pfeffer et al., 2000, Pfeffer, 2001, 2002). Other scales have been developed to assess the seriousness of suicidal attempts in ideation (Beck et al., 1974, 1979); some of these have been adapted for use in children (Jacobsen et al., 1994). At present, few self-administered scales have been adequately tested in child and adolescent populations and their psychometric properties and clinical utility have not been established (Goldston, 2000; Prinstein et al., 2001). Whatever their potential usefulness for research purposes, these scales cannot take the place of a careful clinical evaluation with its attention to rapport, clinical and family context, and use of multiple informants.

## The relevance of risk factors

Assessment of suicidal behavior implies not only the identification of the presence and characteristics of suicidal ideation or suicide attempts, but also the profile of risk and protective factors that influence the degree of probability that a suicidal state will occur. In recent years, many empirical studies utilizing such research methods as psychological autopsy, cross-sectional, and longitudinal designs have validated types of factors that elevate or diminish risk for suicidal behavior among children and adolescents (Pfeffer, 1989). These factors are discussed extensively in other chapters of this book and will be discussed in this chapter with regard to their pertinence in evaluating suicidal behavior.

In addition to the fact that past history of suicidal ideation and suicidal behavior increases risk for future suicidal ideation or suicidal acts (Pfeffer et al., 1993), factors that influence the likelihood for suicidal states can be classified into domains involving: (1) affects, behaviors, and psychiatric disorders; (2) interpersonal relationships; (3) ego functions; and (4) developmental events (Pfeffer, 1986). Each domain contains factors that have been empirically shown to be significantly associated with suicidal behavior among children and adolescents.

The affects, behaviors, and psychiatric disorders domain involves symptoms of depression, anxiety, aggression, as well as such psychiatric disorders as mood disorders, disruptive disorders, substance-abuse disorders, and psychotic disorders including schizophrenia (Pfeffer, 1986). Empirical studies, for example, indicate that the presence of a mood disorder in prepubertal children is associated with a 3.5 times increased risk for a suicide attempt, compared to an absence of a mood disorder (Pfeffer et al., 1993). Adolescents who have a history of a suicide attempt have also been identified as having a high comorbid prevalence of oppositional or conduct disorders (Apter et al., 1988). Substance abuse is significantly associated with suicide among adolescents and young adults, when compared to factors associated with suicide among middle-aged and older adults (Rich et al., 1988).

The domain involving interpersonal relationships includes issues pertinent to social adjustment factors (Pfeffer, 1986). These factors involve features of social roles that people carry out in their daily lives. Social roles include competencies and problems with relationships in the family, with peers, and at school/work. Prospective investigation of prepubertal children suggested that poor social adjustment, especially problems within family relationships, increases risk for a future suicide attempt four times (Pfeffer et al., 1993). Family discord has also been associated with youth suicide and suicide attempts (Brent et al., 1988; Pfeffer et al., 1994). Often these issues are triggers or precipitant for suicidal behavior.

Ego functions are indicators of coping domains and include features of impulsivity, logical, realistic thinking, and mechanisms of defense (Pfeffer, 1986). They are to a large extent biologically based and many have a long-term quality that is highly involved in characteristics of personality profiles. Systematic research suggests that individuals who are impulsive are significantly likely to exhibit suicidal behavior (Coccaro et al., 1989). Ego mechanisms of defense, a psychoanalytical paradigm, have been related to suicidal behavior among children and adolescents (Pfeffer et al., 1995; Ricklitis et al., 1992), with ego defenses such as projection, regression, and reaction formation being significantly associated with suicidal risk, and ego defense such as repression being considered a protective factor against suicidal behavior (Pfeffer et al., 1995). Confusion and inability to realistically appraise current situations increases risk for suicidal behavior (Pfeffer et al., 1995).

The fourth domain involves environmental and developmental events that increase vulnerability for suicidal behavior (Pfeffer, 1986). These may include developmental disorders that increase children's difficulty in coping with academic and psychosocial issues, periods of life transitions (such as entry to adolescence) that may increase suicidal tendencies, and specific severe stresses, such as deaths and losses of emotionally important people, parental psychiatric disorders, or physical or sexual abuse.

Not only is the presence of these factors important in determining the degree of risk for suicidal behavior, but the nature of the interaction between these factors is essential to evaluate regarding the degree of imminent risk for suicidal acts. The following examples illustrate the interactions of factors and their effects on risk for childhood and adolescent suicidal behavior:

Example 1. Sam, a seven-year-old boy, was a diligent student who was compulsive about doing his homework and active in after-school activities. His younger brother, Seth, age four years, suffered from terminal cancer and required intensive treatments at home and in the hospital. Sam's working parents were overwhelmed by the stresses concerning their son, Seth. They were assisted by Sam's maternal grandmother, who lived with the family. She helped Sam with homework and advised him about tensions he sometimes felt with friends. Sam's teacher was supportive of Sam but thought that he was often sad and worried that his brother would die soon. She noticed that in the previous two months Sam had not been able to concentrate on his schoolwork and had needed assistance in completing the work. Suddenly one night, Sam's grandmother had a fatal stroke. Shocked by this, Sam withdrew from his after-school activities, in part because he had no one to accompany him to these activities. He could not concentrate on homework because he was preoccupied with thoughts of his grand-mother's death and wishes to be with her. He wished that he could have cancer, so that he would soon die and be with his grandmother. He exhibited intense frustration when his parents took him with his brother to visit the doctor. Sam uncharacteristically began to fight with his brother. One day, when alone, Sam took an overdose of aspirin and three other medications he found in the family medicine cabinet. Within several hours, he told his mother about this and about his wishes to die and be with his grandmother. His mother took him immediately to the psychiatric emergency room of a nearby hospital.

Sam's serious suicide attempt was precipitated by his intense sense of loss of his grandmother, his envy of his brother for having extensive parental attention, and the possibility that his brother would soon die and be with his grandmother. Of note, Sam's academic standing diminished and he withdrew from enjoyable activities. The increased intensity of lonely feelings was triggered by his parents' act of leaving Sam home alone. He was no longer able to cope and impulsively overdosed on medications that were available in the home. The interaction of increasing and cumulative stresses on a child who had been trying to cope with the serious illness of his younger sibling led to his suicidal state.

Example 2. Jane, a 16-year-old girl, had been depressed for at least two years. When she was nine years old, she was psychiatrically hospitalized after she attempted suicide by cutting her wrists. After discharge from the hospital, she was treated with psy-chotherapy for three years and, because she appeared improved, she stopped her treatment. As a teenager, she joined a group of friends who were truant from school and used marijuana and alcohol. In the previous year, she had developed an intense relationship with a boy but when he told her he wanted to see other girls, she became despondent and wanted to die. She fantasized that if she threatened to kill herself, he would remain with her. However, he had a fight with her about her threats and no longer wanted to see her. Her friends tried to help her with her depressed, hopeless feelings. However, one evening while thinking that nothing would work out for her, she drank a large quantity of alcohol and took an overdose of medication found in the home. She was found comatose on her bedroom floor by her mother at 3 a.m. and was rushed to the hospital where she was admitted to the intensive care unit.

This example illustrates the confluence of risks imparted by a past history of a suicide attempt, chronic depression, and poor social adjustment in an adolescent girl. Her recent serious suicide attempt was precipitated by her acrimonious relationship with her boyfriend. Her depression intensified, her hopelessness was pervasive, and her thinking became constricted and impulsive. Her suicide attempt was facilitated by the influence of alcohol and her intense loneliness. The fortuitous discovery of her condition by her mother was possible because she chose to attempt suicide in her home where the likelihood of discovery was increased.

Example 3. James, an 18-year-old late adolescent boy, had begun the second semester of his first year at college, where he found it difficult to adjust to being away from home. He made several friends and worked consistently to achieve good semester grades. He had wanted to live away from home because he found it unbearable to be in the presence of his alcoholic father, with whom he fought. However, being away from home generated intense anxiety and feelings of panic, especially severe at times of exams. He was very distraught during his final exams and could not relax during winter vacation. While home, he obtained the gun that his father kept in the basement. At times, James contemplated suicide and thought that if his anxieties got too intense he would kill himself. He refused to seek psychological help because he did not believe it had helped his father. He confided to his roommates that he was overwhelmed with family and other personal problems and they told the college dean of students, who arranged an appointment to discuss matters with James. This process proved effective in enabling James to turn in the gun and to begin a trial of psychiatric treatment and psychopharmacological therapy.

Risk of suicide in late adolescent males who have access to guns is quite high and intensified if they are prone to act impulsively. This example illustrates that, despite high risk, danger can be diminished when specific interventions are offered. It is essential to establish a trusting relationship as a means of evaluating risk and promoting intervention.

## Summary

Assessment of suicidal behavior in children and adolescents is based on a comprehensive developmental understanding of emotional, cognitive, and social contexts. Methodical inquiry is essential to appraise suicidal risk and this is best conducted within an atmosphere of empathy, trust, and hopefulness. Empirical research has highlighted numerous risk factors for suicidal behavior in children and adolescents. Of utmost importance is the appreciation of the dynamic equilibrium between multiple risk factors and shifts in them as provocations of suicidal tendencies. Careful assessment usually takes time to identify salient issues that require specific intervention. However, within the context of emergency situations, where little time is available, the prime issue to establish is the immediate degree of danger and to provide a plan that will impede acting out suicidal tendencies.

## REFERENCES

American Academy of Child and Adolescent Psychiatry (2001). Practice parameter for the assessment and treatment of children and adolescents with suicidal behavior. *Journal of the American Academy of Child and Adolescent Psychiatry,* **40** [Suppl. 7]:24S–51S.

Angold, A., Weissman, M. M., John, K. et al. (1987). Parent and child reports of depressive symptoms in children at low and high risk of depression. *Journal of Child Psychology and Psychiatry,* **28,** 901–915.

Apter, A., Bleich, A., Plutchik, R., Mendelsohn, S., and Tyano, S. (1988). Suicidal behavior, depression, and conduct disorder in hospitalized adolescents. *Journal of the American Academy of Child and Adolescent Psychiatry,* **27,** 696–699.

Beck, A. T., Schuyler, D., and Herman, I. (1974). Development of suicidal intent scales. In Beck, A. T., Resnik, H. L. P., Lettieri, D. J. (eds.) *The Prediction of Suicide* (pp. 45–56) Bowie, MD: Charles Press.

Beck, A. T., Kovacs, M., and Weissman, A. (1979). Assessment of suicide intention: the Scale for Suicide Ideation. *Journal of Consulting and Clinical Psychology,* **47,** 343–352.

Brent, D. A., Perper, J. A., Allman, C. J. (1987). Alcohol, firearms, and suicide among youth: temporal trends in Allegheny County, Pennsylvania, 1960–1983. *Journal of the American Medical Association,* **257,** 3369–3373.

Brent, D. A., Perper, J. A., Goldstein, C. E., et al. (1988). Risk factors for adolescent suicide: a Comparison of adolescent suicide victims with suicidal inpatients. *Archives of General Psychiatry,* **45,** 581–588.

Cicchetti, D., and Cohen, D. J. (1995). Perspectives on developmental psychopathology. In Cicchetti, D., Cohen, D. J. (eds.) *Developmental Psychopathology.* New York City, NY: Wiley & Sons, Inc.

Coccaro, E. F., Siever, L. J., Klar, H. M., et al. (1989). Serotonergic studies in patients with affective and personality disorders: correlates with suicidal and impulsive aggressive behavior. *Archives of General Psychiatry,* **46,** 587–599.

Forgas, J. P., Burnham, D. K., and Trimboli, C. (1988). Mood, memory, and social judgments in children. *Journal of Personality and Social Psychology,* **54,** 697–703.

Freud, A. (1963). The concept of developmental lines. *Psychoanalytic Study of the Child,* **18,** 245–265.

Goldston, D. B. (2000). Assessment of suicidal behaviors and risk among children and adolescents. Technical report submitted to NIMH under contract 263-MD-909995; http://www.nimh.nih.gov/research/measures.pdf [accessed September 24, 2000].

Gothelf, D., Apter, A., Brand-Gothelf, A., Offer, N., Ofek, H., Tyano, S., and Pfeffer, C. R. (1998). Death concepts in suicidal adolescents. *Journal of the American Academy of Child and Adolescent Psychiatry,* **37**(12), 1279–1286.

Gregory, R. L. (1987). *The Oxford Companion To The Mind.* Oxford, England: Oxford University Press.

Jacobsen, L. K., Rabinowitz, I., Popper, M., Solomon, R. J., Sokol, M. S., and Pfeffer, C. R. (1994). Interviewing prepubertal children about suicidal ideation and behavior. *Journal of the American Academy of Child and Adolescent Psychiatry*, **4**, 439–452.

Kazdin, A. E., French, N. H., Unis, A. S., and Esveldt-Dawson, K. (1983). Assessment of childhood depression: correspondence of child and parent ratings. *Journal of the American Academy of Child Psychiatry*, **22**, 157–164.

Peller, L. E. (1954). Libidinal phases, ego development and play. *Psychoanalytic Study of the Child*, **9**, 179–198.

Pfeffer, C. R. (1986). *The Suicidal Child*. New York City, NY: Guilford Press.

Pfeffer, C. R. (ed.) (1989). *Suicide Among Youth: Perspectives on Risk and Prevention*. Washington, D.C.: American Psychiatric Press, Inc.

Pfeffer, C. R. (2001). Diagnosis of childhood and adolescent suicidal behavior: unmet needs for suicide prevention. *Biological Psychiatry*, **49**(12), 1055–1061.

Pfeffer, C. R. (2002). Suicidal behavior in children and adolescents: causes and management. In Lewis, M. (ed.) *Child and Adolescent Psychiatry: A Comprehensive Textbook* (3rd edn.) (pp. 796–805).

Pfeffer, C. R., and Richman, J. (1991). Human figure drawings: an auxiliary diagnostic assessment of childhood suicidal potential. *Comprehensive Mental Health Care*, **1**, 77–90.

Pfeffer, C. R., Plutchik, R., and Mizruchi, M. S. (1983). Suicidal and assaultive behavior in children: classification, measurement, and interrelations. *American Journal of Psychiatry*, **140**, 154–157.

Pfeffer, C. R., Newcorn, J., Kaplan, G., Mizruchi, M. S., and Plutchik, R. (1989). Subtypes of suicidal and assaultive behaviors in adolescent psychiatric inpatients: a research note. *Journal of Child Psychology and Psychiatry*, **30**, 151–163.

Pfeffer, C. R., Klerman, G. L., Hurt, S. W., Kakuma, T., Peskin, J. R., and Siefker, C. A. (1993). Suicidal children grow up: rates and psychosocial risk factors for suicide attempts during follow-up. *Journal of the American Academy of Child and Adolescent Psychiatry*, **32**, 106–113.

Pfeffer, C. R., Normandin, L., and Kakuma, T. (1994). Suicidal children grow up: suicidal behavior and psychiatric disorders among relatives. *Journal of the American Academy of Child and Adolescent Psychiatry*, **33**, 1087–1097.

Pfeffer, C. R., Hurt, S. W., Peskin, J. R., and Siefker, C. A. (1995). Suicidal children grow up: ego functions associated with suicide attempts. *Journal of the American Academy of Child and Adolescent Psychiatry*, **34**, 1318–1325.

Pfeffer, C. R., Jiang, H., and Kakuma, T. (2000). Child-Adolescent Suicidal Potential Index (CASPI): a screen for risk for early onset suicidal behavior. *Psychological Assessment*, **12**(3), 304–318.

Piaget, J. (1952). *The Origins of Intelligence in Children*. New York City, NY: International Universities Press.

Prinstein, M. J., Nock, M. K., Spirito, A., and Grapentine, W. L. (2001). Multimethod assessment of suicidality in adolescent psychiatric inpatients: preliminary results. *Journal of the American Academy of Child and Adolescent Psychiatry*, **40**(9), 1053–1061.

Reich, W., Herjanic, B., Welner, Z., and Gandhy, P. R. (1982). Development of a structured psychiatric interview for children: agreement on diagnosis comparing child and parent interviews. *Journal of Abnormal Child Psychology*, **10**, 325–336.

Rich, C. L., Young, D., and Fowler, R. C. (1988). San Diego Suicide Study. I: Young versus old subjects. *Archives of General Psychiatry*, **43**, 577–582.

Ricklitis, C. J., Noam, G. G., and Borst, S. R. (1992). Adolescent suicide and defensive style. *Suicide and Life-Threatening Behavior*, **22**, 374–387.

Singh, G. K., Kochanek, K. E., and MacDorman, M. F. (1996). *Advanced Report of Final Mortality Statistics, 1994. Monthly Vital Statistics Report*; vol. 45, no. 3, suppl. Hyattsville, MD: National Center For Health Statistics.

Waelder, R. (1933). The psychoanalytic theory of play. *Psychoanalytic Quarterly*, **2**, 208–224.

Weissman, M. M., Wickramaratne, P., Warner, V., et al. (1987). Assessing psychiatric disorders in children: discrepancies between mother's and children's reports. *Archives of General Psychiatry*, **44**, 747–753.

Winnicott, D. W. (1971). *Playing and Reality*. New York City, NY: Basic Books.

Zalsman, G., Netanel, R., Fischel, T., Freudenstein, O., Landau, E., Orbach. I., Weizman, A., Pfeffer, C. R., and Apter, A. (2000). Human figure drawings in the evaluation of severe adolescent suicidal behavior. *Journal of the American Academy of Child and Adolescent Psychiatry*, **39**(8), 1024–1031.

# 10

# Suicide prevention for adolescents

Israel Orbach

Suicide and suicide attempts among adolescents are growing at an alarming rate (Diekstra and Garnefski, 1995). Suicide in adolescents, as it is in adults, is an escape from intolerable mental pain, hopelessness, and meaninglessness of their lives into an illusion of peacefulness (Baumeister, 1990; Orbach, 1988; Range, 1992; Shneidman, 1985, 1996). Adolescence, with the dramatic, transitional changes it brings, is the time in life when self-destruction erupts for the first time as an epidemic. This fact can be attributed to the many risks that accompany this transition. Many risk factors for suicide have been identified in adolescents: past suicide attempts, depression, feelings of hopelessness, drug abuse, alcoholism, sexual abuse, mental disorders, isolation, suicide in the family or by a friend, accumulation of negative life events, problems with anger control, low self-esteem, school failure, homosexuality, identity problems, family problems, learning difficulties, difficulties in problem solving, and others (Maris, 1991; Orbach, 1997). The eruption of the suicide epidemic at adolescence is of great concern and has led the efforts to initiate programs for prevention for the young. This chapter presents major approaches, principles, and techniques of suicide prevention programs prevalent in schools and prevention centers. Before the presentation of these, however, we need to gain some understanding into the experiences of the suicidal person as well as into some aspects of the adolescents' inner world. I will focus on these mostly from a psychodynamic perspective.

## The experience of the suicidal person – theories of suicide

Many theories provide insights into the painful experience that might lead to the wish to end one's life. I will focus here on a selection of theories with an emphasis on those which provide insights into the subjective experience of the suicidal individual rather than on objective or sociological analyses.

## The escape from mental pain

Shneidman (1985, 1996) asserts unequivocally that suicide is an escape from psychological pain. Psychological pain is the accumulation of negative emotions due to thwarted or distorted and frustrated psychological needs resulting in unbearable anguish, disturbance, or perturbation. This unbearable pain takes hold of the mind. When the suicidal person believes that their most important needs which define them as a unique person cannot be met and therefore the mental pain (shame, guilt, fear, anxiety, loneliness, angst, dread) will never cease, they will go on to commit suicide. Behind every suicide, Shneidman claims, there is a frustrated need that causes unbearable pain. A similar variation of the pain escape theory has been suggested by Baumeister (1990), who believes that suicide is an end result of a progressive, painful, negative self-awareness and increasing negative affect due to accumulative failures attributed to the self and self-disappointments. The peak of the pain occurs when the person realizes that there is neither any escape from these painful perceptions of the failing self nor any way to change this experience. Consistent with this view of suicide is the empirical finding that adolescents most frequently name mental pain as the cause for their suicidal behavior (Kienhorst et al., 1995). This approach suggests that one key to suicide prevention is the immediate reduction in mental pain.

## Loss and intrapunitiveness

Freud (1917) and later on Menninger (1938) viewed suicide as an end result of a long, self-destructive process beginning with the loss of an ambivalently viewed person. Anger directed toward such a lost person is redirected toward oneself in a self-punitive action and is experienced as anger, revenge, guilt, and lost love. The basic unconscious motive behind suicide is the wish to rejoin or regain the lost person through identification and death. The therapeutic or preventative approach implied here is mourning, acceptance of the loss, and learning to express anger.

## Depression and regulation of anger

The psychiatric medical model depicts major depression as the main cause for suicide. Depression from this perspective is a perturbation of neurobiological systems. These biological disturbances are characterized by anxiety and/or aggression disregulation and are precipitated by various stressors in individuals that are susceptible to the psychologically disrupting effects of psychologically traumatic events (van Praag, 1986). This neurobiological perspective implies that suicide can be prevented by pharmacologically or otherwise rebalancing the underlying neurobiological disturbances, thereby reinstituting the sense of self-control over aggression.

## The suicidal career

Maris (1981) views suicide as an end result of a suicidal career. At the heart of the suicidal career are the inability and unwillingness to accept the condition of one's life. Suicidal people have difficulties in coping with life difficulties and their efforts at adjustment have repeatedly failed. They tend to use coping strategies which are in themselves self-destructive, such as alcohol, drugs, promiscuity, suicide attempts, aggression, negative interactions, etc. After repeated failures, they escape the pain through death. Only learning to accept the limitations of life conditions, compromising the demand for full satisfaction in life, and better coping with life as a whole can prevent and reduce suicidal behavior.

## Hopelessness and cognitive dysfunctions

Suicide is associated with depression and mediated by a deep sense of hopelessness. Hopelessness – the negative expectations of oneself and one's future with no belief in the possibility of a change for the positive – is produced by cognitive dysfunctions such as negative automatic thoughts, distorted perceptions, overgeneralizations, inexact labeling, selective abstractions, and negative biases. These lead the individual to the conviction that there is no cure for his or her suffering and to a strong sense of hopelessness (Beck, 1967; Beck et al., 1993). One expansion of this theory has depicted suicidal individuals as suffering from a more specific deficiency in problem-solving skills, especially an impaired ability to generate new alternative solutions (Schotte and Clum, 1987). Poor problem-solving skills in social situations lead to accumulated failures and increase frustration. This, in turn, leads to both an increase in stress and progressive hopelessness and a sense of lack of personal efficacy. A further development of this theory focuses on negative self-appraisal in problem-solving ability as a cause for hopelessness, rather than the actual ability to solve problems (Dixon et al., 1994). This approach suggests that the focus should be on the experience of hopelessness, changing cognitive dysfunctions and attributional processes, and teaching step-by-step problem-solving skills as the main strategy of suicide prevention (Ellis, 1986).

## Loneliness, alienation, and lack of social support

Jacobs (1971) believes that the route to suicide involves a gradual decline into total social isolation. The suicidal youngster slowly comes to feel that he or she is no longer a part of society. This may start with experiences of loneliness and alienation within the family. Little by little the youngster may attenuate his or her social ties, become more introverted, and lose social support and social satisfaction. Eventually they may come to believe that their problems and personality are so different from those of other youngsters and that they cannot be affiliated socially at all. Feeling stripped from social support and self-love the youngster may come to the point of believing that social norms, including the norms against suicide, do not apply to them. The loosening of these norms may facilitate suicidal acting out. From this theoretical standpoint, the main preventative principle is reconnection to the social support system and a gradual emergence from social alienation.

## The irresolvable problem

Orbach (1986, 1988, 1989) has suggested that suicidal tendencies in young people are directly linked to familial situations and demands that pressure the child or adolescent to solve irresolvable problems. These situations and demands are reminiscent to some degree of concepts such as the double bind and scapegoating. Some typical characteristics of the irresolvable problem include confrontation with problems that are irresolvable by their very nature (e.g., to excel beyond one's capability), confrontation with a family problem that is disguised as a problem of the child (e.g., avoiding divorce by one parent exacerbating the child's problem and using it as a lever to keep the other parent in the family home), limiting alternatives for solutions or behavioral options, and creating a new problem whenever the old one is resolved. In a recent empirical test of this theory (Orbach et al., 1999), four factors have emerged as basic components of the experience of facing irresolvable problems: unattainable demands; commitment to parental happiness; need to be problematic; and giving up individuality for the sake of parents. The irresolvable problem is a subjective state of mind introjected from actual family situations and results in feelings of confusion, being trapped and incapacitated; feelings that all life problems are irresolvable; and hopelessness. The therapeutic and preventive principles implied by this approach include the exploration of the inner state of confusion and emotional processes, the exploration of life situations that are associated with the inner confusion, and increasing options of coping with resolvable and irresolvable problems.

## Self-deterioration and loss of inner control

Ackerly (1967) views children's and adolescents' suicide as an outcome of fear of loss of control over emotions and impulses and of the sense of total inner deterioration. The youngster feels that he or she loses control over aggressive and sexual desires aimed at the surrounding adults. Sadistic parenting may further heighten the danger of losing control. Suicide for such a youngster may offer a release from tyranny of the youngster's impulses. Ackerly describes a severely deteriorated mental state in which ego-strength is insufficient for self-control and the youngster experiences disorganization bordering on psychosis. Accordingly, prevention efforts must rely on a combination of medical treatment with a gradual therapeutic process of gaining self-control and learning to manage intense emotions and acting out tendencies.

## Low self-esteem

Self-esteem is the cornerstone for mental health adjustment and happiness (Kohut, 1977). This is especially true during the formative years of adolescence. Lack of self-esteem is to be found in every pathological state including suicidal behavior. Often, low self-esteem takes on the negative form of experiencing oneself as totally unworthy and as being bad. Youngsters who suffer from this malignant form of low self-esteem feel worthless, but also that they do not deserve to live. Low self-esteem can also turn out to be an active self-destructive process through active self-devaluation (Orbach, 1997) (see also Chapter 6).

Self-devaluation in the form of habitual minimization of one's self-worth and the tendency to withdraw, undermine oneself and minimize one's needs are typical of some suicidal individuals. The findings of several clinical and empirical studies highlight the self-destructive processes implied in self-devaluation. For example, negative self-evaluation distinguished suicidal from nonsuicidal adolescents (Tatman et al., 1993). Brevard et al. (1990) analyzed notes of suicide completers, which evidenced significantly more self-blame and negative self-esteem references compared with notes of suicide attempters. Moreover, low self-esteem correlated significantly in adolescents with suicidal intent and suicidal ideation (Duke and Lorch, 1989). The self-esteem approach to suicide advocates techniques of increasing self-esteem and self-love as the major strategy for suicide prevention.

## Critical vulnerabilities in adolescence development

There are several critical aspects in adolescence development that interact with dynamics of self-destructive behavior which may facilitate suicide or suicide attempts. Some of these aspects are described below.

### Separation-individuation

One of the major tasks to be achieved by any maturing adolescent is the balance between attachment or relatedness and individuation (Blatt, 1995). Over-attachment and lack of individuation may lead to preoccupation with issues of interpersonal relatedness and dependency at the expense of individuation. In contrast, an overconcern with issues of separateness and the dangers of over-attachment leads to a preoccupation with issues of individuation, control, and self-worth. Both of these imbalances may be critical for pathology and self-destructive behavior. Inability to separate makes the youngster vulnerable to anaclitic depression, while overemphasis on individuality may lead to a self-critical depression; both kinds of depression are linked to suicidal behavior. Both types of imbalances are of critical importance to the well-being of adolescents, as they are required on one hand to establish an independent life and, on the other, to be able to form relational intimacy and support systems. Difficulties in these areas may combine with other typical and atypical problems at this stage of development and hasten self-destructive and suicidal behavior.

### Egocentrism

At adolescence, youngsters develop the cognitive capability for formal operational thinking, yet they are not completely free of egocentrism (Elkind, 1967). While adolescents may differentiate between their thoughts and those of other people, there may still be a failure to differentiate between other's views of the youngster and the youngster's own focus of concern. An adolescent may easily assume, for example, that other people are as obsessed with his or her appearance as he or she is. In actual or impending social situations, the young person anticipates the reaction of others to him or herself to be identical to the adolescent's own reaction. The adolescent is continually constructing or reacting to an imaginary audience, thus amplifying the self-consciousness and self-criticism characteristic of this age. Elkind (1967) adds that, while adolescents may fail to differentiate between their own concern about themselves and others' perception of them, they tend at the same time to overdifferentiate their own feelings to the point of perceiving themselves as being unique in their negative self-experience. Thus, the sense of loneliness and deviance may be increased to an extreme degree.

### Self-identity

The adolescent is flooded by psychological, physical, and sexual changes as well as various social demands which produce external and internal conflicts (Erikson, 1950). This particular stage is viewed as a time of searching for an identity, but not of having one yet. One of the difficulties in the construction of identity is the need to change coping styles. At this time in life, adolescents mourn the loss of their childhood and its brevity, their infantile beliefs and wishes, and their idealized parents. Thus, a total reorganization of the self, ego, and identity is required. When this goes well, a sense of self-continuity and sameness between youngsters' past, present, and future in face of the changes they go through is a source of resilience. A sense of self-continuity, persistence, and uniqueness eventually helps youngsters to commit themselves to new strategies and new goals in life. Chandler (1994) argues that a sense of selfhood requires that as adolescents go through changes in life, they should be able (for the sense of self-continuity) to explain the changes that occur to them in a comprehensible way so that they are not experienced as unexplained, strange and estranged. Otherwise they may experience themselves as two different people: the one from the past (before the changes) and the present one (after the changes). The inability to find a sense of perceived continuity over time might hasten self-destructive behavior because youngsters who lack this sense of continuity have no more reason to be committed to their own future well-being than they are to the future of a complete stranger. Chandler argues that if, during such periods of attenuated self-coherence, negative circumstances conspire to make one's life seem intolerable at the moment, then suicide becomes a viable option. A recent study (Orbach and Mikulincer, 1997) has shown that suicidal adolescent inpatients, in contrast to normal and nonsuicidal adolescent inpatients, suffer from a greater degree of inner conflicts and ruptures in their self-representation which endanger their sense of well-being.

### Ego development

Loevinger's (1976) theory of ego development, with its emphasis on impulse control, complexity of self-reflection, and emotional experience, lends itself to the study of suicide in adolescence (see Noam and Borst, 1994). According to Loevinger (1976), each person has a customary orientation to the self and to the world and these frames of reference pass through an expectable series of developmental stages and transitions. At the earliest exploitative stages of ego development, behavior and experiences are characterized as having a stereotyped cognitive style and a preconformist style of externalization. That is, the youngster deals with external and internal problems mostly by externalizing problems onto the world (displacement, regression, identification with the aggressor, etc.), thus tending to attribute failure to external circumstances. Preconformists also tend to show more externalization in psychopathology in cases of developmental failure (e.g., conduct disorders; see Noam and Borst, 1994). Later adolescence is characterized by a more conformist or postconformist frame of reference. Adolescents in these later stages generally cope with inner conflicts with a higher degree of self-awareness, cognitive complexity, mutuality, respect for individual differences, and empathy. The conformist adolescent tends to show more internalization in coping and in psychopathology. These may take the form of principalization, rationalization, and attributing the negative to the self rather than to others. Therefore, compared with preconformists, postconformist adolescents may be more prone to depression and suicidal behavior.

### Coping with success and failure

The ability to sustain a failure is a reflection of mental resilience. Adolescence is a time in which the youngsters start to take responsibility for their performance and attribute success and failure in all spheres of life to themselves rather than to circumstances. Self-esteem as well as social esteem are established on the basis of success and failure. For the adolescent, failure can be immediately perceived as a shameful and humiliating experience and perceived as a blow to the self. The youngster does not have the perspective of viewing failure as potentially having an adaptive value, that it can stimulate resourcefulness and constructive striving and that every failure can be utilized for new learning about oneself and about life. Overdemanding parents fail to teach their children that mistakes can be utilized for self-exploration, seeking new and better ways to achieve blocked goals, and that there is always more than one way to achieve important goals. In a society that lives by a Calvinistic philosphy, success is identical to love, failure is identical to rejection, and striving for achievement is substituted for the yearning for love. The fear of failure can lead to fear of making mistakes and to paralysis as well as to regressive functioning. Thus, a vicious cycle of self-defeating behavior may take place. Learned optimism in the face of failure is one way of helping youngsters stay resilient in the face of failure.

The inability to cope with success is the other side of the same coin and may result in the same self-defeating cycle. Driven high achievers tend to constantly raise their self-demands and standards of what is defined as success. These never-ending self-demands make them very vulnerable to even a single failure. A single failure can completely erase the history of a successful past. The reservoir of past successes does not turn into a stable sense of self-esteem. Further, the danger of easy success is that it may distort the realistic perception of one's abilities and limits. Thus, the pathologically ambitious young achiever may be vulnerable to depression even after a single failure. Blatt (1995) has discussed these issues extensively, examining the relationship between perfectionism and self-destruction. He suggests that for the perfectionist who is driven by an intense need to avoid failure, nothing seems good enough and he or she is unable to derive satisfaction from even a job well done. This perfectionism may be particularly relevant to suicide in adolescents because of these youngsters' tendencies toward idealism during this period in life (see Blos, 1979).

## What makes suicide prevention possible?

Understanding the theory and causes of suicide is not enough to ensure an efficient suicide prevention program. It is necessary to identify what in the suicidal process itself and in its dynamics permits reversing the self-destructive behavior.

One of the inherent features of self-destruction which opens possibilities for intervention is the understanding that suicidal behavior is rooted in a multidimensional conflict. At the same time that the suicidal individual experiences an intense wish to die, he or she also wants to go on living. Along with the perception of death as attractive, there exists an intense fear of death (cf. Orbach et al., 1991). This delicately balanced conflict provides an opportunity to shift the suicide conflict toward a nonsuicidal conflictual balance.

Suicide is also a temporary state of mind. The intense feelings of despair, pessimism, and perception of death as the only solution are usually short-lived. If a person can be helped to live through the suicidal state of mind, he or she may come out of immediate danger. This fact makes it possible to intervene successfully. Similarly, predisposing factors (e.g., early losses) and precipitating factors (e.g., disciplinary crisis or romantic disappointment) for suicide can both be changed or dealt with effectively, thus reducing the danger of suicidal acting out.

Another nonspecific factor that often serves as a successful barrier against suicide is social support. Social support serves as a stress alleviator that moderates the effects of internal and external stress.

Finally, vulnerability to stress can be decreased and resilience can be directly bolstered through a variety of psychological techniques, such as problem-solving skills training, management of negative emotions, and increase of self-esteem, all of which are important protective resources against stress related to suicidal behavior.

## Strategies of suicide prevention

Silverman and Maris (1995) have extended Haddon's (1980) injury control models for public health into suicide prevention. This involves the classical tripartite model of primary, secondary, and tertiary intervention.

*Primary* intervention is aimed at preventing dangerous hazards and reducing existing hazards. Applied to suicide prevention, this entails limiting the use of or access to the means of suicide or preliminary antecedents of suicidal behavior, such as reducing the toxic content of domestic gasses, controlling the availability of firearms, limiting the number of pills per bottle sold over the counter, or providing adolescents with training in conflict resolution and anger management.

*Secondary* intervention refers to intervention during the injury phase for people who are generally defined as an at-risk group. The preventative means used here are aimed at creating a distance between hazards and individuals who are at risk, and strengthening the resistance of persons at risk (e.g., individual tablet packaging, confiscation of firearms and medication from suicide attempters, prevention of access to rooftops and high buildings, psychological intervention for the psychiatrically ill, early detection of distress, and initiation of psychoeducational programs and community support).

*Tertiary* prevention, which is usually defined as the postinjury phase, is aimed at individuals who have already seriously attempted suicide. These preventative measures are designed to rapidly detect and limit damage that has already occurred and to initiate immediate and long-term reparative actions. These measures include interventions such as improved assessment of suicidal risk, treatment of suicidal individuals, hospitalization of suicide attempters, follow-up for behavioral problems seen in the emergency room, proper media coverage of suicide stories, and postintervention teams for survivors.

Some of the secondary and tertiary prevention strategies have been described by Potter et al. (1995), Berman and Jobes (1995), and Gould and Kramer (2001), and are summarized in the AACAP Practice parameter (2001) and Center for Disease Control (1992) and Centers for Disease Control and Prevention (1994) recommendations and resources guide. These include the following:

## School and community gatekeeper training

These programs are provided to school personnel such as counselors, teachers, coaches, cafeteria workers, clergy, police, physicians, and nurses in order to teach them how to identify at-risk students and refer them to professional mental health services. The training program includes teaching warning signs for suicide and referral procedures.

Adolescents themselves have been identified as an important gatekeeping group, as troubled youngsters often turn first to their peers and friends (Ross, 1985). Hence, some prevention programs target youngsters themselves, to teach them how to identify, talk, and refer their suicidal friends, with a special emphasis on managing issues of confidentiality requested by the troubled youngster.

## General suicide education

In addition to facts, warning signs, and community resources, these programs focus on problem-solving skills, stress management, social coping, and increased self-esteem tactics. The focus in these modes of intervention is usually on: (1) the correction of common misconceptions about youth suicide, (2) the *identification* of self-destructive warning signs (e.g., teen depression, school behavior, making final arrangements), (3) first-aid *helping steps* (e.g., listen, be honest, share feelings, get help), (4) *practicing* communicating effectively with a distressed/suicidal friend (e.g., initiating discussion, showing caring and empathy, asking for clarification, giving support and lending perspective), and (5) *finding help* (school and community resources for teens, in crisis).

## Screening programs

These programs are aimed at early detection, assessment, and referral. The typical school screening program administers a questionnaire on psychological problems related to suicide, such as symptoms of depression, to all students. Those who score higher than a predetermined cut-off score are referred to the school counselor for additional interviews and, if needed, for treatment.

## Peer support programs

These programs take place at school or community settings and foster peer relationships, coping competencies, and networking among at-risk youths.

## Postintervention and cluster prevention

These programs consist of strategies aimed at coping with the aftermath of suicide in the community or school (Center for Disease Control, 1992, Centers for Disease Control and Prevention, 1994). They are designed to help prevent or contain suicide clusters and to help youth to cope with the experience of loss.

# Suicide prevention tactics

Various suicide prevention programs employ different tactics (Center for Disease Control, 1992). These tactics follow from the major theoretical principles believed to reduce the mental anguish and suffering of the suicidal youngster and to increase his or her resilience. Several major principles can be identified as underlying themes of suicide prevention programs:

1. Facilitation of open communication and enhancement of group support in order to gain emotional relief.
2. Enhancement of self-management skills.
3. Enhancement of problem-solving skills.
4. Increasing self-esteem and competence by changing cognitions.

5.    Increasing personal growth.
6.    Increasing resilience by heightening awareness of inner experiences in face of internal and external stress.

Almost all existing prevention programs utilize the above tactics of prevention to some degree, but each emphasizes one principle or tactic as its major focus. The various tactics will be described in some detail.

### Emotional relief through group support and communication

This tactic is utilized by almost every existing suicide prevention program. The aim behind this preventative approach is to reduce emotional distress and mental pain immediately. This goal is usually facilitated by an accepting group atmosphere of encouraging open communication, empathy, and sharing. The tone for such an atmosphere is set by the group leader who proposes a common goal for the group, emphasizes the universality of the problems of young people, encourages self-expression without criticism, and sets the structure and limits for the group. Tellerman (1993), who devised a suicide prevention program based primarily on cathartic outlet, group cohesion, empathy, and problem-solving approaches, proposes several devices to facilitate group cohesion and emotional expression, as well as problem solving. First, she defines the common goal as a creation of a safe environment to help members find something wonderful about themselves and then more specifically to use the group for sharing feelings and problems, and to learn to meet the challenges of living and to master life problems; to learn that they have the ability to solve life's problems, and to learn to integrate feelings, thinking, behaviors, and social awareness. The group cohesion atmosphere is further enhanced by emphasizing the need for reciprocity, a nonjudgmental approach, and encouragement (e.g., "That's a good question; a lot of people wonder about it; I am glad you were able to take the risk"). For example, Tellerman (1993) sets the general tone for the group through a poem she reads to the group in the first session: "This group is for each of you to feel better about yourself ... to get stronger ... to solve problems better ... to show your hurt and not to be afraid ... when you give out, you'll get back many times over ...." Tellerman uses some powerful techniques to encourage self-expression and empathy. In the ten-step, problem-solving program she proposed, each participant is asked to recognize a problem he or she has, to identify (define) the problem, and to bring the problem to the group. Each member of the group is asked to pretend that the problem presented is his or her own, to brainstorm for possible solutions, to discuss the pros and cons of the suggested solutions, to choose a good solution, to plan in detail to carry it out, to carry out the plan, and to report the outcome to the group.

The fact that participants agree that each one will present a problem facilitates openness and emotional sharing. When participants are asked to pretend that a presented problem is their own, mutual empathy, sharing, and group cohesion are enhanced. The presentation of the problems and the many solutions offered by the group members help the youngsters realize not only that they are not different from their peers because of their problems, but also that there are many more alternative solutions than they have realized before.

Another tactic for increasing emotional expression has been proposed by Hames (1997). She employs a graphic technique in which participants are given a sheet of paper with a boldly drawn circle at the top. Each participant is asked to think of the six to eight most prominent feelings he or she has been having recently and list these in no particular order. With multicolored crayons the participants are asked to choose a color that represents each feeling. Next they are asked to draw lines through the circle, so that each feeling is depicted as a piece of pie, appropriately colored and sized according to how predominant the feeling is for each one. Then they are asked to share their productions with the group. This approach helps the participants to identify their feelings and talk about the commonality, uniqueness, power, and range of feeling they experience.

## Enhancement of self-management and emotional regulation skills

Increased affective self-awareness or expression are not therapeutic goals in themselves. Many adolescents are all too aware or expressive of their intense negative affects. The purpose of greater awareness is in the service of enhanced self-management and emotional regulation skills. Distress and emotional flooding may result in the inability to contain negative feelings and increase negative self-perceptions and psychological pain to an unbearable degree. Emotional flooding may eventually lead to impulsive acting out of self-destructive behavior. Learning how to manage feelings of anger, anxiety, and depression through techniques of self-soothing may reduce the level of pain and the danger of acting out. Linehan (1993) offers a program of systematic learning of skills of self-management and self-regulation of negative emotions, as well as managing stressful situations. Although these are offered on an individual basis, they could easily be adapted to a group setting.

One way to manage negative emotion is to get to know the emotion by noting it, identifying it, and observing it. Linehan (1993) suggests trying to experience it like a wave coming and going without fighting it and without acting on it. Participants are often required to record their observations in a daily log, beginning with naming the emotion, identifying its intensity, identifying the precipitating event, defining how this event was interpreted by them, noticing the bodily changes that accompany the emotional state, noticing the immediate urge for a specific action, and what was actually done. At the end, the participant is asked to record what the after-effect of the emotion was, and, in an overall summary, to try to understand the meaning and function of the particular emotion. This emotional awareness and its recording help provide the person with a sense of inner control.

In a different training exercise, this program teaches how to control and manage negative emotions by counteracting them. For feelings of fear, it is suggested to actively engage in the frightening activity (over and over again), to approach the event/places/task that arouse fear, to control the action by making a small step/list/plan to approach the goal and to take the first step in the list. For feelings of justified guilt and shame, it is suggested to repair the transgression, to apologize, to make things better, to avoid future mistakes, to accept the consequences gracefully, and to let go. For handling anger, the participants are instructed to gently avoid the person with whom one is angry rather than attack, to avoid thinking about him or her, to do something nice rather than mean, to imagine sympathy and empathy for the other person rather than blame them.

Yet another exercise teaches the participants to exercise self-soothing through increased sensitivity of the senses. Vision is sensitized by buying a beautiful flower for oneself or watching the stars at night. Hearing is sensitized by listening to soothing music, and paying attention to nature's sounds. For smell, it is suggested to use a favorite perfume or lotion or bake cookies. Sensations of taste are increased by having a favorite drink (no alcohol) and dessert. For touch sensations, it is suggested to take a bubble bath, put clean sheets on the bed, have a massage, soak your feet, etc. The leading idea here is to treat oneself with pleasant, self-loving activities, rather than ruminate about negative emotions. The program suggests similar self-management skills for handling stress, improving the moment for increasing positive emotions, and so on.

## Enhancing problem-solving skills

D'Zurilla and Nezu (1990) have described the several successive stages of the problem-solving process:

1. Problem orientation. This encompasses the individual's general awareness that he or she has a problem and that he or she has the ability to solve it.
2. Problem definition. This relates to factual information about the problem, the clarification of its nature, and delineation of a *realistic* problem-solving goal. This entails an examination of the problem area, defining its extent and limits, and describing it in a way that makes sense to the individual. The clear definition

of a problem usually raises the level of motivation and enhances a sense of self-efficacy.

3.   Generation and evaluation of alternative solutions. This is a most critical stage of problem solving, as individuals who suffer from problem-solving deficiencies are usually blocked at this stage and cannot find alternative solutions and their evaluation.

4.   Make a decision about the best solution to be implemented by a structured plan.

5.   Monitor and evaluate the outcome and self-reinforcement for the accomplishment.

Almost all prevention programs use these stages in a more or less structured manner to teach problem-solving skills. The five stages are enhanced by group work and the leader, in clarifying the exact nature of the problem, in generating as many solutions as possible offered by the individual and the group members, and in discussing how the various solutions helped or did not help the different members. A further step is helping the individual to assess the pros and cons of each solution in reference to the defined goal and to choose the best solution with an option for other alternatives in line. The group approach to problem solving is most efficient, as it exposes each specific individual to many possible alternatives that they were not aware of before as well as to a systematic way of approaching the definition of the problem and assessment of the alternatives. An individual in such a group may also derive satisfaction from realizing that, although one feels incapable at times of solving his or her problem, one is still able to offer solutions more easily to someone else's problem.

This problem-solving approach is well-demonstrated in Tellerman's (1993) program and that of Orbach and Bar-Joseph (1993). In addition, Orbach and Bar-Joseph offer a somewhat different approach to problem-solving skill learning. They discuss positive and negative aspects of various problem-solving approaches (e.g., negative self-attribution, self-blame, rigidity, openness to alternatives, focusing on doing, emotional orientation, compromises, etc.). Then each participant is asked to fill out a coping questionnaire describing his or her own coping style and to analyze his or her own strengths and weaknesses. At a third stage, participants are presented with several made-up life problems and are asked to present their approach and solution to the presented problem and analyze them.

## Increasing self-esteem and competence by changing cognitions

Attitudes toward oneself and the social environments can be changed for the positive by changing cognitive functioning and content. Klingman and Hochdorf (1993) have utilized behavior cognitive functioning principles in their suicide prevention program. They have used Ellis' (1985) ABC (activating event, belief and consequence) technique for training students to cope with stress by changing cognitions. They employ written exercises for examining distress-activating events and their associated feelings, cognitions, and actions in order to change the meaning of events, irrational thinking, and negative automatic thoughts. For example, the students analyze a vignette of an event – failure in an exam – in terms of the elicited or automatic thoughts ("I am worth nothing") leading to a feeling (shame, fear), and resulting in an action (escape, cheating). The participants are taught the substitution of the irrational negative thoughts by positive and encouraging ones: Event – separation from partner; thought – I will overcome; feeling – pain; action – talk to a close person. Participants get to exercise describing a real life event, substituting the irrational with an optimistic positive approach. Finally, they learn that feelings and actions can be self-controlled through the generalization that "I do + I think + I feel = my mood."

At a later stage, the students utilize the new cognitive approach to expand it to new areas of functioning, such as empathy for distressed friends. One such exercise is a simulation of an editorial board of a youth magazine responsible for an advice column. The participants are asked to respond to "distress letters" and suggest advice along the principles they have learned.

Similar tactics utilize positive self-talk for self-encouragement and enhancement of self-esteem ("Problems are my teachers, they help me learn and grow"; "I am moving forward in the direction of my goals"; "I do not fear problems"; "I know what to do"; "I believe in myself"). (See Hemstetter, 1986.)

Cognitive and behavioral tactics can also be utilized for increasing self-esteem and a positive image by having participants answer affirmatively such questions as: "What is good about myself?," "What do I like about myself and my life?," "What good things have I heard from others about me?," "What do I do best?," "How am I similar to others?," and "How am I unique?."

## Increasing personal growth

Some of the suicide prevention programs go beyond the teaching of problem-solving skills, emotion management, and cognitive transformation. These programs try to extend personal problem management to more general aspects of meaning in life by enhancing personal growth through self-commitment, extended contact with society, and helping others. One such program, suggested by Eggert et al. (1995), consists of two parts. The first part provides teaching of skills and self-management and the second part emphasizes broader school bonding, providing social support for others, participating in school activities and clubs, and expanding participants' interests. The main idea behind such programs is that the ability to create meaning in life, to be involved in self and social commitments, and to help others is one of the most useful educational devices to help the youngster transcend daily difficulties towards a more meaningful approach to life. Such a transcendence may become a most powerful approach to enhancement of life.

## Increasing resilience by increasing awareness of inner experiences in face of internal and external stress

Some suicide prevention programs are based on the therapeutic working hypothesis that an experiential working through of inner pain, distress, anxiety, and depression may increase resilience when faced with a future inner crisis. Intense emotional states have a beginning, a unique developmental process, and an ending. Learning about these inner processes may help remind the participants that they have survived a past crisis and learned from it. The gradual experiential awareness of the inner process that takes place at times of distress and crisis can help in understanding, expressing, controlling, and eventually coping with it more effectively. When a youngster is aware, for example, of the inner process of depression – how it begins, how it changes, how it is experienced, what the signs of distress are, what makes him/her feel worse or better, how it was dealt with – the unpleasant experience becomes less frightening, more controlled, and more comprehensible so that in future occurrences it can be handled more effectively. The inner experiences tapping the internal processes involved are usually elicited by questions such as: "If you can remember a time when you felt really 'down' and can return in your minds to that time, what words come to mind to describe the way you felt then?".

- How would you describe the way your behavior changed at that time?
- What kinds of thoughts occurred to you when you were feeling so "low?".
- Did you ever think that you would always feel that way – that things would never get better?
- What kinds of things were said to you at that time that were helpful? That weren't helpful?
- Feeling as you did, how did you deal with the situation?
- Considering your feelings at that time, whom would you choose to talk to? Why? Whom wouldn't you talk to? Why?

One such program that is based on introspective discussion and sharing was introduced by Ross (1985) and expanded by Orbach and Bar-Joseph (1993). In the latter program, the guided discussion focuses on critical issues for adolescents. Emphasis is put on negative and positive aspects, sharing of experiences, universality and similarity of the experiences, coping and learning alternative ways to solve problems, and encouraging a self-help and peer-help approach.

The workshop consists of seven weekly meetings of two hours' duration. Each meeting is devoted to one of the following topics: (1) depression and happiness; (2) the adolescent and their family; (3) feelings of helplessness; (4) coping with failure; (5) the personal perspectives on coping with stress and problem-solving; (6) coping with suicidal urges; (7) summary and feedback. An additional workshop session on separation and loss is optional.

Each meeting is semi-structured and centers on three phases of discussion: description of the experience (e.g., Can you tell us about such an experience?, What kinds of problems arose between you and your family?); working through the discussed experience (e.g., How do these feelings change over time?, How does it get better or worse?, What made you have thoughts about suicide?, Can you distinguish between different types of failure?); and coping with the problem or with the inner experience (e.g., What did you do?, What would you like to change in the situation or in yourself?, Who helped you most?, How did you get over it?, What is the best thing to do in such a situation?).

The leader is provided with guidelines for each meeting, including information and facts about the topic under discussion, clues about how to handle problems such as resistance, negativistic responses, or anxiety, and how to promote the discussion.

A different approach to enhancement of awareness of the inner emotional experiences has been proposed by Bradley and Rotheram-Borus (1990). They have termed their technique "the feeling thermometer" as an aid for the participants to describe what happens to them emotionally and physically in various situations. It consists of asking teenagers to view their emotions as a thermometer and identifying situations in which they are the hottest (most upset, depressed, or angry), the coolest (most relaxed, feeling good), warm (upset, but not terribly), and cool (feeling OK). Participants are encouraged to describe what happens emotionally and physically under each condition (temperature). One adolescent may describe anger, violent feelings, loss of control, sweating, and shaking when most upset. A second may withdraw, start to feel nothing, feel edgy, or cry. They are also taught to relate these experiences to specific life situations and their specific behavioral response. A visual aid is helpful to the participants to understand the concept of the feeling thermometer.

## The integrative approach to suicide prevention

There is a growing awareness among researchers of suicide prevention programs (Center for Disease Control, 1992; Dryfoos, 1990; Kalafat and Elias, 1995; King et al., 2001; Silverman and Felner, 1995) that high-risk behaviors are interrelated and that a customized integrative package of different comprehensive services and programs is required in each school or community. Further, preventative efforts cannot constitute a "one-shot" effort; rather continuing preventative efforts are needed. Silverman and Felner (1995) emphasize that no single program may be appropriate for all populations; rather research efforts should focus on which suicide prevention program will be most appropriate for which population and under what conditions. Kalafat and Elias (1995) advocate a comprehensive prevention program that provides an integrative bonding experience in the community or school, including strategies for providing students with tactics for handling internal and external stress, opportunities for increased decision-making about rules, enhanced interactions with teachers and other students, and with opportunities to take on responsibilities. In other words, to use the school as a bridge for preparation to cope with life itself. Some efforts for suicide prevention have even included the extensive involvement of parents in these programs (Sharlin, 1987). Kalafat and Elias (1995) provide one example of several existing integrative models, detailing the principles to be implemented in a comprehensive suicide prevention model.

One example of a suicide prevention program based on an integrative approach is that of Eggert et al. (1995), who also accompanied it with an evaluation study. The at-suicide-risk students participating were assigned to one of three groups:

- Group 1: assessment protocol plus a one-semester Personal Growth Class (PGC 1)
- Group 2: assessment protocol plus a two-semester Personal Growth Class (PGC2)
- Group 3: an assessment protocol only

In addition, a control group of students – defined as not at risk for school failure – served as a comparison group for changes observed between preintervention and at follow-up.

The program started with a three-staged case identification process which was used to identify the sample of suicide-risk youth. The first step was to identify the sample pool on the basis of: (1) below expected credits earned for current grade level; (2) in the top 25th percentile for days absent per semester; (3) grade point average (GPA) < 2.3 with a pattern of declining grades, or a precipitous drop in GPA > 0.07; (4) prior school dropout status; and (5) referral from school personnel for being in serious jeopardy of school failure or dropout.

The participants completed a questionnaire containing items used for screening purposes, measuring suicide-risk behaviors, depression, and drug involvement. Suicide-risk status was based on levels and combinations of these variables.

All youth identified as at suicide risk were then contacted by a trained psychosocial nurse specialist or counselor. The nurse / counselor conducted an in-depth assessment of each youth's suicide potential using a structured interview. Each youth, whether in an experimental or comparison group, was personally introduced to a school "case manager" following the interview for appraisal of the youth's status and needs. Further, each student's parent of choice (or guardian) was contacted by telephone and similarly advised of the child's status and needs.

The prevention program was structured as an elective high school offering, called the Personal Growth Class (PGC). Youth were encouraged to take the one-semester class, PGC1, or add another semester, the PGC2.

PGC was conducted in small groups of 12 students, with one group per high school. The intervention was delivered by trained school personnel. The class was taught as one of the student's five assigned daily classes. PGC groups met daily for 55-minute periods in regular classrooms, and students received an elective credit each semester for course completion.

The fundamental program components in both PGC1 and PGC 2 were: (1) a small-group work component characterized by social support and help exchanged in group-leader-to-student and peer-to-peer relationships; (2) weekly monitoring of activities targeting changes in mood management, school performance and attendance, and drug involvement; and (3) life skills training in self-esteem enhancement, decision-making, personal control (skills training in anger, depression, and stress management), and interpersonal communication. Group support and skills training were integrated, and the skills training was applied in response to specific real-life problems emerging from the youth.

Specific attitudes toward suicide (e.g., beliefs that suicide is a viable solution to life problems) and suicidal behaviors (thoughts, threats, attempts) were addressed in the decision making skills unit (e.g., by teaching depression and anger management skills), and in the interpersonal communication unit (e.g., by engaging external support networks).

PGC2 emphasized broader school bonding, training youth to transfer their skills and provide and seek social support by joining and participating in existing school clubs and activities that match their interests. In addition, PGC2 extended skills acquisition by encouraging the transfer and application of skills learned in PGC1 to more difficult real-life situations at home and school. PGC2 also fostered the development of pleasant, health-promoting recreation and social activities to counter suicidal thoughts and behaviors, anger and/or depression, and drug involvement.

The outcome evaluation of this study indicated that after a 5- and 10-month follow-up, all groups showed decreased suicide risk behaviors, depression, hopelessness, stress, and anger. All groups also reported increased self-esteem and network social support. Increased personal control was observed only in the experimental groups. These short-term positive results are similar to findings found in research of other suicide prevention programs. But the long-term effectiveness of prevention programs in reducing actual suicides has not been studied yet and is awaiting sophisticated longitudinal studies.

## Conclusion

There is no single dynamic or explanation for self-destructive behavior and there is no one way to cope with this tragic phenomenon. Suicide is probably a part of our existential being in the world and some still believe that self-destruction may be a biological given in the form of instinct, genes, or a built-in potential of our dynamic physiological system. Even if we differ from such an extreme pessimistic view, suicide is still a problem – for the specific individual and for society and culture in general, in particular for the western culture which emphasizes individuality and personal achievement. From this broader perspective, it is clear that suicide prevention should go beyond existing programs that integrate various strategies and tactics aimed at increasing personal resilience and well-being. Suicide prevention should become a public health issue and concern not only for the health profession, but for social political leadership. Prevention programs should be based on national policies and cultural values integrating enhancement of life in everyday living.

## REFERENCES

Ackerly, W. C. (1967). Latency-age children who threaten or attempt to kill themselves. *Journal of the American Academy of Child Psychiatry*, **6**, 242–261.

American Academy of Child and Adolescent Psychiatry (2001). Practice parameter for the assessment and treatment of children and adolescents with suicidal behavior. *Journal of the American Academy of Child and Adolescent Psychiatry*, **40** (Suppl. 7) 24S–51S.

Baumeister, R. F. (1990). Suicide as escape from self. *Psychological Review*, **97**, 90–113.

Beck, A. T. (1967). *Depression: Clinical Experimental and Theoretical Aspects*. New York City, NY: Harper and Row.

Beck, A. T., Steer, R. A., Beck, J. S., and Newman, C. F. (1993). Hopelessness, depression, suicidal ideation, and clinical diagnosis of depression. *Suicide and Life-Threatening Behavior*, **23**, 139–145.

Berman, A. L., and Jobes, D. A. (1995). Suicide prevention in adolescents (ages 12–18). *Suicide and Life-Threatening Behavior*, **25**, 143–154.

Blatt, S. J. (1995). The destructiveness of perfectionism: implications for treatment of depression. *American Psychologist*, **50**, 1003–1020.

Blos, P. (1979). *The Adolescent Passage: Developmental Issues*. New York City, NY: International Universities Press.

Bradley, J., and Rotheram-Borus, M. J. (1990). *Evaluation of Imminent Danger for Suicide: A Training Manual.* University of Oklahoma Youth Services.

Brevard, A., Lester, D., and Young, B. (1990). A comparison of suicide notes written by suicide completers and suicide attempters. *Crisis*, **11**, 7–11.

Center for Disease Control (1992). *Youth Suicide Prevention Programs: A Resource Guide.* Atlanta, GA: Atlanta Center for Disease Control.

Centers for Disease Control and Prevention (1994). Prevention Guidelines Database (1994). *Suicide Contagion and the Reporting of Suicide: Recommendations From a National Workshop.* MMWR 43 (RR-6):9–18. *http://aepo-xdv-www.epo.cdc.gov/wonder/prevguid/m0031539/m0031539.asp*

Chandler, M. (1994). Self-continuity in suicidal and nonsuicidal adolescents. In Noam, U. G., and Borst, S. (eds.) *Children, Youth and Suicide: Developmental Perspectives* (pp. 55–70). San Francisco, CA: Jossey-Bass.

Diekstra, R. F. W., and Garnefski, N. (1995). On the nature, magnitude, and causality of suicidal behavior: an international perspective. *Suicide and Life-Threatening Behavior*, **25**, 36–57.

Dixon, W. A., Heppener, P. P., and Rudd, M. D. (1994). Problem solving appraisal, hopelessness and suicide ideation: evidence of a mediational model. *Journal of Counseling Psychology*, **41**, 91–98.

Dryfoos, J. G. (1990). *Adolescents at Risk: Prevalence and Prevention.* New York City, NY: Oxford University Press.

Duke, R. L., and Lorch, B. D. (1989). The effects of school, family, self-concept, and deviant behavior on adolescents' suicide ideation. *Journal of Adolescence*, **12**, 239–251.

D'Zurilla, T. J., and Nezu, A. M. (1990). Development and preliminary evaluation of the Social Problem Solving Inventory. *Psychological Assessment: A Journal of Consulting and Clinical Psychology*, **2**, 156–163.

Eggert, L. L., Thompson, E., Herting, J. R., and Nicholas, L. J. (1995). A prevention research program: reconnecting at risk youth. *Issues in Mental Health Nursing*, **15**, 107–135.

Elkind, D. (1967). Egocentrism in adolescence. *Child Development*, **38**, 1025–1034.

Ellis, A. (1985). Expanding the ABC's of RET. In Mahoney, M., and Freeman, A. (eds.) *Cognition and Psychotherapy* (pp. 313–324). New York City, NY: Plenum Press.

Ellis, T. E. (1986). Towards a cognitive therapy for suicidal individuals. *Professional Psychology: Research and Practice*, **17**, 125–130.

Erikson, E. H. (1950). *Childhood and Society.* New York City, NY: Norton.

Freud, S. (1917). Mourning and melancholia. In Strachey, J. (ed. and translator) *The Standard Edition of the Complete Psychological Works of Sigmund Freud*, Vol. 14 (pp. 243–258). London: Hogarth Press. (Original work published 1917.)

Gould, M. S., and Kramer, R. A. (2001). Youth suicide prevention. *Suicide and Life-Threatening Behavior*, **31** [Suppl], 6–31.

Haddon, W. Jr. (1980). Advances in epidemiology of injuries as a basis for public policy. *Public Health Reports*, **95**, 411–421.

Hames, C., (1997). *Helping Teens Identify Feelings and Positive Coping: A Graphic Technique.* Kingston, RI: University of Rhode Island, College of Nursing.

Hemstetter, S. (1986). *What To Say When You Talk To Yourself.* Scottsdale, AZ: Griddle Press.

Jacobs, J. (1971). *Adolescent Suicide*. New York City, NY: Wiley International.

Kalafat, J., and Elias, M. (1995). Suicide prevention in the broad and narrow foci. *Suicide and Life-Threatening Behavior*, **25**, 10–21.

Kienhorst, I. W. M., De Wilde, E. J., Diekstra, R. F. W., and Walters, W. H. G. (1995). Adolescents' image of their suicide attempt. *Journal of the American Academy of Child and Adolescent Psychiatry*, **43**, 623–628.

King, R. A., Schwab-Stone, M., Flisher, A. J., Greenwald, S., Kramer, R. A., Goodman, S. H., Lahey, B. B., Shaffer, D., and Gould, M. S. (2001). Psychosocial and risk behavior correlates of youth suicide attempts and suicidal ideation. *Journal of the American Academy of Child and Adolescent Psychiatry*, **40**(7), 837–846.

Klingman, A., and Hochdorf, Z. (1993). Coping with distress and self-harm: the impact of primary prevention programs among adolescents. *Journal of Adolescence*, **16**, 121–140.

Kohut, H. (1977). *The Restoration of the Self*. New York City, NY: International Universities Press.

Linehan, M. (1993). *Skill Training Manual for Treating Borderline Personality Disorder*. New York City, NY: The Guilford Press.

Loevinger, J. (1976). *Ego Development: Conceptions and Theories*. San Francisco, CA: Jossey-Bass.

Maris, R. W. (1981). *Pathways to Suicide: A Survey of Self-destructive Behavior*. Baltimore, MD: Johns Hopkins University Press.

Maris, R. W. (1991). Introduction to assessment and prediction of suicide. *Suicide and Life-Threatening Behavior*, **21**, 1–17.

Menninger, K. (1938). *Man against Himself*. San Diego, CA: Harcourt Brace.

Noam, G. G., and Borst, S. (1994). Developing meaning, losing meaning: understanding suicidal behavior in the young. In Noam, G. G., and Borst, S. (eds.) *Children, Youth and Suicide: Developmental Perspective* (pp. 39–54). San Francisco, CA: Jossey-Bass.

Orbach, I. (1986). The insolvable problem as a determinant in the dynamics of suicidal behavior in children. *American Journal of Psychotherapy*, **XL**, 511–520.

Orbach, I. (1988). *Children Who Don't Want to Live*. San Francisco, CA: Jossey-Bass.

Orbach, I. (1989). Familial and intrapsychic splits in suicidal adolescents. *American Journal of Psychotherapy*, **XLIII**, 356–367.

Orbach, I. (1997). A taxonomy of factors related to suicidal behavior. *Clinical Psychology: Theory and Practice*, **4**, 208–224.

Orbach, I., and Bar-Joseph, H. (1993). The impact of a suicide prevention program for adolescents on suicidal tendencies, hopelessness, ego identity, and coping. *Suicide and Life-Threatening Behavior*, **23**, 120–129.

Orbach, I., and Mikulincer, M. (1997). Self-representation of suicidal adolescents [unpublished manuscript]. Ramat-Gan, Israel: Department of Psychology, Bar-Ilan University.

Orbach, I., Milstein, E., Har-Even, D., Apter, A., Tyano, S., and Elitzur, A. (1991). A multi-attitude suicide tendency scale for adolescents. *Psychological Assessment: A Journal of Consulting and Clinical Psychology*, **3**, 398–404.

Orbach, I., Mikulincer, M., Blumenson, R., Mester, R., and Stein, D. (1999). The subjective experience of problem irresolvability and suicidal behavior: dynamics and measurement. *Suicide and Life-Threatening Behavior*, **29**(2), 150–164.

Potter, L., Powell, E. K., and Kachur, P. (1995). Suicide prevention from a public health perspective. *Suicide and Life-Threatening Behavior*, **25**, 82–91.

Range, L. (1992). Suicide prevention guidelines for schools. *Educational Psychology Review*, **5**, 1–20.

Ross, C. P. (1985). Teaching children the facts of life and death: suicide prevention in schools. In Peck, M. L., Farberow, N., and Litmund, R. E. (eds.) *Youth suicide* (pp. 147–169). New York City, NY: Springer.

Schotte, D. E., and Clum, G. A. (1987). Problem-solving skills in suicidal psychiatric patients. *Journal of Consulting and Clinical Psychology*, **55**, 49–54.

Sharlin, S. (1987). *A Suicide Prevention Program for the Young*. Haifa, Israel: Department of Social Work, Haifa University.

Shneidman, E. S. (1985). *Definition of Suicide*. New York City, NY: Wiley & Sons.

Shneidman, E. S. (1996). *The Suicidal Mind*. New York City, NY: Wiley & Sons.

Silverman, M. M., and Felner, R. D. (1995). Suicide prevention programs: issues of design, implementation, feasibility, and developmental appropriateness. *Suicide and Life-Threatening Behavior*, **25**, 92–104.

Silverman, M. M., and Maris, R. W. (1995). The prevention of suicidal behavior: an overview. *Suicide and Life-Threatening Behavior*, **25**, 10–21.

Tatman, S. M., Greene, A. L., and Karr, L. C. (1993). Use of the Suicide Probability Scale (SPS) with adolescents. *Suicide and Life-Threatening Behavior*, **23**, 188–203.

Tellerman, S. J. (1993). *Talking Troubles*. Alexandria, VA: The American Counselling Association.

van Praag, H. M. (1986). Biological suicide research: outcome and limitation. *Biological Psychiatry*, **21**, 1305–1323.

# 11

# Cognitive behavioral therapy after deliberate self-harm in adolescence

Richard Harrington and Younus Saleem

## Circumstances of suicidal attempts

The kinds of cognitive behavioral interventions that are provided for adolescents who have taken a deliberate overdose, or who have deliberately harmed themselves in other ways, will depend to a large extent on the circumstances in which attempts occur. These include (1) acute problems that are faced by the young person; (2) the chronic problems that they face; (3) the presence of psychiatric disorders such as depression; and (4) the thoughts associated with suicidal attempts.

### Acute problems

Many episodes of self-poisoning or self-harm in young people are preceded by stressful events. In a study in Manchester, England, adolescents who had deliberately poisoned themselves were found to have experienced a much greater level of personal difficulties in the three months prior to the episode than matched subjects from the general population (Kerfoot et al., 1995). In particular, they were more often reported to have problems with friendships, to be poor school-attenders, and to be having arguments with members of their families. Very commonly, there was some kind of quarrel with a key person in the young person's life. An example was an adolescent girl who had a chronically poor relationship with her mother. She had been out late repeatedly. One morning her mother confronted her and was very critical of her. The girl took a large overdose of paracetamol later that day.

### Chronic problems

Many of the problems that adolescent suicide-attempters must deal with are chronic, that is, have been present for several months. The most common long-standing problems are summarized in Table 11.1.

**Table 11.1.** Chronic problems experienced by adolescents who deliberately harm themselves (Kerfoot et al., 1996)

| Problems | Adolescent overdose ($n = 40$) % | Community control ($n = 40$) % |
|---|---|---|
| Broken home | 57 | 15 |
| Parental psychiatric disorder | 35 | 30 |
| Poor relationship with mother | 57 | 10 |
| Family stressful event in the past year | 70 | 35 |
| Parent has criminal conviction | 42 | 27 |
| Family on benefits | 77 | 30 |

**Broken home**

Kerfoot and colleagues (Kerfoot et al., 1996) found that more than half of adolescents who have deliberately poisoned themselves came from broken homes. In some cases, the parents' relationship had broken down shortly before the suicidal attempt. However, more commonly the break-up of the relationship had occurred several years before. It was quite common to find that the adolescents had experienced unsatisfactory arrangements for continuing contact, usually with the father. Often, the parents would be involved in severe and ongoing relationship difficulties. Adolescent suicide-attempters were often exposed to role models of violence or arguments within the family.

**Parental psychiatric disorder**

In the same study, approximately one-third of the adolescents who harmed themselves had parents with psychiatric problems. The most common psychiatric problem was depression in the mother. Parental personality problems were also relatively common. Severe psychiatric disorders such as schizophrenia were, however, relatively rare.

**Family functioning**

There were also high levels of unhealthy family functioning (Kerfoot et al., 1996). These were assessed using a standardized questionnaire, the Family Assessment Device (Miller et al., 1985). In comparison with community controls, adolescent overdose cases reported significantly more unhealthy family functioning. For example, they rated their families as being less able to communicate effectively, showing less warmth, and being more inconsistent. Similar trends were found for parental reports of family functioning, though these reached statistical significance on only one scale.

All in all, these findings suggest that adolescents who have poisoned themselves tend to come from families with a wide range of relationship difficulties.

### Other family difficulties

It was common to find that the families of adolescents who had poisoned themselves were subject to stresses of one kind or another. Stresses experienced during the previous year included bereavement, parental unemployment, rehousing, and being burgled. These stresses commonly occurred against a background of deprivation and poverty. Around three-quarters of overdose cases came from families where at least one member was on benefits (Kerfoot et al., 1996).

## Psychiatric disorder

In over 80% of community and referred cases of suicide attempts, there are associated psychiatric disorders, most often depressive, anxiety, and behavioral disorders (Brent, 1997). For example, in the study of Kerfoot and colleagues patients were assessed with a standardized psychiatric interview, the Schedule for Affective Disorders and Schizophrenia – Child Version (Puig-Antich and Chambers, 1978). Major depressive disorder was found in around two-thirds of cases. Although this proportion may seem high, a very similar rate was found in another much larger study (Harrington et al., 1998b). Behavioral disorders were also relatively common: 35% of overdose cases were found to have oppositional disorder, and 22% conduct disorder (Kerfoot et al., 1996).

The patients seen in the study of Kerfoot et al. (1996) were followed up six weeks later. Only 6 of the 16 overdose cases with major depressive disorder on the first assessment still had major depression at the second assessment. Similar findings were reported by Harrington et al. (1998b). Thus, although many young patients who take overdoses meet the criteria for major depression shortly after the overdose, for most of these patients the depression is mild. It is possible that in such patients it is secondary to the kinds of difficulties described above. Nevertheless, it is important to note that a significant minority of adolescent suicide-attempters have persistent depressive disorder (Harrington et al., 1998b).

## Thoughts associated with suicidal attempts

It seems, then, that deliberate self-harm in young people is strongly associated with acute and chronic life problems, and with psychiatric disorders such as depression. To plan cognitive-behavioral treatment programs, however, it is also important to know about the motivational aspect of self-poisoning, about the thoughts that precede attempts, and the styles of thinking that are associated with attempts.

### Premeditation

Most episodes of deliberate self-harm in young people appear to involve little planning. For example, in the study of Kerfoot and colleagues (1996), in only 20% of cases was there evidence of planning for more than three hours before the overdose. Most commonly, the overdose was taken on impulse, usually with tablets that were most easily available (containing paracetamol in more than 60% of cases). In most cases intent to die seemed low. For example, only three left suicide notes, and just six took the overdose when there was no-one nearby. The implication is that the decision to take the overdose was often made with little or no planning, or appraisal of the likely consequences.

### Hopelessness

Several studies have found an association between adolescent suicidal behavior and hopelessness (Burgess et al., 1998; Kerfoot et al., 1996). It is important to assess hopelessness for two main reasons. First, hopeless patients are more likely to drop out of treatment. Second, hopelessness may be a predictor of completed suicide after a suicidal attempt (Hawton and Catalan, 1982).

## Rationale for the use of cognitive behavioral therapy in suicidal adolescents

Cognitive behavioral therapies (CBT) have a number of features that make them particularly useful in the treatment of suicidal adolescents. First, the cognitive component of CBT includes many techniques to deal with the negative cognitions that are strongly associated with self-harm in adolescence, such as hopelessness. Second, the behavioral component of CBT includes techniques that can be used to help the adolescent to overcome the social and personal problems that are commonly associated with self-harm in this age group. Techniques such as social problem-solving and facilitation of communication are an integral part of many CBT programs. Third, CBTs are an effective treatment for some of the psychiatric disorders that are strongly associated with deliberate self-harm, such as depressive disorder (Harrington et al., 1998a). For instance, Wood and colleagues (Wood et al., 1996) found that CBT was significantly more effective than relaxation training in a clinical sample of depressed adolescents. In another clinical study, Brent and colleagues (Brent et al., 1997) showed that cognitive therapy was superior both to family therapy and supportive treatments for clinically depressed adolescents. As assessed at follow-up two years later, however, there were no significant differences in outcome between the

**Table 11.2.** Key questions to be addressed in the assessment of adolescents after deliberate self-poisoning

---

1. What was the extent of suicidal intent?
2. What is the risk of suicide now, or of further self-harm?
3. What is the reason for the adolescent's attempt in terms of mental state, psychiatric disorder, and/or social context?
4. What acute, chronic, personal or environmental problems must the adolescent deal with?
5. Does the adolescent have a psychiatric disorder and, if so, what is its nature?
6. What kind of help is most appropriate, and is the patient willing to accept such help?
7. What strengths does the adolescent and/or the family have?

---

CBT, systematic behavioral family therapy, and nondirective supportive therapy groups (Birmaher et al., 2000). Cognitive-behavioral techniques, such as interpersonal problem-solving, may also be useful in adolescents with behavioral disorders (Kazdin, 1997). This is important because, as described above, suicidal behavior in adolescence is often associated with behavioral disturbance of some kind. Finally, as Brent describes (Brent, 2001; Brent and Lerner, 1994), the collaborative and educational approach of CBT may be particularly useful in this patient group. Most adolescents who harm themselves do not actively request treatment, and are often distrustful of adult authority. Cognitive-behavior therapists actively seek the collaboration of the young person and, at the same time, foster self-efficacy on the part of the client.

## General assessment

The general assessment of adolescents who harm themselves, such as the assessment of suicidal risk, is dealt with in Chapter 9. The following points, however, are particularly relevant to the planning of CBT with this patient group (Table 11.2).

### Precipitants of deliberate self-harm

As described earlier, many adolescent suicidal-attempters have experienced acute stresses in the weeks preceding the attempt. Many of these stresses involve interpersonal difficulties with peers, problems in the family, or both. Exploration of the nature of these difficulties is important before deciding what kind of help may be appropriate. For example, it may not be appropriate to give CBT to the adolescent, when the main precipitating problem is chronic stress within the family. On the other hand, techniques such as social problem-solving may help the adolescent to deal with acute stresses such as problems with relationships.

## Chronic problems

Adolescent suicidal behavior often occurs in the context of chronic problems. Indeed, discord between the adolescent and a peer (girlfriend or boyfriend, or a row over a friendship), or with the family, is very common. An assessment must be made at an early point as to whether the peer or family problems are so severe as to make it difficult for the patient to benefit from cognitive treatment. In some cases, it may be better to have a few sessions with the adolescent and family together (see below) in order to explore family communication and problem-solving. However, it should be stressed that it can be very difficult to change chronically dysfunctional families. In such circumstances, it can be appropriate to undertake individual work with the adolescent, even when it is obvious that the adolescent's problems occur in the context of chronic intrafamilial difficulties.

## Assessment of psychiatric disorders

Most suicidal adolescents show some psychiatric symptoms, particularly symptoms of depression. As discussed earlier, in the majority of cases, depression remits rapidly within a few weeks. However, a minority of adolescents suffer from clinically significant degrees of major depression that require treatment in their own right. A small proportion of adolescents who self-harm suffers from other disorders. Examples include post-traumatic stress symptoms or eating disorders. Occasionally, self-harm presages serious psychiatric disorders such as schizophrenia, though this is relatively uncommon.

## The young person's family and motivation for help

Almost all studies have found that self-harming adolescents and their families comply poorly with conventional forms of outpatient treatment (Trautman et al., 1993). Many adolescents who harm themselves do not necessarily expect help and, contrary to popular belief, their suicidal attempt is rarely a "cry for help." Furthermore, some will not have been told by the accident and emergency staff that they are due to be seen by a mental health professional. It is therefore very important, from an early stage in the assessment, that attempts are made to establish rapport with the adolescent and family. A decision needs to be made early on about the degree of suicidal risk, and about admission to hospital. Similarly, one occasionally encounters suicidal adolescents whose home situation is so chaotic that compulsory admission to care is indicated. However, as a general rule, it is much better to try to work with the adolescent and the family rather than against them.

### Strengths of the adolescent and the family

It is important to identify at an early stage the strengths that the adolescent and family have. For instance, are there areas in the adolescent's life, such as school, peer relationships, or family, that are particularly strong? Who does the adolescent turn to at times of crisis? Is there someone in the family, or outside of the family, who might be able to help? Does the adolescent or family have a professional who is likely to be helpful, such as a social worker or general practitioner?

The initial assessment should also establish how the adolescent has coped with crises in the past. It is quite common to find that adolescents have dealt with previous problems more effectively. Understanding the adolescent's coping abilities, and the reasons why they failed to cope at around the time of the overdose, can be very important in planning treatment.

## Cognitive behavioral techniques

Cognitive behavior therapists use a variety of different techniques when working with suicidal adolescents. The choice of technique depends on many factors, including the young person's developmental level, the nature of the problem being treated, and the therapist's psychological model of the causes of the adolescent's problems. However, most of the cognitive behavior therapies have the following features in common.

### Therapist stance

The attitude or mental posture of the cognitive behavior therapist working with young people has been described using terms such as consultant and educator (Kendall, 1991). The therapist is active and involved but does not have all the answers. Rather, the therapist seeks to develop a collaborative relationship that stimulates the adolescent to think for him or herself. The idea is not to tell the young person what to do but rather to give him or her the opportunity to try things out and to develop skills. There is an emphasis on the adolescent learning through experience. Thus, as in CBT with adults, there are homework assignments in which the adolescent carries out tasks that are agreed in the session. These are often framed as an experiment. For example, the adolescent may feel that she is disliked by her friend because she, the adolescent, has harmed herself. The adolescent and therapist may conclude that the best way of finding out is for the adolescent to try and talk to her friend.

## Cognitive behavioral formulation

The cognitive behavioral formulation is based on information from the initial assessment. It should be a written explanation of the problem that highlights the key cognitive and behavioral factors that are thought to play a role in the onset or maintenance of the adolescent's suicidal behavior. It should also reflect the role of external factors, such as family difficulties or peer problems, in the young person's views of self and the world. The formulation is likely, then, to be multi-layered and to outline several priorities for treatment. The development of a formulation is an essential part of CBT with suicidal young people.

## Education and engagement of the adolescent and family

All forms of CBT should begin with an explanation of the formulation and the model of treatment for the adolescent and family. The nature of this explanation depends on the child's level of cognitive development. Young people who have developed what Piaget (Piaget, 1970) called formal thinking skills can usually understand the kind of explanation of CBT that would be given to adults. Such an explanation might, for instance, include the relationship between the way people think about themselves and their environment, and their suicidal feelings. Many young adolescents find it difficult however to think about thinking and require explanations that are more appropriate for their developmental stage. For example, the therapist might present to the adolescent a story about a social situation that could have several different interpretations (e.g., a stranger knocking at the door) and explore with the adolescent the various different thoughts and feelings that could occur. How would the young person feel, for example, if he or she thought the stranger looked like the murderer shown on the evening news? What if it was the adolescent's birthday and the stranger was wearing a postman's uniform and carrying a large parcel? Stories such as the *The Emperor's New Clothes* can also be a useful way of getting over ideas such as the power of thought and belief in determining how we behave (Wilkes et al., 1994).

Although the CBTs are usually viewed as individual or group treatments there is a growing trends towards encouraging parents to have a role. Parental involvement is important for several reasons. First, parents or significant others can often be very helpful in implementing a therapeutic program. For instance, they can help to reinforce homework assignments. Moreover, they can provide information about ongoing stresses in the child's life and about the continuation of certain symptoms that the child may be reluctant to talk about (e.g., peer relationship problems, antisocial behavior). Second, there is the practical reason that it will often be the parents who bring the child for therapy. Third, parental behaviors and attitudes may be important predisposing or maintaining factors for the child's problems. For example, it is quite common to find that parents of suicidal adolescents can be very critical of the adolescent for taking an overdose, and thereby inadvertently reinforcing the adolescent's negative self image.

## Problem-solving

A basic ingredient of both cognitive and behavioral approaches to suicidal behavior in young people is problem-solving. Although the immediate antecedents of many suicidal episodes in young people can often be identified as specific cognitions or affects, these are usually provoked by some kind of external problem. As described earlier, these problems are commonly of an interpersonal nature, involving either the family or peers. Training adolescents in problem-solving helps them to deal with these external problems and also provides a useful model for many cognitive behavioral procedures.

Problem-solving with suicidal adolescents involves much the same steps as in suicidal adults (Hawton and Catalan, 1982). In the first step the adolescent is encouraged to identify a solvable problem. Some problems require a choice between alternatives (e.g., shall I stop seeing my boyfriend?), others require the attainment of a specific goal (e.g., how can I get on better with my mother?). Next, the adolescent is helped to choose a realistic and defined goal that can be achieved in a short period of time. For example, a realistic goal for an adolescent who wants to improve her relationship with her mother might be to go shopping with her once a week (though, clearly, the attainment of this goal will involve negotiation with the mother). It is very important that the adolescent is helped to choose an attainable goal, because the failure to resolve problems that cannot easily be remedied (e.g., a mother with alcoholism, a father whose contact visits have always been most inconsistent) can itself lead to depression and suicidality.

The third stage of problem-solving is to clarify the steps necessary to achieve the goal. At this point, the therapist and adolescent will often need to review the methods that the adolescent has previously used to try to solve the problem. Which methods seemed to help and which did not? The likely or actual consequences of each method should be established.

The fourth stage is to draw up a plan to carry out the strategy. The tasks should be clear. For example, the adolescent who has been having problems with peer relationships might have the goal of going to the youth club at least once before the next session. It is sometimes helpful to frame these tasks as experiments (e.g., "there can be no guarantee that it will work, but you won't know until you have tried it"). Tasks are often set as homework, for discussion at the next session.

The final stage is to review progress. Adolescents who have achieved their goals should be praised for doing so and plans made for the next goal. If the adolescent has not completed the task, the reasons for this should be explored. One common reason is that the task set was too demanding. In such cases, it is sometimes possible to break the task up into smaller components.

The therapist must of course recognize that not all problems have solutions. It may not be possible, for instance, for the adolescent to maintain a harmonious relationship with a parent who has severe personality problems. At the same time, however, the therapist should try to identify inappropriately negative attitudes that can block progress in therapy. Commonly encountered negative styles of thinking are low self-esteem (e.g., "nothing I do ever succeeds") and catastrophizing (e.g., "I tried to say hello and she did not reply. The whole relationship is going to fail"). Problem-solving may prove difficult in the presence of such negative attitudes. Patients may therefore need to be helped in modifying such attitudes using cognitive techniques.

## Cognitive techniques

At the core of most of the cognitive therapies used with young people are techniques for eliciting and monitoring cognitions and for correcting distorted conceptualizations and beliefs about the world.

### Self-monitoring

At all ages there is an emphasis on *self-monitoring*, that is on charting thoughts and on recording the relationship between thoughts and other phenomena such as behaviors or recent experiences. In older adolescents cognitions can be elicited using much the same techniques as in adults. For example, the young person might be asked to keep a diary charting the relationship between emotions (e.g., depression), events (e.g., a row at home) and thoughts associated with these events (e.g., "this always happens. It will never get any better"). The idea of such exercises is to get over the idea that there may be links between events, thoughts, and emotions. If the adolescent cannot keep a diary, then it can sometimes help to ask what he or she was thinking before coming to the appointment. Most report thoughts about the therapist, the hospital, or the treatment. The therapist then labels these as "automatic thoughts" or "the things you say to yourself." In younger adolescents it is often necessary to use more developmentally appropriate methods. For instance, cartoon drawings such as the *Thought Detective* (Stark, 1990) can help to communicate the idea that the child is actively involved in the understanding of thinking and behavior.

### Cognitive restructuring

*Cognitive restructuring* forms an important part of many CBT programs. The first step is to identify the thought. The thought itself should be noted down. Next, arguments and evidence to support the thought should be considered. Then arguments and evidence that cast doubt on the thought should be identified. Finally, patients should reach a reasoned conclusion based on the available evidence, both for and against their thinking.

Problematic thoughts are often underpinned by characteristic attitudes and assumptions about the self or about the world. Typical examples include the view that in order to be happy the patient must be liked by everyone; or that aggression is a legitimate way of dealing with interpersonal conflicts. These attitudes cannot usually be identified using the approach used to identify problem thoughts because they are not fully articulated in the patient's mind. Rather, they are implicit rules that often can only be inferred by the person's behavior. In the later stages of therapy with older adolescents it may be possible to encourage the patient to look for patterns in his or her reactions to situations that betray these *underlying assumptions*. These techniques may be particularly useful in preventing repetition of self-harm.

## Core behavioral techniques

In parallel with cognitive methods the therapist also uses relevant behavioral techniques. Many programs include a system of behavioral contingencies in which a system of rewards is set up to reinforce desirable behaviors. Reward systems for younger adolescents usually involve the parents, but in some programs there is an emphasis on self-reinforcement in which the adolescent rewards him or herself.

Most mental problems are worsened by inactivity. Activity scheduling involves the scheduling of goal-directed and enjoyable activities into the adolescent's day. The adolescent, therapist, and caretakers collaborate to plan the young person's activities for a day on an hour-by-hour basis. Specific behavioral techniques are also used to treat certain symptoms. For example, sleep disturbance may be reduced by sleep hygiene measures. Relaxation training may be useful for somatic anxiety symptoms.

## Cognitive behavioral treatment of specific mental disorders

Cognitive behavioral techniques can also be used to treat the mental disorders that are sometimes associated with suicidal behavior in adolescents, particularly depressive disorders and conduct disorders.

## Depressive disorders

Many slightly different cognitive behavioral approaches have been developed for depressed children and adolescents (Harrington et al., 1998d). Most programs have the following features. First, the therapy often begins with a session or sessions on emotional recognition and self-monitoring. The aim is to help the young person to distinguish between different emotional states (e.g., sadness and anger) and to start linking external events, thoughts, and feelings. Second, behavioral tasks may be used to reinforce desired behaviors and thence to help the young person to gain control over symptoms. Self-reinforcement is often combined with activity scheduling, in which the young person is encouraged to engage in a program of constructive or pleasant activities. Patients are taught to set realistic goals, with small steps towards achieving them, and to reward themselves at each successful step on the way. At this stage, it is quite common to introduce other behavioral techniques to deal with some of the behavioral or vegetative symptoms of depression. For example, many depressed youngsters sleep poorly and will often be helped by simple sleep hygiene measures. Third, various cognitive techniques are used to reduce depressive cognitions. For example, adolescents may be helped to identify cognitive distortions and to challenge them using techniques such as pro-con evaluation. Techniques to reduce negative automatic thoughts, such as "focus on object," are also employed.

## Conduct disorders

Cognitive behavioral programs for young people with conduct disorder and aggression usually have a strong focus on social cognitions and interpersonal problem-solving. The aim of therapy is to remedy the cognitive distortions and problem-solving deficits that have been identified in empirical research. Several programs have been developed and most have the following features in common. Self-monitoring of behavior enables adolescents to identify and label thoughts, emotions, and the situations in which they occur. Social perspective taking helps them to become aware of the intentions of others in social situations (Chandler, 1973). Use is made of case vignettes, role-play, modeling, and feedback. For example, adolescents might be asked to describe what is going on in a picture. Anger control training aims to increase awareness of the early signs of hostile arousal (e.g., remembering a past grudge) and to develop techniques for self-control. Problem-solving skill training attempts to remedy the deficits in cognitive problem-solving processing abilities that are often found in aggressive young people.

## Contraindications

Although the cognitive behavior therapies may be useful in the aftercare of suicidal adolescents, there are several relative contraindications to their use.

### Developmental stage

Some of the techniques that are used in CBT require that the patient has knowledge about cognition, or is able to use executive processes such as planning or monitoring learning, or both. For example, many programs require that the young person completes homework assignments that may involve some degree of planning (e.g., phoning a friend to see if she is really cross). Younger adolescents are likely to find this difficult as they are less likely to plan activities before carrying them out. Similarly, a key task in some cognitive programs is to evaluate the evidence for and against a particular belief, such as that "my friends don't want to know me." However, the ability to hold mental representations of "theory" versus the "evidence" emerges only gradually during adolescence (Kuhn et al., 1988). Children less than ten years tend to ignore evidence against their beliefs. It is only by middle adolescence that most individuals develop the skill of separating theory from evidence.

It will be appreciated that since metacognitive abilities are thought to be the result of experience as well as constitution, some of them can be learned. Nevertheless, it is clear that adolescence is a transitional period in cognitive development. Developmental stage is therefore an important determinant of the best technique for the patient. As a general rule, older adolescents respond better to cognitive treatments than younger children (Durlak et al., 1991). Different techniques may therefore need to be applied to children of different ages. Preadolescent children may need behavioral procedures or simple cognitive techniques such as self-instruction training. Adolescents are more likely to benefit from cognitive techniques such as changing automatic thoughts.

### Severity of disorder

One of the criticisms that is often made of the cognitive behavior therapies is that they may not be effective in the most severe cases of disorder. Several researchers are now starting to address this issue and CBT has been used, for example, as part of treatment programs for very severe cases of conduct disorder (Kazdin, 1997). Nevertheless, it has to be said that much of the research that has been conducted up to now with the CBT has been based on young people with relatively mild problems. Moreover, for some conditions there is evidence that severe cases respond less well to CBT than mild cases. For instance, Jayson and colleagues reported that increased severity of social impairment was associated with a reduced response to CBT in adolescents with major depression (Jayson et al., 1998), many of whom had suicidal behavior.

### Social context

Suicidal behavior in young people is deeply imbedded in a social context. This has implications both for how the problems should best be managed and for the likely response to treatment. No treatment for the adolescent is likely to succeed if basic needs such as adequate educational opportunities or security of family placement are not met. For instance, adolescents who are moved frequently from one home to another are unlikely to be helped by CBT, or indeed by any other kind of psychological intervention.

## Organizing treatment

### Types of CBT program

The ideal treatment plan depends on the nature of the adolescent's problems but can include individual work, group sessions, or both. Individual programs are particularly useful in settings where the numbers of cases referred with a particular problem (e.g., depressed suicidal adolescents) are not great enough to sustain a group. One-to-one work is often necessary with adolescents whose problems are so severe that they may disrupt a group. Certain kinds of techniques, such as cognitive restructuring, are better carried out with the individual patient.

Group CBT programs provide supervised practice of a number of skills, such as social problem-solving, in a peer setting. Practising skills with peers may increase the likelihood of skills transfer to real-world peer interactions. The group also provides a good opportunity to practise problem-solving skills with real life dilemmas that arise in the group. This is, arguably, better than having to rely on staged situations such as role play. Wood and Traynor (unpublished manuscript) have developed a program for groups of adolescents who have repeatedly harmed themselves called Developmental Group Psychotherapy. The first group involves six sessions in which there is an emphasis on dealing with the acute problems that these adolescents face. There is much emphasis on techniques such as problem-solving. This is followed by a long-term group in which there is more emphasis on the principles of psychodynamic psychotherapy.

## Involving parents

The extent of parental involvement depends on the problem that is presented. Parental attitudes towards the child may be crucial in determining the outcome of treatment. Thus, negative attitudes towards the child, as shown by high levels of hostility and criticism, are highly predictive of the outcomes of a wide variety of psychiatric problems (Vostanis et al., 1994). It may be possible to work with the parent/s to produce changes in beliefs about the child.

It is sometimes helpful to see the family together in order to improve communication within the family. Kerfoot and colleagues (Kerfoot et al., 1995) describe a five-session home-based program for the families of adolescents who have deliberately poisoned themselves. The first assessment session is followed by sessions that help the family to (1) understand the episode, (2) communicate more effectively, (3) solve problems more effectively, and (4) understand the problems that adolescents experience.

Parents may also be directly involved in cognitive behavioral programs for disorders such as depression. Probably the best developed parallel parental course for children with depression is that of Clarke and Lewinsohn (Lewinsohn et al., 1990). This course involves a mixture of parental group sessions that aim to reinforce CBT with the child and conjoint behavioral family sessions.

## Common technical problems

There are several common problems that can occur during CBT with suicidal young people.

### Therapist factors

One of the most common mistakes made by trainees is taking on patients who are unsuitable for CBT. Most research studies of cognitive therapy have been based on selected cases. Clinical practice should generally be confined to the kinds of cases that have been included in these studies. Thus, for example, the effectiveness of therapy with depressed adolescents has been demonstrated in samples with relatively low rates of comorbidity with other problems (Harrington et al., 1998c). It cannot be assumed that adolescents with, say, depression and severe conduct disorder will respond to treatment in the same way as those with "pure" depression. Another common problem is the failure to construct an adequate cognitive behavioral formulation of the young person's difficulties. This can lead to the application of techniques in a "cookbook" fashion, which is not tailored to the needs of the individual.

The attitudes of the therapist may lead to problems. For example, many suicidal adolescents who are referred for therapy are in difficult life situations and believe that their predicament cannot be resolved. In such cases the therapist may be drawn into the belief that "anyone would feel like that" in the same situation. This view is generally incorrect. It is important that the therapist adopts an optimistic problem-solving approach and does not catastrophize the problem.

### Patient factors

The patient's beliefs can also lead to difficulties during therapy. Some young people come to treatment with the belief that all of their problems will be cured by psychological therapy. It is important that they understand the limitations of cognitive therapy. Therapists must ensure that specific and realistic goals are set at the start of the course. Other youngsters denigrate the therapy in statements such as "I've had five visits and nothing has changed at all." In such cases the therapist should explain that treatment often follows a variable course, with downs as well as ups.

Many technical problems can arise during CBT with young people. One of the most common is failure to complete homework assignments. In such cases the therapist must first think back to the previous session to ensure that the homework tasks were adequately discussed. With younger patients, for example, it is important to get them to repeat the task back to ensure that they have understood it. Homework problems can often be prevented. The therapist must model persistence and not simply give up if homework has not been completed. Another common problem is the adolescent who does not talk in a session. In such cases the therapist should try to take the pressure off the young person by, for example, saying that "I will do the talking for a while." Once the adolescent starts talking the therapist can try to understand the source of the problem.

### Parent factors

Parental attitudes can be a powerful determinant of the outcome of treatment. Some parents believe that their adolescent is simply "making it up" and does not really have a problem. "He will grow out of it." Some take the opposite view, and believe that the child's problems are so severe and so much part of the personality that nothing can be achieved in therapy. Careful exploration of these beliefs by the therapist, followed by an appropriate explanation, can help to modify these attitudes.

### Length of treatment and follow-up

Length of treatment varies considerably according to the nature of the presenting problem. Programs for adolescents who repeatedly harm themselves are often lengthy, taking up to 20 weekly sessions. Programs for adolescents whose self-harm is associated with depression tend to be shorter, at around 12–16 sessions within eight weeks (Clarke et al., 1990). Versions of CBT as brief as eight sessions have been shown to be effective for depressive disorder in adolescents (Wood et al., 1996). Many adolescents who have harmed themselves need not come for lengthy courses of treatment. Sometimes one or two visits for simple advice and encouragement are all that is required.

## Efficacy

The evidence base on the efficacy of interventions for young people who harm themselves can be divided into studies in which the main focus of treatment was suicidality, or studies of the efficacy of treatments for disorders that are often associated with suicidality, particularly depression.

### Suicidal behavior

There have been no published randomized trials of CBT for adolescents presenting with suicidal behavior. However, studies with suicidal adults suggest that techniques such as problem-solving may be of benefit, though studies thus far have generally been far too small to detect an effect on repetition (Hawton et al., 1998).

### Depression

There have been at least six randomized controlled studies of cognitive behavior in samples of children with depressive symptoms recruited through schools (Harrington et al., 1998c). The design has usually been to screen all children with a depression questionnaire and then to invite those with a high score to participate in a group intervention. In four of the trials cognitive therapy was significantly superior to no treatment.

Encouraging results have also been obtained for clinically diagnosed cases of depressive disorder. A quantitative meta-analysis of six studies found a significant improvement in the CBT group over the comparison interventions (Harrington et al., 1998a). The pooled odds ratio in an intent to treat analysis was 2.2.

There are few data regarding the factors that influence treatment outcome. The most consistent finding thus far has been that children with severe depressive disorders respond less well than children with mild or moderately severe conditions. Research has also examined the role that changes in negative cognitions might have in predicting outcome. Cognitive therapy is not differentially more effective in cases with high cognitive distortion. Parallel parental sessions do not significantly enhance the beneficial effect of cognitive therapy with the child (Lewinsohn et al., 1990).

Published research has several limitations. First, it is based on samples with mild or moderately severe depression. CBT may not be effective in severely depressed children. Second, much of the research has compared CBT with inactive comparison conditions such as remaining on a waiting list or psychological placebo. It is not known how CBT compares with other recognized forms of intervention, such as medication. Third, it is unclear whether cognitive or behavioral processes correlate with a better outcome. The therapeutic basis for change is therefore uncertain. Even so, CBT is a highly promising treatment for juvenile depression with replicated beneficial effects.

## Conclusions

Although the CBTs have not yet been evaluated in the aftercare of suicidal adolescents, they are a promising form of intervention. Problem-solving techniques are likely to be of value in helping adolescents to deal with the stresses that are commonly associated with deliberate self-harm in this age group. Cognitive techniques may be particularly useful when the suicidal adolescent is also depressed. Large randomized trials are required, however, to establish whether these interventions reduce the risk of repetition.

## Acknowledgements

Portions of this article are based in a chapter to be published in the *Oxford Textbook of Psychiatry*, and we are grateful for permission to reproduce them here. We are also grateful for permission from the *British Journal of Psychiatry* to reproduce Table 11.1.

## REFERENCES

Birmaher, B., Brent, D. A., Kolko, D., Baugher, M., Bridge, J., Holder, D., Iyengar, S., and Ulloa, R. E. (2000). Clinical outcome after short-term psychotherapy for adolescents with major depressive disorder. *Archives of General Psychiatry*, **57**(1), 29–36.

Brent, D. A. (1997). The aftercare of adolescents with deliberate self-harm. *Journal of Child Psychology and Psychiatry*, **38**, 277–286.

Brent, D. A. (2001). Assessment and treatment of the youthful suicidal patient. *Annals of the New York Academy of Sciences*, **932**, 106–128; discussion 128–131.

Brent, D. A., and Lerner, M. S. (1994). Cogntive therapy with affectively ill, suicidal adolescents. In Wilkes, T. C. R., Belsher, G., Rush, A. J., and Frank, E. (eds.) *Cognitive Therapy for Depressed Adolescents* (pp. 298–322). New York City, NY: Guilford Press.

Brent, D., Holder, D., Kolko, D. et al. (1997). A clinical psychotherapy trial for adolescent depression comparing cognitive, family, and supportive treatments. *Archives of General Psychiatry*, **54**, 877–885.

Burgess, S., Hawton, K., and Loveday, G. (1998). Adolescents who take overdoses: outcomes in terms of changes in psychopatholgy and the adolescents' attitudes to care and to their overdose. *Journal of Adolescence*, **21**, 209–218.

Chandler, M. J. (1973). Egocentrism and anti-social behavior: the assessment and training of social perspective-taking skills. *Developmental Psychology*, **9**, 326–332.

Clarke, G., Lewinsohn, P., and Hops, H. (1990). *Leaders Manual for Adolescent Groups. Adolescent Coping with Depression Course.* Eugene, OR: Castalia Publishing Company.

Durlak, J. A., Fuhrman, T., and Lampman, C. (1991). Effectiveness of cognitive-behavior therapy for maladaptive children: a meta-analysis. *Psychological Bulletin*, **110**, 204–214.

Harrington, R., Whittaker, J., Shoebridge, P. et al. (1998a). Systematic review of efficacy of cognitive behaviour therapies in child and adolescent depressive disorder. *British Medical Journal*, **316**, 1559–1563.

Harrington, R. C., Kerfoot, M., Dyer, E. et al. (1998b). Randomized trial of a home based family intervention for children who have deliberately poisoned themselves. *Journal of the American Academy of Child and Adolescent Psychiatry*, **37**, 512–518.

Harrington, R. C., Whittaker, J., and Shoebridge, P. (1998c). Psychological treatment of depression in children and adolescents: a review of treatment research. *British Journal of Psychiatry*, **173**, 291–298.

Harrington, R. C., Wood, A., and Verduyn, C. (1998d). Clinically depressed adolescents. In Graham, P. (ed.) *Cognitive Behaviour Therapy for Children and Families* (pp. 156–193). Cambridge: Cambridge University Press.

Hawton, K., and Catalan, J. (1982). *Attempted Suicide.* Oxford: Oxford Medical Publications.

Hawton, K., Arensman, E., Townsend, E. et al. (1998). Deliberate self harm: systematic review of efficacy of psychosocial and pharmacological treatments in preventing repetition. *British Medical Journal*, **317**, 441–447.

Jayson, D., Wood, A. J., Kroll, L. et al. (1998). Which depressed patients respond to cognitive-behavioral treatment? *Journal of the American Academy of Child and Adolescent Psychiatry*, **37**, 35–39.

Kazdin, A. E. (1997). Practitioner review: psychosocial treatments for conduct disorder in children. *Journal of Child Psychology and Psychiatry*, **38**, 161–178.

Kendall, P. C. (1991). *Child and Adolescent Therapy. Cognitive-Behavioural Procedures.* New York City, NY: Guilford Press.

Kerfoot, M., Harrington, R. C., and Dyer, E. (1995). Brief home-based intervention with young suicide attempters and their families. *Journal of Adolescence*, **18**, 557–568.

Kerfoot, M., Dyer, E., Harrington, V. et al. (1996). Correlates and short-term course of self-poisoning in adolescents. *British Journal of Psychiatry*, **168**, 38–42.

Kuhn, D., Amsel, E., and O'Loughlin, M. (1988). *The Development of Scientific Thinking Skills*. San Diego, CA: Academic Press.

Lewinsohn, P. M., Clarke, G. N., Hops, H. et al. (1990). Cognitive-behavioural treatment for depressed adolescents. *Behavior Therapy*, **21**, 385–401.

Miller, I. V., Epstein, N. B., Bishop, D. S. et al. (1985). The McMaster Family Assessment Device: reliability and validity. *Journal of Marital and Family Therapy*, **11**, 345–356.

Piaget, J. (1970). Piaget's theory. In Mussen, P. H. (ed.) *Carmichael's Manual of Child Psychology*, Volume 1 (pp. 703–732). New York City, NY: Wiley.

Puig-Antich, J., and Chambers, W. (1978). The Schedule for Affective Disorders and Schizophrenia for school-aged children [unpublished interview schedule]. New York City, NY: New York State Psychiatric Institute.

Stark, K. D. (1990). *Childhood Depression: School-based Intervention*. New York City, NY: Guilford.

Trautman, P. D., Stewart, N., and Morishima, A. (1993). Are adolescent suicide attempters non-compliant with outpatient care? *Journal of the American Academy of Child and Adolescent Psychiatry*, **32**, 89–94.

Vostanis, P., Nicholls, J., and Harrington, R. C. (1994). Maternal expressed emotion in conduct and emotional disorders of childhood. *Journal of Child Psychology and Psychiatry*, **35**, 365–376.

Wilkes, T. C. R., Belsher, G., Rush, A. J. et al. (1994). *Cognitive Therapy for Depressed Adolescents*. New York City, NY: Guilford Press.

Wood, A. J., Harrington, R. C., and Moore, A. (1996). Controlled trial of a brief cognitive-behavioural intervention in adolescent patients with depressive disorders. *Journal of Child Psychology and Psychiatry*, **37**, 737–746.

## 12

# Follow-up studies of child and adolescent suicide attempters

Julie Boergers and Anthony Spirito

## Introduction

Suicide attempts are a substantial public health problem among children and adolescents. In the U.S., suicide is the third-leading cause of death among adolescents (National Center for Health Statistics, 1993). It is estimated that approximately 9% of adolescents in the U.S. attempt suicide each year, and rates of completed suicide among U.S. adolescents increased 28.3% from 1980 to 1992 (Centers for Disease Control, 1995). In most developed countries, youth suicide has increased dramatically and is one of the leading causes of death among young people (Diekstra and Golbinat, 1993).

Adolescents who attempt suicide are at high risk for continued problem behaviors and repeat suicide attempts. Approximately 30% of adolescents who complete suicide have made a prior attempt (Shaffer et al., 1988). Thus, it is critical to better understand the postattempt course of adolescent suicide attempters, in order to inform both treatment and secondary prevention efforts. This chapter will summarize findings from follow-up studies of adolescent suicide attempters. Four major areas will be reviewed: (1) continued psychiatric disturbance, (2) rates of repeat attempts, (3) rates of completed suicide, and (4) treatment compliance.

There are several different ways to study the outcomes of adolescent suicide attempts. First, retrospective studies compare the characteristics of first-time suicide attempters with repeat attempters, or study individuals who have completed suicide via "psychological autopsies." While these types of studies contribute important information, they are not follow-up studies, per se, and are beyond the scope of this chapter. In contrast, prospective studies identify suicide attempters and follow them across time. Prospective studies allow for an examination of psychosocial factors and eliminate the bias of hindsight, but are typically quite difficult to accomplish because of high attrition over the course of the study. Thus, most follow-up studies have been conducted over short periods of time.

Table 12.1 presents summaries of these studies in order of the length of the follow-up period.

In another type of follow-up study, common in Finland and Sweden, official registries and/or records are reviewed. In other countries, such as Great Britain, hospital re-admission rates for suicide attempts are reported. These types of studies allow researchers to trace an entire cohort, and thus may provide better estimates on rates of re-attempt and rates of completed suicide. However, they are limited in the descriptive information they can provide. In addition, privacy laws in many countries prohibit access to such data. Table 12.2 summarizes follow-up studies which utilize reviews of hospital admission or national health service data. As in Table 12.1, these studies are presented by length of follow-up period.

Many studies present data on combined adolescent and adult samples, but adult findings are probably not generalizable to adolescents (Safer, 1997). Thus, studies which report findings on combined adolescent-adult populations will not be discussed in detail in this chapter but, for the reader's reference, are summarized in Table 12.4. Similarly, although adolescent suicide attempters often have a very different course than suicide ideators, the two groups are sometimes included together in follow-up studies without examining for group differences. Again, these types of studies will not be reviewed in detail, but are summarized in Table 12.3.

## Psychosocial functioning at follow-up

Little information is available regarding the long-term adjustment of adolescent suicide attempters. Nonetheless, the literature suggests that many young suicide attempters remain at risk for continued psychosocial dysfunction in various domains, regardless of the severity of their initial attempt (e.g., Rauenhorst, 1972). Key findings from the studies compiled in Tables 12.1 through 12.4 will be highlighted in this section, including data on general adjustment, academic functioning, social functioning, behavior, and psychopathology.

Most follow-up studies draw general conclusions about the overall adjustment of adolescents following a suicide attempt. For example Hawton et al. (1982) interviewed 50 adolescents one month following their attempt, with about half describing their overall adjustment as improved, and about 40% reporting no change. Angle et al. (1983) derived an overall adjustment score based on school, work, and interpersonal functioning. At the 9-year follow-up, all 24 adolescent suicide attempters who were re-contacted described higher levels of life satisfaction and better interpersonal functioning, but functional status was not related to number of repeat attempts.

**Table 12.1.** Prospective follow-up studies of adolescent suicide attempters

| Reference | Sample | Age at attempt | Setting | Control group | FU Period | % Recontacted | % Attempt at FU | % Complete at FU | Adjust. data | Treat. data |
|---|---|---|---|---|---|---|---|---|---|---|
| Taylor and Stansfield (1984) | n = 50 (82%F) | 8–17 | GH | None | Not reported | 100% | Not reported | 0 | N | Y |
| Trautman and Rotheram (1987) | n = 76 | <17 yrs. | GH | None | Not reported | Not reported | Not reported | 0 | N | Y |
| Spirito et al. (1992) | n = 100 (87%F) | 13–18 (x = 15) | GH/PH | None | 1 mo. & 3 mo. | 80% | 6% at 1 mo. 10% at 3 mo. | 0 | Y | Y |
| Spirito et al. (1994) | n = 62 (85%F) | 13–17 (x = 15) | ED | None | 3 mo. | Not reported | 7% | 0 | Y | Y |
| Donaldson et al. (1997) | n = 23 (83%F) (Treatment group) | 12–17 (x = 15) | GH | n = 78 suicide attempters in "standard care" | 3 mo. | 100% | None in treatment group; 9% in comparison group | 0 | Y | Y |
| Pillay and Wassenaar (1995) | n = 39 (65%F) | 15–20 | GH | n = 36 medical; n = 37 healthy | 6 months | 98% of attempters; 91% of controls | Not reported | 0 | Y | Y |
| Brent et al. (1993) | n = 48 (46%F) | 13–18 (x = 16) | PH | n = 33 ideators; n = 53 psychiatric | 4–14 months (x = 6.7 mo.) | 67% | 15% of attempters; 15% of 2% ideators; of psychiatric | 0 | Y | Y |
| White (1974) | n = 40 (82%F) | 13–19 | GH | None | 1 year | 80% | 12% | 0 | Y | Y |

(cont.)

**Table 12.1.** (*cont.*)

| Reference | Sample | Age at attempt | Setting | Control group | FU Period | % Recontacted | % Attempt at FU | % Complete at FU | Adjust. data | Treat. data |
|---|---|---|---|---|---|---|---|---|---|---|
| Hawton et al. (1982) | n = 50 (90%F) | 13–18 | GH | None | 1 mo. & 1 year | 100% | 14% at 1 yr. | 0 | Y | N |
| Kienhorst et al. (1991) | n = 48 (85%F) | 14–21 (x = 17) | PH | n = 66 Depressed | 1 year | 83% of attempters; 85% of controls | 12.5% of attempters; 5.4% of controls | 0 | Y | N |
| McIntire et al. (1977) | n = 26 (80%F) | 14–18 | PH | None | 6–24 mo. (x = 17 mo.) | 52% | 31% | 0 | Y | Y |
| Cohen-Sandler et al. (1982) | n = 20 (37%F) | 5–14 | PH | n = 21 depressed; n = 35 psychiatric | 5–36 mo. (x = 17 mo.) | 96% | 20% of attempters; none of controls | 0 | Y | Y |
| Barter et al. (1968) | n = 45 | <21 | PH | None | 4–44 mo. (x = 21 mo.) | 71% | 42% | 0 | Y | N |
| Stanley and Barter (1970) | n = 44 (68%F) | 10–21 | PH | n = 25 psychiatric controls | x = 22 mo. | 100% of attempters; 66% of controls | 50% of attempters; 19% of controls | 0 | Y | N |
| Nardini-Maillard and Ladame (1980) | n = 130 (67%F) | 14–19 | GH | None | 6 yrs. | 10% | 15% | 3.8% of original sample | Y | N |
| Farbstein et al. (2002) | n = 216 (71%F) | 14–18 | GH | Matched controls FU in at Israeli Army | 1 mo. to 5 yrs. | 100% | 3% | 1% | Y | N |

| Study | n | Age | Setting | Controls | FU duration | | | | | |
|---|---|---|---|---|---|---|---|---|---|---|
| Kerfoot and McHugh (1992) | n = 41 (80%F) | 8–16 | GH | None | 14 mo. & 7 yrs. | 90% at 14 mo.; 41% at 7 yrs. | 7% at 14 mo.; 20% at 7 yrs. | 0 | Y | Y |
| Pfeffer et al. (1991, 1993, 1994, 1995) | n = 25 | 5–15 (x = 11) | PH | n = 28 ideators; n = 16 psychiatric; n = 64 nonpatients | 6–8 yrs. (x = 7.1 yrs.) | 64% | 32% of attempters; 21% of ideators; 12% psychiatric controls; 6% of nonpatients | 0 | Y | Y |
| Mehr et al. (1982) | n = 7 | x = 15 | GH | n = 10 accidents; n = 12 illness | 2–8 yrs. | 9% of attempters; 14% of controls | 26% of attempters; 19% of accident; 10% of illness* | 0 | Y | Y |
| Angle et al. (1983) | n = 15 (93%F) | 12–18 (x = 14.5) | PH | None | 9 yrs. | 32% | 47% | 0 | Y | N |
| Granboulan et al. (1995) | n = 127 (64%F) | x = 16 | PH | None | 7–17 yrs. (x = 11.5 yrs.) | 48% | 31% | 3.9% of subjects traced | Y | Y |

*Note:* GH, General Hospital; PH, Psychiatric Hospital; ED, Emergency Department; Adjust., adjustment; Treat., treatment; FU, follow-up.

*Re-attempt broadly defined as "self-destructive behavior" in this study.

**Table 12.2.** Retrospective record reviews of adolescent suicide attempters

| Reference | Sample | Age at attempt | Setting | Control group | FU period | % Repeat attempts | % Completed suicides |
|---|---|---|---|---|---|---|---|
| Litt et al. (1983) | n = 27 (78%F) | 10–17 (x = 15) | ERR | None | 1 yr. | Not reported | Not reported |
| Goldacre and Hawton (1985) | n = 2492 (74%F) | 12–20 | GHR | None | 1–5 yrs. (x = 2.8 yrs.) | 6.3% within 1 yr.; 9.5% within 5 yrs. | 0.2% (0.1% of females; 0.7% of males) |
| Sellar et al. (1990) | n = 3034 (71%F) | 12–20 | GHR | None | 1–6 yrs. (x = 3.6 yrs.) | 6.6% within 1 yr.; 10.2% within 6 yrs. | 0.3% (0.1% of females; 0.8% of males) |
| Kotila and Lonnqvist (1988) | n = 362 (68%F) | 15–19 | GHR | None | 1–10 yrs. (x = 5 yrs.) | Not reported | 2.2% (1.2% of females; 4.3% of males) |
| Paerregaard (1975) | n = 27 (63%F) | <19 | NHS | None | 10 yrs. | Not reported | None |
| Otto (1972) | n = 1547 (79%F) | <21 | NHS | n = 1547 | 10–15 yrs. | Not reported | No completed suicides among controls. Among attempters: 4.3% (2.9% of females; 10% of males) |
| Hawton et al. (1996) | n = 755 (85%F) | <16 | GHR | None | 1–17 yrs. | 9.4% within 1 yr.; 19.3% within 17 yrs. | Not reported |

*Note:* GHR, General Hospital records; ERR, Emergency Room records; NHS, National Health Service; FU, follow-up.

**Table 12.3.** Follow-up studies combining adolescent suicide ideators with suicide attempters

| Reference | Sample characteristics | Age at attempt (yrs.) | Setting | Control group | Follow-up period | % Recontact | % Attempt at follow-up | Adjustment data | Treatment compliance data |
|---|---|---|---|---|---|---|---|---|---|
| King et al. (1995) | n = 100 (59%F) | x = 15.1 | PH | None | 6 mo. | 67.50% | 18% | Y | Y |
| Morrison and Collier (1969) | n = 34 (60%F) | <17 | EPC | None | 1 yr. | Not reported | 0 | N | Y |
| Gutstein and Rudd (1990) | n = 47 (53%F) | x = 14.4 | Varied | None | 12–18 mo. | Not reported | 4.30% | Y | Y |
| Mattson et al. (1969) | n = 75 (73%F) (64% attempters) | <18 | EPC | n = 95 Psychiatric | 3–34 mo.; x = 17 mo. | Not reported | 4% of suicidals; none of controls | Y | Y |
| Deykin et al. (1986) | n = 319 (62%F) | 13–17 | ER | None | 2 yrs. | Not reported | 6.60% | Y | Y |
| Myers et al. (1991) | n = 38 (51%F) | 7–17 | OPD | n = 23 depressed | 3 yrs. | 65% of suicidal; 88% of depressed | "suicidality": 32% (17% of controls) | Y | N |
| Pfeffer et al. (1992) | n = 53 | 5–15 | PH | n = 16 psychiatric; n = 64 nonpatients | 6–8 yrs. | 64% | 26% suicidals; 12% psychiatric; 6% nonpatients | Y | Y |
| Motto (1984) | n = 335 (64%F) (62% attempters) | 10–19 | PH | None | 4–10 yrs. (x = 7 yrs.) | Not reported | 4.5% (9% males, 1.9% females) | Y | N |

*Note:* ER, emergency room; EPC, emergency psychiatric clinic; OPD, outpatients department; PH, psychiatric hospital.

**Table 12.4.** Follow-up studies combining adolescent and adult suicide attempters

| Reference | Sample | Age at attempt (yrs.) | Setting | Control group | FU period | % Re-contacted | % Attempt at FU | % Complete at FU | Adjust. data | Treat. data |
|---|---|---|---|---|---|---|---|---|---|---|
| Rauenhorst (1972) | n = 38 (100%F) | 16–30 | GH | n = 44 (medical) | x = 18 mo. | 76% of attempters; 88% of controls | Not reported | 0 | Y | Y |
| Nordstrom et al. (1995) | n = 1573 (64%F) | 14–92 (50%< 35) | ED | None | 1–8 yrs.; x = 5 yrs. | Not applicable | Not reported | M < 35: 9.7% F < 35: 2.5% | N | N |
| Hawton and Fagg (1988) | n = 1959 (66%F) | 10–60 | GH | None | 6–9 yrs.; x = 8 yrs. | Not applicable | Not reported | 2.8% | N | N |
| DeMoore and Robertson (1996) | n = 223 (67%F) | 13–73 | Varied | None | 18 yrs. | Not applicable | Not reported | M: 8.2% F: 6.0% | N | N |
| Mehlum (1994) | n = 51 (100%M) | 18–25 (x = 20) | MR | None | 20 yrs. | Not applicable | Not reported | 3.9% | N | N |

*Note:* GH, General Hospital; ED, Emergency Department; MR, Military Records; Adjust., adjustment; Treat., treatment; FU, follow-up.

Granboulan et al. (1995) obtained information on adjustment from a wide range of sources, from the patients themselves, to their parents or physicians. They found that 29% of their sample had improved, 22% seemed to be unchanged, and 33% presented with lower levels of functioning 11 years after the initial adolescent suicide attempt. Similarly, McIntire et al. (1977) reported that only 23% of 26 adolescents demonstrated improvements in functional adaptation as reflected by clinician ratings of adjustment completed 6 months to 2 years following discharge from a psychiatric hospital. Improvements in overall adjustment were more likely if adolescents' living conditions improved after the initial hospitalization. Studying a sample of suicide attempters who were not admitted to a psychiatric hospital, White (1974) made a significantly higher estimate of improvement (56%), based on clinician ratings at one year. Cohen-Sandler et al. (1982) found that about two-thirds of the psychiatrically hospitalized suicidal children and adolescents followed at 18 months demonstrated behavioral and social functioning that was within normal limits on the Child Behavior Checklist.

In a more recent study, Farbstein et al. (2002) identified 216 Israeli adolescents who had made a suicide attempt and were evaluated in one of five general hospitals. They examined the military records of these adolescents when they served in the army as young adults between 18 and 21 years of age. A matched comparison group was selected from other soldiers without any history of suicide attempts. Compared to the controls, the male attempters had higher rates of premature discharge from military service and shorter military service. Their physical and mental health fitness ratings while in the army were also lower than controls. Female attempters had shorter service stays, more jail sentences and more hospitalizations than matched female controls.

Other markers of adjustment have also been examined. Spirito and colleagues (1992) found that about one-third of suicide attempters seen in a general hospital and one-fifth of suicide attempters seen in a psychiatric hospital sample did not attend school regularly when contacted at three-month follow-up. Long-term follow-ups have found lower rates of educational achievement than would be normally expected (Angle et al., 1983; Laurent et al., 1998).

Family difficulties persist at follow-up for many of these adolescents. In one study, 14% of adolescent suicide attempters described both their family and peer relationships as "not good" to "very bad" at three-month follow-up (Spirito et al., 1992). Hawton and colleagues (1982) found that while improvement was likely in the areas of peer and romantic relationships, family problems were less likely to improve one month following the suicide attempt. Barter et al. (1968) found that while most nonattempter controls were living at home, less than half of suicide attempters were living at home with their parents at the 21-month follow-up.

Similarly, when psychiatrically hospitalized suicide attempters were compared to child and early adolescent psychiatric controls, suicide attempters were more likely to be placed outside the home after discharge (Cohen-Sandler et al., 1982). As young adults, suicide attempters have been found to marry less frequently and divorce more often than controls with no history of a suicide attempt (Otto, 1972).

Behavioral problems are often noted in the follow-up literature. About one-quarter of adolescent suicide attempters were involved in physical fighting, and 14% reported having run away when re-contacted at three months (Spirito et al., 1992). In a seven-year follow-up of 41 subjects, Kerfoot and McHugh (1992) found that 37% reported substance abuse during the years following their suicide attempt and 29% had been convicted of a crime.

Other self-destructive behaviors are often reported by suicide attempters compared to adolescents who have not attempted suicide. Mehr et al. (1982) found that adolescent suicide attempters were more likely to report a drug overdose than were adolescents who were followed after a hospitalization for injury or illness. In Sweden, adolescents followed for 10–15 years following a suicide attempt reported greater frequency of conduct-disordered behavior and alcoholism when compared to age-matched controls with respect to extensive government records (Otto, 1972). The suicide attempters had more recorded sick days, were more likely to receive disability pensions, and were more likely to be declared unfit for military service. Approximately one-third of the males were arrested more than once in the 10–15 years following their suicide attempt (Otto, 1972). Laurent et al. (1998) also found high rates of contact with the criminal justice system.

Adolescent suicide attempters are also at greater risk for injuries and death by other causes. In one study, Mehr et al. (1982) found that five of the seven adolescent suicide attempters they followed had been in a motor vehicle crash in the eight years following their attempt. Spirito et al. (1992) found that 9% of a general hospital sample and 14.6% of a psychiatric hospital sample had been involved in a motor vehicle crash at three months following their attempt. Furthermore, 15.4% of the general hospital sample and 31.8% of the psychiatric hospital sample had emergency department (ED) visits for injury within the three months following the initial suicide attempt. Granboulan and colleagues (1995) found that while 3.9% of attempters they were able to trace in an 11-year follow-up had committed suicide, an additional 7% had died of "unnatural or violent causes," such as homicide, substance abuse, or motor vehicle crashes.

Whether adolescent suicide attempters have a higher incidence of maladjustment than other psychiatric patients is unclear. Cohen-Sandler et al. (1982) compared child and adolescent suicide attempters with depressed and mixed psychiatric controls group 18 months after hospitalization. Suicide attempters were more likely to experience stressors, such as school changes (74%), change in parental marital status (21%), and change in parental financial status (32%) than the controls. However, the overall number of stressful life events did not differ significantly from the two psychiatric comparison groups. There were also no differences on parental behavior ratings at follow-up, but the suicide attempters demonstrated better social functioning than the depressed adolescents (Cohen-Sandler et al., 1982). Stanley and Barter (1970) found no significant difference in peer relationships, school performance, or living arrangements between adolescent suicide attempters and psychiatrically hospitalized adolescents who had not made an attempt. However, adolescents with repeat suicide attempts did have a poorer academic performance and fewer peer relationships than the comparison group.

## Repeat suicide attempts

A significant percentage of adolescent suicide attempters will make a repeat attempt at some point. Estimates of re-attempt are summarized in Tables 12.1 through 12.4, and information about risk factors for repeat attempts among adolescents will also be highlighted in this section. As is readily apparent, there is considerable variability in estimates of re-attempts, and this variability appears to be associated with several factors: (1) length of follow-up, (2) type of study (e.g., prospective or retrospective), and (3) characteristics of the sample (e.g., patients who present to a general hospital as opposed to a psychiatric hospital).

Despite the fact that fewer adolescents are re-contacted in longer follow-up studies, higher repetition rates are typically reported. In prospective studies, rates range from 12% to 14% at one year (Hawton et al., 1982; Kienhorst et al., 1991; White, 1974) and from 20% to 50% at two- to three-year follow-up (Cohen-Sandler et al., 1982; McIntire et al., 1977; Stanley and Barter, 1970). It seems likely that the rates in some of the longer studies may be underestimates, since patients become much more difficult to contact as the follow-up period lengthens. As can be seen in Table 12.1, re-contact rates in prospective studies of adolescent suicide attempters range from 98% at six months (Pillay and Wassenaar, 1995) to 9% at eight years following the index attempt (Mehr et al., 1982).

Studies using hospital re-admission rates have reported one-year re-attempt rates ranging from 6% (Goldacre and Hawton, 1985; Sellar et al., 1990) to 9% (Hawton et al., 1996). When patients are re-contacted directly, rates range from 10% within three months following the index attempt (Hawton et al., 1982; Spirito et al., 1992), to 12% at one year (Kienhorst et al., 1991; White, 1974).

Finally, higher re-attempt rates have been found among those adolescents who had been psychiatrically hospitalized than those seen in general hospital samples (e.g., Spirito et al., 1992).

There has been an effort to identify factors which can predict which individuals will make repeat attempts. With each attempt, there is an increase in relative risk for re-attempt. Based on data from a representative sample of 1508 high-school students, Lewinsohn et al. (1994) estimated that adolescents who make suicide attempts are 8.1 times more likely to make a future attempt than those who have never made a suicide attempt. In another study, psychiatrically hospitalized preadolescent suicide attempters were six times more likely to attempt suicide during a six- to eight-year follow-up than a control group (Pfeffer et al., 1993).

Regarding demographic factors, males are more likely than females to re-attempt, and older teens are more likely than younger teens to re-attempt suicide (Cohen-Sandler et al., 1982; Goldacre and Hawton, 1985). Suicidal intent or lethality of a suicide attempt is typically predictive of repeat attempts (Cohen-Sandler et al., 1982; Cotgrove et al., 1995; Hawton et al., 1982; McIntire et al., 1977; Otto, 1972; Pfeffer et al., 1991). Notably, Brent and colleagues (1993) did not find a link between lethality and repeat attempts in a sample of psychiatrically hospitalized adolescents; however, psychiatric hospitalization may be confounded with lethality of attempt.

Regarding psychosocial factors which may contribute to repeat attempts, environmental stress during the follow-up period has been implicated (Cohen-Sandler et al., 1982; McIntire et al., 1977). Adolescents who make a repeat attempt at follow-up have poorer social adjustment (Barter et al., 1968; Pfeffer et al., 1993; Stanley and Barter, 1970), poorer academic performance (Stanley and Barter, 1970), and are less likely to be living with a parent (Barter et al., 1968; Cohen-Sandler et al., 1982) than those who do not make repeat suicide attempts. Other predictors of repeat attempts at follow-up include affective disorders (Brent et al., 1993; Pfeffer et al., 1993), depressive symptoms (Kienhorst et al., 1991), and chronic difficulties such as conduct problems and behavior disturbance (Hawton et al., 1982).

Some researchers have attempted to identify periods of highest risk following the initial attempt. For example, Goldacre and Hawton (1985) have suggested that adolescents are at greatest risk for re-attempt during the first few months following the initial attempt. In their examination of British hospital admission data, they found that 69% of boys and 41% of girls who made a repeat attempt within the first year did so during the first three months. Similarly, Hawton et al. (1982) found that five of the seven repeat attempts in their sample of 50 adolescent suicide attempters occurred within the first three months following the index attempt. Both of these studies used hospital re-admission data. Therefore, it is unlikely that the rates are inflated by increased enrollment rates in the early period following the attempt. It should be noted that although there is an early period of greater risk for re-attempt, repeat attempts do appear to decline after 18 years of age (Angle et al., 1983).

More research is needed on those factors that increase the likelihood of repeat attempts, in order to improve treatment. Brent and colleagues (1993) found that psychiatrically hospitalized adolescents who re-attempted during the six-month follow-up period were somewhat less likely to have received family therapy than those patients who did not re-attempt at 18-month follow-up. Cohen-Sandler et al. (1982) also found that repeat attempters were half as likely to have received family therapy as those who did not make a repeat attempt. These studies suggest that family therapy may be a useful way to reduce repeat suicide attempts among adolescents.

## Completed suicide

Adolescent suicide attempters are at relatively high risk for eventual death by suicide. In 1992, 7% of those who committed suicide in the U.S. were under 20 years old (Kachur et al., 1995). The percentage of suicide attempters who go on to complete suicide appears to be related to the length of the follow-up period in adult samples (Lester, 1996). Follow-up studies of adolescent suicide attempters over relatively short periods of time rarely find completed suicides (see Table 12.1), whereas studies conducted over five years have found substantial rates of completed suicide. In a six-year follow-up, Nardini-Maillard and Ladame (1980) found that 3.8% of 130 adolescent suicide attempters had died by suicide. In another French study, 3.9% of 127 patients traced had committed suicide when the average follow-up time was 11.5 years (Granboulan et al., 1995). In a prospective study which included adolescents who had been psychiatrically hospitalized for either suicidal ideation or a suicide attempt, Motto (1984) found a 4.5% completed suicide rate over a four- to ten-year period. Because some of the adolescents who were untraceable in these studies may have died, these rates may underestimate the true incidence of completed suicide.

As Table 12.1 illustrates, however, attrition becomes more of a difficulty as the follow-up period lengthens. For this reason, studies which review official registries or records have the potential to provide more accurate estimates of the rates of completed suicide. Even these types of studies may underestimate suicide rates, due to incomplete or inaccurate information on death certificates (e.g., Goldacre and Hawton, 1985). Rates of suicide in studies which utilize a long-term follow-up by review of records range from 2.2% at five years (Kotila and Lonnqvist, 1988) to 4.3% at 10–15 years (Otto, 1972).

One of the strongest predictors of completed suicide is a previous suicide attempt (Spirito et al., 1989). Safer (1997) reviewed 14 studies of adolescents psychiatrically hospitalized for either suicidal ideation or suicide attempts, and found an average rate of completed suicide of 0.15% per year across studies with an average follow-up length of 3.6 years. This rate is almost four times greater than that found for psychiatrically treated outpatient adolescents, and 14 times greater than the rates for youths 15–19 years old in the U.S. About 30% of adolescents who complete suicide have made a prior attempt (Shaffer et al., 1988). Adolescents who make multiple repeat attempts are approximately three times more likely to eventually complete suicide than those who make a single attempt (Kotila and Lonnqvist, 1989).

There is also a clear gender difference in completed suicide among adolescents. Male attempters are at substantially higher risk for eventual death by suicide (Goldacre and Hawton, 1985; Kachur et al., 1995; Kotila and Lonnqvist, 1988; Motto, 1984; Otto, 1972; Sellar et al., 1990). On average, the rate is five times greater for male suicide attempters than for female suicide attempters (Safer, 1997). These gender differences may be even more pronounced during the first three months following an attempt (Sellar et al., 1990). In a sample that included a broad age range (DeMoore and Robertson, 1996), teenage substance-abusing males were at highest risk for completed suicide at follow-up.

A number of other variables have been associated with eventual completed suicide. An active method of attempt, such as hanging or use of a firearm, has a higher likelihood of resulting in an eventual completed suicide than a passive method of attempt, such as ingestion (Granboulan et al., 1995; Otto, 1972). A number of variables assessed during an initial psychiatric hospitalization were found to be predictive of eventual completed suicide in males at four- to ten-year follow-up (Motto, 1984). These included clear communication of suicidal intent, actively seeking assistance after the initial attempt and symptoms of depressed mood, such as hopelessness, apathy, and psychomotor retardation. None of the adolescents who were judged to have good verbal communication skills went on to commit suicide (Motto, 1984).

Attention has also been paid to identifying critical periods during which adolescent suicide attempters are at highest risk for completed suicide. While most completed suicides occur within the first year postattempt, the average time elapsed is about three years. In one study (Otto, 1972), about one-quarter of attempters who subsequently committed suicide did so within the first year, but the median time elapsed between the index attempt and completed suicide was

3.5 years. Similarly, Motto (1984) found that in his sample, the time from the index attempt to completed suicide ranged from six weeks to seven years, with a mean of three years from time of attempt.

Adolescents who eventually succeed in committing suicide also tend to manifest greater psychiatric disturbance at the time of their initial attempt. For example, two of the five individuals who committed suicide in the Granboulan et al. (1995) study had been diagnosed as psychotic at the time of the initial attempt. In a nonpsychiatric sample of young male suicide attempters in the military, substance abuse at the time of attempt was associated with a higher risk of eventual completed suicide (Mehlum, 1994). In contrast, young men who were not depressed or psychotic at the time of attempt had a greater chance of long-term survival (Mehlum, 1994).

## Treatment compliance

The relatively high re-attempt rate and the risk of eventual completed suicide makes appropriate intervention with these high-risk adolescents critical. However, these adolescents typically have very poor compliance with outpatient treatment. While even nonsuicidal adolescents tend to attend relatively few psychotherapy sessions (Tolan et al., 1988), psychotherapy attendance may be worse among those adolescents who have attempted suicide. Trautman et al. (1993) found that about three-quarters of adolescent suicide attempters and nonsuicidal adolescents terminated treatment "against medical advice." However, the suicide attempters dropped out much more quickly than nonsuicidal adolescents, attending a median of three sessions before dropping out of treatment compared to 11 sessions for the nonsuicidal adolescents.

Rates of treatment compliance at follow-up range from 23% of patients presenting to a psychiatry emergency clinic (Morrison and Collier, 1969) to 84% of psychiatrically hospitalized patients (Cohen-Sandler et al., 1982). Many attempters fail to attend even one psychotherapy session after their attempt. At least three studies have found that almost half of adolescent suicide attempters failed to keep their initial psychotherapy appointment (Pillay and Wassenaar 1995; Rauenhorst, 1972; Taylor and Stansfield, 1984).

Even those adolescent suicide attempters who follow through with a psychotherapy referral often fail to receive an adequate course of treatment. McIntire et al. (1977), for example, found that about one-third of the attempters they followed remained in treatment for two months or more. In an 11-year follow-up study of psychiatrically hospitalized adolescent suicide attempters, Granboulan et al. (1995) found that about one-third did not comply with any postdischarge treatment, and about one-fifth attended treatment irregularly or prematurely discontinued treatment. In a review of the literature, Spirito and colleagues (1989) estimated that about one-half of all adolescent suicide attempters receive either no treatment or inadequate treatment; that is, they attend only one or two psychotherapy sessions.

Treatment follow through seems to vary depending on the setting in which the adolescent is initially treated. In emergency departments (EDs), for example, poor rates of treatment compliance have often been documented among adult suicide attempters (see Krulee and Hales, 1988, for a review). With one exception (Burgess et al., 1998), most follow-up studies suggest that this is an issue of concern regarding adolescent suicide attempters as well. Litt et al. (1983) found that only one-third of 14 adolescent suicide attempters seen in a general hospital ED and discharged home received any follow-up care. Similarly, Spirito et al. (1992) studied 78 adolescent suicide attempters seen in a general hospital and discharged home, and found that 18% never kept an outpatient appointment, 14% went only once or twice, and 23% had attended three or four sessions by the time of the three-month follow-up. In a sample of 76 female adolescent suicide attempters presenting to an urban hospital ED, Trautman and Rotheram (1987) found that 14.5% never attended an outpatient therapy appointment, 38% attended one or two appointments, and only 32% attended three or more appointments. Although adolescents who have been psychiatrically hospitalized are somewhat more likely to attend outpatient treatment than adolescents seen in a general hospital after a suicide attempt and discharged home (Brent et al., 1993; Spirito et al., 1992), treatment compliance is a significant problem in the psychiatrically hospitalized population as well.

Follow-up studies have also shown other factors characterizing those who are noncompliant with treatment. Characteristics of the family, such as socioeconomic status and family size, typically do not distinguish those attempters who attend treatment from those who do not attend (Spirito et al., 1994; Taylor and Stansfield, 1984). Adolescent suicide attempters with higher levels of suicidality and depression may be more likely to follow through with the first psychotherapy visit (Taylor and Stansfield, 1984). Whether a history of a prior suicide attempt is associated with treatment noncompliance is unclear. In a small sample of adolescents, Litt et al. (1983) found that patients with a history of previous suicide attempts were much more likely to be noncompliant with treatment. Trautman et al. (1993) found no relation between number of previous suicide attempts and treatment dropout. In contrast, Spirito et al. (1994) found that a history of prior attempt, greater planning of the attempt, and alcohol use at the time of attempt were all associated with *better* treatment compliance. These factors may have resulted in greater concern among parents, who therefore made greater efforts to ensure that these adolescents complied with treatment (Spirito et al., 1994). Family factors have also been related to treatment compliance (Spirito et al., 1994; Taylor and Stansfield, 1984; Trautman and Rotheram, 1987). Parents with a positive attitude toward psychiatric treatment are more likely to ensure their adolescent attends a first psychotherapy visit (Taylor and Stansfield, 1984).

Adolescents who drop out of treatment are at greater risk for re-attempt or completed suicide. Rates of referral failure are particularly high among re-attempters (Litt et al., 1983; White, 1974). Without treatment, the risk factors associated with their initial attempt usually remain unaddressed. One study demonstrated that at six months following the attempt, feelings of hopelessness were reduced among those who received psychotherapy, while an untreated group remained as hopeless as they had been at the time of the attempt (Pillay and Wassenaar, 1995).

Several studies have been designed to address treatment noncompliance. Deykin et al. (1986) provided a social work outreach intervention consisting of community education about adolescent suicidal behavior, as well as direct service to adolescents who had attempted suicide. The direct service component of the intervention included providing support, acting as an advocate for the adolescent, helping the adolescent to obtain social and financial supports, and ensuring that they kept therapy appointments. The adolescents who received the outreach intervention were more likely to attend outpatient treatment appointments and had fewer subsequent visits to the ED than the attempters who did not receive outreach intervention. However, after controlling for prior history of suicidal behavior, there was no difference in repeat suicide attempts between the experimental and control group. Rotheram-Borus et al. (1996) included training workshops for ED staff, an on-call family therapist, and a videotape for families about what to expect in psychotherapy as part of their compliance enhancement intervention. Adolescent suicide attempters who received this intervention were more likely to attend their first therapy session at the hospital clinic (95%) than a comparison group of suicide attempters (83%).

Donaldson et al. (1997) developed a psychotherapy compliance enhancement intervention that included a verbal agreement between the adolescent and parent to attend at least four psychotherapy sessions in the community, and three brief telephone interviews over an eight-week period to problem-solve about suicidal ideation and treatment compliance. Only 9% of the suicide attempters who received the intervention did not attend any treatment sessions. Furthermore, no repeat attempts were reported in the experimental group ($n = 23$), while 9% of the comparison group made a repeat attempt within three months

(Donaldson et al., 1997). In a follow-up to this study, Spirito et al. (2002) randomly assigned adolescents to the compliance enhancement program described above or to standard disposition planning. The compliance enhancement program resulted in the adolescents' attending significantly more therapy sessions than the standard disposition planning group, after controlling for the barriers to service encountered in community treatment centers.

## Summary and conclusions

Several major conclusions can be drawn from studies reviewed in this chapter on the follow-up course of adolescent suicide attempters. There is a high level of continued behavioral dysfunction among adolescent suicide attempters, suggesting that, for most, the suicide attempt is not an isolated problem. There is also a much higher rate of both repeat attempts and eventual completed suicide among adolescent suicide attempters compared to adolescents without prior suicidal behavior. The risk factors for repeat attempts include gender, severity of the initial attempt, affective and conduct disorders, and family conflict. However, adolescent suicidal behavior has multiple contributing factors, so our ability to predict repeat attempts and especially completed suicide will always be limited.

In the literature on adult suicidal behavior, the use of survival analysis has been recommended in order to clarify risk factors (Leon et al., 1990). For example, statistical techniques such as Cox's proportional hazards model can be used to estimate the significance of different risk factors at different points in time (Leon et al., 1990). These techniques could be applied to studies of adolescent suicidal behavior, in order to identify differential risk periods. For example, some risk factors may exert their effects over a relatively brief period of time, while others may persist for years.

More studies are needed about *protective* factors. For example, McIntire et al. (1977) found that moving from a foster home to a permanent home greatly reduced the risk for repeat attempt. Other protective factors against repeat attempts include adequate social relationships and social support (Angle et al., 1983; Barter et al., 1968) and the use of repression, rather than more immature defense mechanisms (Pfeffer et al., 1995).

Follow-up studies have also revealed that many adolescent suicide attempters receive little or no treatment. This finding has led to several systematized programs designed to enhance treatment compliance, with promising results. Still, there are very few empirical trials of treatment with this population, so little is known about which type of psychotherapy is most helpful in improving their postattempt course. For example, Ross and Motto (1984) conducted a 35-session therapy group with ten adolescent suicide attempters and seven suicide ideators, and found that within a two-year period, none of them had re-attempted or completed suicide. However, their sample was small and there was no control group. In contrast, Rudd and colleagues (1996) did have a control group for their trial of group therapy for adolescents and young adults with a history of suicidal behavior. The experimental treatment took place in a day treatment program, and components included psychoeducation, problem-solving, and traditional experiential-affective techniques. The treated group demonstrated improvements in suicidal ideation and behavior, but the control group improved as well.

Particularly in the current health care climate, it will be important for follow-up studies to direct more attention to treatment in order to effectively address the negative sequelae of adolescent suicide attempts. Because of the potentially serious consequences of a false-negative prediction, we need to provide at least a minimal intervention to all adolescent suicide attempters, and intensive intervention to some proportion of this group. To improve the cost-effectiveness of interventions, studies which provide a more in-depth investigation of the postattempt course are also needed. However, the existing follow-up literature provides us with an important starting point for assessment and treatment planning for these adolescents.

## REFERENCES

Angle, C. R., O'Brien, T. P., and McIntire, M. S. (1983). Adolescent self-poisoning: a nine-year follow-up. *Developmental and Behavioral Pediatrics*, **4** (2), 83–87.

Barter, J. T., Swaback, D. O., and Todd, D. (1968). Adolescent suicide attempts: a follow-up study of hospitalized patients. *Archives of General Psychiatry*, **19**, 523–527.

Brent, D. A., Kolko, D. J., Wartella, M. E., Boylan, M. B., Moritz, G., Baugher, M., and Zelenak, J. P. (1993). Adolescent psychiatric inpatients' risk of suicide attempt at 6-month follow-up. *Journal of the American Academy of Child and Adolescent Psychiatry*, **32**, 95–105.

Burgess, S., Hawton, K., and Loveday, G. (1998). Adolescents who take overdoses: outcome in terms of changes in psychopathology and the adolescent's attitude to care and to their overdose. *Journal of Adolescence*, **21**, 209–218.

Centers for Disease Control (1995). Suicide among children, adolescents, and young adults – United States, 1980–1992. *Morbidity and Mortality Weekly Report*, **44**, 289–291.

Cohen-Sandler, R., Berman, A. L., and King, R. A. (1982). A follow-up study of hospitalized suicidal children. *Journal of the American Academy of Child and Adolescent Psychiatry*, **21**, (4), 398–403.

Cotgrove, A., Zirinsky, L., Black, D., and Wesson, D. (1995). Secondary prevention of attempted suicide in adolescence. *Journal of Adolescence*, **18**, 569–577.

DeMoore, G. M., and Robertson, A. R. (1996). Suicide in the 18 years after deliberate self-harm: a prospective study. *British Journal of Psychiatry*, **169**, 489–494.

Deykin, E. Y., Hsieh, C., Joshi, N., and McNamarra, J. J. (1986). Adolescent suicidal and self-destructive behavior: results of an intervention study. *Journal of Adolescent Health Care*, **7**, 88–95.

Diekstra, R. F., and Golbinat, W. (1993). The epidemiology of suicidal behavior: a review of three continents. *World Health Statistics Quarterly*, **46**, 52–68.

Donaldson, D., Spirito, A., Arrigan, M., and Aspel, J. W. (1997). Structured disposition planning for adolescent suicide attempters in a general hospital: preliminary findings on short-term outcome. *Archives of Suicide Research*, **3**, 271–282.

Farbstein, I., Dycian, A., King, R., Cohen, D. J., Kron, A., and Apter, A., (2002). A follow-up study of adolescent attempted suicide in Israel and the effects of mandatory general hospital admission. *Journal of the American Academy of Child and Adolescent Psychiatry*, **41**, 1342–1349.

Goldacre, M., and Hawton, K. (1985). Repetition of self-poisoning and subsequent death in adolescents who take overdoses. *British Journal of Psychiatry*, **146**, 395–398.

Granboulan, V., Rabain, D., and Basquin, M. (1995). The outcome of adolescent suicide attempts. *Acta Psychiatrica Scandinavica*, **91**, 265–270.

Gutstein, S. E., and Rudd, M. D. (1990). An outpatient treatment alternative for suicidal youth. *Journal of Adolescence*, **13**, 265–277.

Hawton, K., and Fagg, J. (1988). Suicide and other causes of death following attempted suicide. *British Journal of Psychiatry*, **152**, 359–366.

Hawton, K., O'Grady, J., Osborn, M., and Cole, D. (1982). Adolescents who take overdoses: their characteristics, problems and contacts with helping agencies. *British Journal of Psychiatry*, **140**, 118–123.

Hawton, K., Fagg, J., and Simkin, S. (1996). Deliberate self-poisoning and self-injury in children and adolescents under 16 years of age in Oxford, 1976–1993. *British Journal of Psychiatry*, **169**, 202–208.

Kachur, S. P., Potter, L. B., and Powell, K. E. (1995). *Suicide in the U.S., 1980–1992*. Atlanta, CA: National Center for Injury Prevention and Control.

Kerfoot, M., and McHugh, B. (1992). The outcome of childhood suicidal behavior. *Acta Paedopsychiatrica*, **55**, 141–145.

Kienhorst, C. W. M., DeWilde, E. J., Diekstra, R. F. W., and Wolters, W. H. G. (1991). Construction of an index for predicting suicide attempts in depressed adolescents. *British Journal of Psychiatry*, **159**, 676–682.

King, C. A., Segal, H., Kaminski, K., Naylor, M. W., Ghaziuddih, N., and Radpour, L. (1995). A prospective study of adolescent suicidal behavior following hospitalization. *Suicide and Life-Threatening Behavior*, **25**, 327–337.

Kotila, L., and Lonnqvist, J. (1988). Adolescent suicide attempts: sex differences predicting suicide. *Acta Psychiatrica Scandinavica*, **77**, 264–270.

Krulee, D., and Hales, R. (1988). Compliance with psychiatric referrals from a general hospital psychiatry outpatient clinic. *General Hospital Psychiatry*, **10**, 339–345.

Laurent, A., Foussard, N., David, M., Boucharlat, J., and Bost, M. (1998). A 5-year follow-up study of suicide attempts among French adolescents. *Journal of Adolescent Health*, **22**, 424–430.

Leon, A. C., Friedman, R. A., Sweeney, J. A., Brown, R. P., and Mann, J. J. (1990). Statistical issues in the identification of risk factors for suicidal behavior: the application of survival analysis. *Psychiatry Research*, **31**, 99–108.

Lester, D. (1996). The mortality of attempted suicides in follow-up studies of male suicide attempters. *Perceptual and Motor Skills*, **83**, 530.

Lewinsohn, P. M., Rohde, P., and Seeley, J. R. (1994). Psychosocial risk factors for future adolescent suicide attempts. *Journal of Consulting and Clinical Psychology*, **62**, 297–305.

Litt, I. F., Cuskey, W. R., and Rudd, S. (1983). Emergency room evaluation of the adolescent who attempts suicide: compliance with follow-up. *Journal of Adolescent Health Care*, **4**, 106–108.

Mattson, A., Seese, L. R., and Hawkins, J. W. (1969). Suicidal behavior as a child psychiatric emergency: clinical characteristics and follow-up results. *Archives of General Psychiatry*, **20**, 100–109.

McIntire, M. S., Angle, C. R., Wikoff, R. L., and Schlicht, M. L. (1977). Recurrent adolescent suicidal behavior. *Pediatrics*, **60**, 605–608.

Mehlum, L. (1994). Young male suicide attempters 20 years later: the suicide mortality rate. *Military Medicine*, **159**, 138.

Mehr, M., Zelter, L. K., and Robinson, R. (1982). Continued self-destructive behaviors in adolescent suicide attempters, Part II-A Pilot study. *Journal of Adolescent Health Care*, **2**, 183–187.

Morrison, G. C., and Collier, J. G. (1969). Family treatment approaches to suicidal children and adolescents. *Journal of the American Academy of Child and Adolescent Psychiatry*, **8**, 140–153.

Motto, J. A. (1984). Suicide in male adolescents. In Sudak, H. S., Ford, A. B., and Rushforth, N. B. (eds.) *Suicide in the Young*. Boston, MA: PSG Inc.

Myers, K., McCauley, E., Calderon, R., and Treder, R. (1991). The 3-year longitudinal course of suicidality and predictive factors for subsequent suicidality in youths with major depressive disorder. *Journal of the American Academy of Child and Adolescent Psychiatry*, **30**, 804–810.

Nardini-Maillard, D., and Ladame, F. (1980). The results of a follow-up study of suicidal adolescents. *Journal of Adolescence*, **3**, 253–260.

National Center for Health Statistics (1993). Advance report of final mortality statistics, 1990. *Monthly Vital Statistics Report*, **41**(7), 1–44.

Nordstrom, P., Samuelsson, M., and Asberg, M. (1995). Survival analysis of suicide risk after attempted suicide. *Acta Psychiatrica Scandinavica*, **91**, 336–340.

Otto, U. (1972). Suicidal acts by children and adolescents: a follow-up study. *Acta Psychiatrica Scandinavica*, **233**, 7–117.

Paerregaard, G. (1975). Suicide among attempted suicides: a 10-year follow-up. *Suicide*, **5**, 140–145.

Pfeffer, C. R., Klerman, G. L., Hurt, S. W., Lesser, M., Peskin, J. R., and Siefker, C. A. (1991). Suicidal children grow up: demographic and clinical risk factors for adolescent suicide attempts. *Journal of the American Academy of Child and Adolescent Psychiatry*, **30**, 609–616.

Pfeffer, C. R., Peskin, J. R., and Siefker, C. A. (1992). Suicidal children grow up: psychiatric treatment during follow-up period. *Journal of the American Academy of Child and Adolescent Psychiatry*, **31**, 679–685.

Pfeffer, C. R., Klerman, G. L., Hurt, S. W., Kakuma, T., Peskin, J. R., and Siefker, C. A. (1993). Suicidal children grow up: rates and psychosocial risk factors for suicide attempts during follow-up. *Journal of the American Academy of Child and Adolescent Psychiatry*, **32**, 106–113.

Pfeffer, C. R., Hurt, S. W., Kakuma, T., Peskin, J. R., Siefker, C. A., and Nagabhairava, S. (1994). Suicidal children grow up: suicidal episodes and effects of treatment during follow-up. *Journal of the American Academy of Child and Adolescent Psychiatry*, **33**, 225–230.

Pfeffer, C. R., Hurt, S. W., Peskin, J. R., and Siefker, C. A. (1995). Suicidal children grow up: ego functions associated with suicide attempts. *Journal of the American Academy of Child and Adolescent Psychiatry*, **34**, 1318–1325.

Pillay, A. L., and Wassenaar, D. R. (1995). Psychological intervention, spontaneous remission, hopelessness, and psychiatric disturbance in adolescent parasuicides. *Suicide and Life-Threatening Behavior*, **25**, 386–392.

Rauenhorst, J. M. (1972). Follow-up of young women who attempt suicide. *Diseases of the Nervous System*, **33** (12), 792–797.

Ross, C. P., and Motto, J. A. (1984). Group counseling for suicidal adolescents. In Sudak, H., Ford, A., and Rushforth, N. (eds.) *Suicide in the Young* (pp. 367–392). Boston, MA: John Wright.

Rotheram-Borus, M. J., Piacentini, J., Roosem, R., Graae, F., Cantwell, C., Castro-Blanco, D., Miller, S., and Feldman, J. (1996). Enhancing treatment adherence with a specialized emergency room program for adolescent suicide attempters. *Journal of the American Academy of Child and Adolescent Psychiatry*, **35**, 654–663.

Rudd, M. D., Rajab, M., Orman, D., Stulman, D., Joiner, T., and Dixon, W. (1996). Effectiveness of an outpatient intervention targeting suicidal young adults: preliminary results. *Journal of Consulting and Clinical Psychology*, **64**, 179–190.

Safer, D. J. (1997). Adolescent / adult differences in suicidal behavior and outcome. *Annals of Clinical Psychiatry*, **9**, 61–66.

Sellar, C., Hawton, K., and Goldacre, M. J. (1990). Self-poisoning in adolescents: hospital admissions and deaths in the Oxford Region 1980–85. *British Journal of Psychiatry*, **156**, 866–870.

Shaffer, D., Garland, A., Gould, M., Fisher, P., and Trautman, P. (1988). Preventing teenage suicide: a critical review. *Journal of the American Academy of Child and Adolescent Psychiatry*, **27**, 675–687.

Spirito, A., Brown, L., Overholser, J., and Fritz, G. (1989). Attempted suicide in adolescence: a review and critique of the literature. *Clinical Psychology Review*, **9**, 335–363.

Spirito, A., Plummer, B., Gispert, M., Levy, S., Kurkjian, J., Lewander, W., Hagberg, S., and Devost, L. (1992). Adolescent suicide attempts: outcomes at follow-up. *American Journal of Orthopsychiatry*, **62**, 464–468.

Spirito, A., Lewander, W. J., Levy, S., Kurkjian, J., and Fritz, G. (1994). Emergency department assessment of adolescent suicide attempters: factors related to short-term follow-up outcome. *Pediatric Emergency Care*, **10**, 6–12.

Spirito, A., Boergers, J., Donaldson, D., Bishop, D., and Lewander, W. (2002). An intervention trial to improve adherence to community treatment by adolescents following a suicide attempt. *Journal of the American Academy of Child and Adolescent Psychiatry*, **41**, 435–42.

Stanley, E. J., and Barter, J. T. (1970). Adolescent suicidal behavior. *American Journal of Orthopsychiatry*, **40**, 87–96.

Taylor, E. A., and Stansfield, S. A. (1984). Children who poison themselves: prediction of attendance for treatment. *British Journal of Psychiatry*, **145**, 132–135.

Tolan, P., Ryan, K., and Jaffe, C. (1988). Adolescents' mental health service use and provider, process, and recipient characteristics. *Journal of Clinical Child Psychology*, **17**, 229–236.

Trautman, P., and Rotheram, M. J. (1987). Referral failure among adolescent suicide attempters. Poster presented at the Annual Meeting of the American Academy of Child Psychiatry, Los Angeles, CA.

Trautman, P. D., Stewart, N., and Morishima, A. (1993). Are adolescent suicide attempters non-compliant with outpatient care? *Journal of the American Academy of Child and Adolescent Psychiatry*, **32**, 89–94.

White, H. C. (1974). Self-poisoning in adolescents. *British Journal of Psychiatry*, **124**, 24–35.

# 13

# Children and adolescents bereaved by a suicidal death: implications for psychosocial outcomes and interventions

Cornelia L. Gallo and Cynthia R. Pfeffer

## Epidemiology of suicide in U.S.

Although the 30 575 Americans who committed suicide in 1998 did not represent a substantial change in the total number of annual deaths, the suicide rate among adolescents aged 15–19 years old in the United States increased 11% from 1980–1997, while the rate among youngsters 10–14 years old increased over the same period by 109% (Centers for Disease Control, 2002). "The increased suicide rates are thought to reflect changes in the social environment, changing attitudes toward suicide and increasing availability of the means to commit suicide," (Kaplan, et al., 1994, p. 1121). Of the nearly 5000 individuals under age 25 years who killed themselves, a large proportion left siblings behind. Furthermore, of the roughly 13 000 people in the 25- to 44-years-old age group who committed suicide in 1998, probably at least half were parents and of the 6000 people 65 years old or older many were grandparents. Thus, it is likely that over 12 000 children and adolescents yearly are affected by suicidal deaths of close family members. This chapter will focus on the psychosocial impact of a family suicide on children and adolescents and discuss intervention strategies at the individual, family, and community level. It will also discuss how these effects may elevate the risk for suicidal behavior of children and adolescents.

An urgent clinical research imperative is to identify factors that elevate or diminish the risk of detrimental outcome for children and adolescents bereaved by the suicide of a relative. Most extant studies have investigated the impact of spousal suicide on surviving spouses. Methodologically rigorous bereavement research involving children and adolescents is only a recent area of study (Pfeffer et al., 2000, 2002). Several factors account for the dearth of information comparing the developmental course of children exposed to loss by suicide to that of control groups of children. First, since suicide is relatively uncommon, it is hard to assemble a large cohort of bereaved child subjects for systematic study. Second, those studies that have been done have focused primarily on white, urban, middle-class children of average or above-average intelligence. Comparing children of different races, religions, ethnicities, and socioeconomic backgrounds may provide a different light. Finally, current knowledge may be biased because bereaved parents often deny the potential pathological effects of suicidal deaths on children (Cain and Fast, 1966).

## Characteristics of children and adolescents who have lost family members to suicide

Despite the paucity of empirical data from controlled studies of children and adolescents who have experienced a suicidal death of a relative, clinical observations suggest that negative sequelae following suicidal deaths are common (Osterweis et al., 1984, p. 87). For example, Cain and Fast (1966) studied mental health clinic records to assess 45 children and adolescents, aged four years to 14 years, whose parent committed suicide approximately four years before clinical assessment, and concluded that these children suffered from depression and/or disruptive behavior problems. Reporting on 36 children and adolescents, aged 2–17 years, who experienced the suicidal death of a parent, Shepherd and Barraclough (1976) found that children experienced anxiety and significant environmental stress both before and after the parent's suicide. This study was limited because the children were not directly interviewed. Data were gathered only from surviving parents within weeks after suicide and again five to seven years later.

Brent and colleagues (1993c) reported that 25 adolescents whose adolescent siblings committed suicide were more likely to report a new onset of major depressive disorder after the suicidal death than 25 demographically matched controls.

Grossman and Clark's (1995) study of 16 prepubertal children whose parent died from suicide indicated that childhood exposure to family violence, threats of suicide and marital strife prior to the suicidal deaths were the most significant factors related to posttraumatic stress disorder (PTSD) symptoms. Specifically, children with PTSD symptoms tended to be those who were dealing with multiple traumatic experiences within a year preceding the suicidal death. Cleiren and Grad (1994) compared bereavement after suicide, traffic accident and illness for spouses and youth siblings. The results indicated that, for adults and children, the influence of mode of death on most aspects of psychosocial health is absent or small. PTSD symptoms were almost as common among the illness-bereaved groups as they were among the accidental and suicide death groups. In a longitudinal study, Cerel et al. (1999) compared 26 children (age 5–17 years old) bereaved by parental suicide to 332 children bereaved by parental deaths due to other causes. No differences in PTSD symptoms were observed between the two groups despite the authors' anticipation that the suicide-bereaved children would exhibit more PTSD symptoms. The authors noted that most of the children in the study had no interaction with the deceased at the immediate time of death. Yet, it is common for children who witness a suicide or discover the death scene to develop persistent bad dreams and intrusive images of the scene and to re-experience sounds or images of the scene (Clark and Goebel, 1996).

Pfeffer and colleagues (1997) interviewed both the caretakers and 22 children in 16 families who had a suicidal death in the family. Compared to children without a history of suicide of a relative, the children with a family history of a suicidal death were found to have higher rates of psychosocial problems, especially of symptoms of posttraumatic stress, depression, and social maladjustment. More specifically, children and adolescents bereaved by the suicidal death of siblings have been reported to have difficulty in school; oppositional, risk taking, and destructive behavior; suicidal ideation; somatic complaints; and increased risk of alcohol and drug use (Clark and Goebel, 1996).

Within 18 months of a parental death due to suicide or cancer, Pfeffer et al. (2000) compared 16 suicide-bereaved children and 64 age-matched cancer-bereaved children. The suicide-bereaved children showed significantly more depressive symptoms, involving negative mood, interpersonal problems, ineffectiveness, and anhedonia.

Cain (1972) described a group of adolescents who lost a sibling to suicide; five years after the death, half of them reported having guilty feelings, crying and trembling episodes upon remembering their sibling and wishes that it had been they who had died instead. Brent and colleagues (1993c) reported that six months after the suicide of a sibling, adolescents were at a sevenfold increased risk for developing a major depression, compared to a group of control subjects unexposed to suicide. Yet, at three-year follow-up (Brent et al., 1996a), the bereaved siblings were less symptomatic than controls. To what extent sibling suicide has pathogenic effects over and above the loss of a sibling to other causes is not clear. Comparing adolescents whose siblings died by car accident and suicide, Clark and Goebel's (1996) five-year study did not observe any "remarkable differences between the quality of grief in siblings bereaved by suicide and siblings bereaved by car accident. This conclusion is consistent with the limited empirical evidence available on the topic but runs counter to prevailing clinical theory" (Clark and Goebel, 1996, p. 376).

Development of children bereaved by suicidal deaths may be impeded by factors that affect their support network, among which are actual and perceived stigma. In the community or school, children and adolescents may be exposed to the social stigma, curiosity, and sensationalism that often surround a suicide. Others' perceived negative feelings about suicide may result in a bereaved child feeling isolated, ineffective, ashamed, or resentful (Osterweis et al., 1984). These stressful experiences adversely affect children's social adjustment and intensify feelings of guilt, worthlessness, sadness and anxiety, and may promote suicidal ideation or suicidal behavior (Osterweis et al., 1984).

## Children and adolescents bereaved by parental death

Bereavement early in life increases children's susceptibility to depression, anxiety, (Kranzler et al., 1990; Raphael 1982; Van Eerdevegh et al., 1982; Weller et al., 1991) and social adjustment problems (Kaffman and Elizur, 1983, 1996) such as school dysfunction and delinquency (Osterweis et al., 1984). Tennant (1988) reviewed the research on the adult psychopathological sequelae of a parent's death during childhood; they concluded that the quality of parenting by the surviving parent following the loss was the most influential factor in a child's adjustment (Tennant, 1988). Ness and Pfeffer (1990) concurred that the eventual development of adult psychopathology reflected the quality of home life and personal adaptation subsequent to the childhood loss of a parent.

Development of children who have experienced the suicidal death of a relative may be impaired by parental emotional unavailability resulting from the parent's own traumatic grief reactions to the suicide. Parents' inability to attend adequately to children's needs may increase children's risk for suicidal acts, mood and anxiety disorders, and impaired social adjustment (Pfeffer et al., 1997). Thus, to understand the effect on children of a family suicide, it is critical to examine the impact of a suicidal death on bereaved parents.

## Adult bereavement after suicidal deaths

In general, epidemiological data suggest that adults are at increased risk for psychological morbidity following bereavement from any cause. Depressive symptoms are very common in widows and widowers in the first months of bereavement and up to 20% of surviving spouses are depressed one year later.

Many studies find increased smoking and alcohol consumption and greater use of tranquilizers among such bereaved adults (Osterweis et al., 1984).

Spousal bereavement after a suicide is often influenced by complex factors such as social stigma, isolation, and circumstances such as financial instability and relocating (Osterweis et al., 1984). When bereavement is the result of suicidal deaths, Constantino and Bricker (1995, p. 132) found that surviving spouses "endure overwhelming biopsychosocial changes which tend to place them at greater health risk compared to individuals who lose their spouses from natural or accidental causes. Furthermore, to the extent that longstanding psychopathology was present in the deceased, the surviving spouse may already be burdened by a prolonged history of marital stress."

In contrast to the results of the above studies, some studies have found few if any differences between bereavement by suicide and by other modes of death. For example, Cleiren and Grad (1996) compared the psychosocial problems of spouses bereaved as a consequence of motor vehicle accidents or suicide in two different countries; they found that "differences between modes of death were minimal or nonexistent for measures related to depression and acceptance of loss. The family history and preceding psychosocial health are usually more important indicators and predictors of adaptation than the cause of death" (Cleiren and Grad, 1996, p. 43).

A recent review by Jordan (2001), however, supports the notion that suicide bereavement is distinctive in several ways: "the thematic content of the grief, the social processes surrounding the survivor, and the impact suicide has on family systems" (p. 91). Jordan also reviews some of the methodological issues involved in comparing bereavement experiences due to different types of death. Clarifying the impact of mode of death on the bereavement process of surviving spouses and parents thus needs further study.

Like bereaved spouses, parents of adolescent suicides were at higher risk for depression than controls, and, at follow-up three years later, mothers of suicide victims were still at an increased risk for recurrent depression (Brent et al., 1996a). Pfeffer et al. (1997) has also reported that the bereaved parents who have lost a relative to suicide have significantly higher levels of psychiatric symptoms, mainly anxiety and depression, than adults in the community. This is a concerning finding since children's reactions and adjustments to parental suicidal deaths are often related to the adjustment of the surviving parents. In contrast, Cerel et al. (2000)'s longitudinal examination of families of suicide- and nonsuicide-bereaved children examined parental and family functioning at intervals up to 25 months after the death; they found that while suicide-bereaved children's families had significant psychopathology and family disruption, the surviving suicide-bereaved parents did not manifest higher levels of psychopathology compared to other bereaved parents and many maintained positive relationships with their children.

Similarly concerning is the impact of adolescent suicidal deaths on peers. Brent and colleagues (1993 a, b) compared a sample of 146 friends and acquaintances of 26 adolescent suicide victims to demographically matched unexposed controls. Compared to controls, the peer group exposed to suicide showed a more than threefold increase in the incidence of major depressive disorder subsequent to exposure and a concomitant increase in suicidal ideation. Yet, there was no increase in suicide attempts in the exposed group. Risk factors for the development of a new-onset major depressive disorder after exposure to peer suicide included previous personal or family history of depression, stressful life events, closeness with the suicide victim, and witnessing the suicide or finding the body. It is not clear how to reconcile Brent et al.'s findings of an increased incidence of depression but not suicide attempts following peer suicide with other epidemiological studies suggesting the occurrence of "contagious" peer suicide and suicide attempts as an aftermath (Gould et al., 1996).

Another systematically studied effect of suicidal deaths is the response of the community toward the bereaved family. "It is suggested that in suicide bereavement, social reactions may be different, more condemning and unsupportive in comparison with reactions to other causes of death" (Cleiren and Grad, 1996, p. 37). Consistent with reports of families bereaved by suicide feeling isolated and ostracized, extended family, friends, colleagues, and neighbors often feel unable to express their reactions or concerns and are frightened by the violence and perceived rage of the suicidal act. People outside the immediate family learn about suicides in many different ways, usually with varying degrees of accuracy, detail, and curiosity. Newspaper and other media reports often sensationalize or stigmatize the situation. To the detached observer, the articles may appear brief and factual, but to the spouses and children they threaten to strip away privacy, make intimate problems public, evoke gossip, or implicitly disparage the deceased or family (Shepherd and Barraclough, 1974). Those close to the victim may experience anger, frustration, helplessness, and guilt as a result of these reports. Calhoun and his group (1976) compared the social impressions of strangers towards hypothetical cases of parents whose child died from natural causes or suicide and towards spouses bereaved by either self-inflicted gunshot or leukemia. The hypothesis was that the type of death would impact how people felt about the bereaved, anticipating that suicidal deaths would precipitate a negative impression of the families. The results suggested "a general pattern of more negative social impressions of the parents of the child who committed suicide and the surviving spouse was seen as more likely to have been to blame in some way for the [suicidal] death, more likely to have been able to do something that might have prevented the death" (Calhoun et al., 1976, p. 216). The types of stigma attached to suicidal deaths and the responses that suicide trigger in people most likely influence the support and responses offered to the families as well as having possible pathogenic effects on the survivors.

## A diagnostic dilemma: distinguishing between symptoms of bereavement and major depressive disorder

Bereavement is generally associated with increased likelihood of mood disorders in children and adolescents (Pfeffer et al., 1997) but distinguishing between the symptoms of bereavement and major depressive disorder is often difficult. Complicating the task of differential diagnosis is the frequency of sad, depressed mood in both disorders. Although the presence of a mood disorder increases the risk for suicidal behavior in children and adolescents (Lewis, 1996), Weller et al. (1991) found that suicidal ideation was also surprisingly common in children who had recently lost a parent through various causes. Brent and his colleagues (1993a, b, 1994) attempted to determine whether the depressive reactions of youth exposed to suicidal deaths were uncomplicated bereavement or major depression by examining the longitudinal risk of recurrent major depression. They compared 146 friends and acquaintances of 26 suicide victims with 146 demographically matched unexposed controls at six months after the suicidal deaths and 1–18 months later. They concluded that "depressive reactions observed in the youth exposed to suicide were most consistent with major depressive episodes on the basis of course and risk of recurrence. Exposure to suicide was associated with an increased risk of recurrent depression but not an increased risk of suicidal behavior" (Brent et al., 1994, p. 231). In Cerel and colleagues' longitudinal study, cited above, comparing children bereaved by suicide to children with a nonsuicide parental death, the suicide-bereaved children showed more overall psychopathological symptoms, including higher levels of behavioral disruption, anxiety, and depressive symptoms at almost every measured time interval. The authors comment that these children "have not yet passed through the age of risk for the development of severe psychopathology. As these children enter adulthood, they might be at increased risk for mental illness and suicidality" (Cerel et al., 2000, p. 679).

### Case example

The case of Amy illustrates the occurrence of a major depressive episode complicating bereavement after a parental suicide. When first seen, Amy, a 13-year-old adolescent, lived with her father and two younger sisters; her mother had overdosed on her own antidepressant medication 16 months earlier. Over the three months prior to bringing Amy for treatment, her father had become increasingly frustrated that Amy was not helping him at home as she previously had. He brought her to treatment asking how to make her resume her old responsibilities. He reported that Amy had been spending more time alone in her room, not helping with the household chores or playing with her sisters. She used to take great pride in making elaborate meals for the family, yet for the past month had eaten only cereal. She had not been doing as well in school in the most recent marking period, and was often late for the bus because she couldn't get up in time. With her friends, she was pleasant and talked on the phone for hours. At home, however, she was angry, defiant, and grouchy most of the time. When asked about her mother, Amy replied that her mother was better off where she was, with less suffering. In fact, Amy commented, she understood why she killed herself. Amy herself had frequent thoughts about her own death and planned to "take pills on [her] mother's next birthday." Once in an ongoing psychotherapy treatment and started on an antidepressant medication, Amy was no longer haunted by her plan to kill herself and gradually resumed her interest in school and home life.

This vignette illustrates the complicated continuum of clinical symptoms between bereavement after a suicidal death and a major depressive disorder. While her initial sadness was a direct reaction to her mother's suicidal death, the later symptoms were more consistent with a major depressive disorder. In this case, recognizing and intervening with her mood disorder improved her functioning and quality of life. The vignette underlines the clinical importance of being alert to the possibility of an ensuing mood disorder complicating the course of bereavement. Depression, however, is not the only condition that can complicate the course of bereavement following a suicidal death.

## Another diagnostic dilemma: distinguishing between symptoms of bereavement and PTSD

As DSM-IV (American Psychiatric Association (APA), 1994) notes, PTSD can result when "a person experienced, witnessed or was confronted with an event that involved actual or threatened death and the person's response involved intense fear, helplessness or horror" (pp. 427–429). Certainly, many of the gruesome experiences children may accidentally encounter around suicidal deaths constitute traumatic experiences.

The potential symptoms or behaviors resulting from such exposure cluster in three major areas: (1) persistent re-experiencing of the traumatic event;

(2) persistent avoidance of stimuli associated with the trauma and/or a general numbing of responsiveness, and (3) persistent symptoms of hyperarousal. Re-experiencing may take the form of repetitive play in which themes or aspects of the trauma are expressed or frightening dreams with unrecognizable content, or trauma-specific re-enactment behaviors. Avoidance behaviors may be seen as efforts to evade thoughts, feelings, activities, and places associated with the trauma. The child may be unable to recall details of the trauma, feel detached or estranged from others, manifest a restricted affect, or experience a sense of a foreshortened future. Insomnia, irritability, difficulty concentrating, exaggerated startle response, or hypervigilance indicate persistent arousal. Children in particular may show disorganized or agitated behavior. To meet the DSM-IV criteria for the diagnosis of PTSD, the duration of the symptoms must be at least one month but can last for months to years (APA, 1994). Briefer episodes may not meet the full DSM-IV criteria, yet still be impairing or distressing. Some children will have some of the signs and symptoms of PTSD, but clinicians or parents may fail to recognize them as related to the trauma.

Since children are often unable to verbalize the nature of the distress they are experiencing, especially around violent and frightening events, understanding their behavior, as part of this clinical picture, is critical for both initiating treatment and symptom relief. Specifically, the children's developmental course can be irrevocably altered by the intrusion of these aberrant behaviors and anxieties. Unidentified and untreated PTSD can lead to further risk of psychopathology, which in turn may be linked to an increased risk of suicidal behavior (Lewis, 1996). Determining when the anxiety and distress of bereavement is compounded by the presence of posttraumatic stress symptoms is a complicated, but essential, clinical task (Brent et al., 1995, 1996b).

### Case example

Todd was a six-year-old boy, living with his parents, who came to clinical attention eight months after his older brother shot himself in the backyard. Todd no longer wanted to play out back and cried or avoided getting in the car when it was parked in the back. He played constantly with a makebelieve gun, shooting everyone wherever he went. He had trouble falling asleep in his own bed and frequently awoke screaming. When there was a loud noise, Todd jumped and often cried, requiring extensive soothing and comforting to calm down. Todd did not want to go anywhere without one of his parents. Todd's mother noticed changes in her son, but she thought they would go away as he got older. She planned to buy him a dog to play with in order to help him get over his fear of the backyard. Todd's school recommended an evaluation for him when he started telling the other children he was having dreams that his brother was going to kill him too.

Todd's mother brought him to a mental health clinic, where he was diagnosed with PTSD. When questioned about the events surrounding the death, Todd's mother reported that her memory was poor, but that Todd was at a friend's home when his brother died and came home hours after the body had been removed. Todd's recollection was strikingly different; he reported arriving home to police cars and an ambulance at his house. He ran through the house looking for his parents and found a circle of people around his brother, who was covered in blood with "his brains on the lawn." He saw his mother was crying and she told him to go back to his friend's house for dinner. When he returned home later, his mother explained that his brother had shot himself, because he was very sad.

Todd started in weekly individual therapy. After a few weeks, he was only slightly improved and hence was started on clonidine. Two weeks later, Todd was able to express his fears that his brother probably shot himself that day because he was so angry with Todd. Todd's brother, who had been irritably depressed, had scolded Todd bitterly the night before for breaking a dish. Todd slowly began being able to go in the backyard with his parents' support and his behavior became less aggressive.

This clinical example is typical of a child whose bereavement process is complicated by the traumatic nature of his experience. Todd's hypervigilance, sleep disturbance, lability, and avoidance behaviors are all consistent with a posttraumatic response. Todd had many previously unexpressed fears and guilty feelings that he had caused his brother's death. Todd's mother herself was having trouble sleeping and avoided the backyard as well. She was not aware of the overall pattern of Todd's symptoms, but rather regarded each behavior as an isolated instance. When confronted with Todd's memories of his brother's death, Todd's mother was able to remember more fully what had happened. Learning that Todd's behaviors were part of a syndrome enabled her to be more aware of Todd's complicated experiences and more attentive to his distress. Recognizing the constellation of symptoms that can be superimposed on a bereavement process and complicate the clinical picture is essential for correct diagnosis and appropriate treatment.

## Studies of bereavement interventions

Although there are numerous reports of clinicians' experiences with bereaved children and families in individual, family and group settings, few systematic studies of postsuicide bereavement interventions for children and adults have been conducted. Treatments that have been described include individual and family therapy, professionally run structured groups, and peer support groups. Constantino and Bricker (1995) compared the effects of two theoretically derived eight-week nursing postvention sessions for 32 spouses bereaved by suicidal deaths. The findings suggested that "both groups experienced an overall reduction in depression and distress" (Constantino and Bricker, 1995, p. 131), but all the subjects were self-selected and this study did not include a group of individuals who did not attend group sessions.

In reviewing the literature, Schneiderman et al. (1994) found only four randomized controlled studies of bereavement programs. Significant methodological flaws existed in all four studies despite the review's conclusions that two studies showed benefit to the participants and two others showed none. The review concluded that "it is entirely likely that social class, premorbid family functioning, social supports, the age of the dead family member and of the survivors as well as the nature of the death (sudden, expected, suicide, etc.) have as much to do with individual and family functioning during the bereavement period as any intervention we might provide . . . . It is entirely possible that bereavement programs may work for some under certain conditions" (p 217). Polak et al.'s (1975) study of crisis intervention services with family members who survived a recent sudden death highlights the complexity of bereavement after suicidal death. They observed a "high correlation between poor outcome (measured by the development of physical or mental illness or serious social disruption in the family) and the following tragic circumstances: (1) degree of suddenness, (2) degree of violence, (3) direct observation of the death and the occurrence of the death in the home, (4) suicidal death, (5) death of a child under 12, and (6) family members directly or indirectly contributing to the death" (p. 147). They concluded that "environmental forces play a much greater role in determining outcome than is often believed. Social systems factors also seem to be important intervening variables in influencing outcome, but existing techniques of crisis intervention are not effective in producing significant change in constructive social systems in situations such as sudden death" (p. 148). Perhaps crisis interventions can only recognize families that are in need of more extensive support and intervention rather than providing the necessary treatment. Further highlighting the complexity of bereavement, Parkes' (1980) review of efficacy of bereavement treatments found that interventions are of value especially when the bereaved perceive their families as unsupportive or unavailable, or for individuals who are possibly at risk for other reasons.

Several clinical researchers have developed specific treatments to address the unique needs and issues for families who have had a suicidal death. Rogers et al. (1982) developed a Survivors Support Program for individual families who had lost a family member to suicide. The intervention was a nonprofessional, time-limited, structured program of support and assistance specifically toward understanding and resolving the stresses of bereavement after a suicidal death. The family members met together with two trained volunteers for a series of eight two-hour issue-directed sessions. The participants were most motivated to feel better about themselves, express their feelings, and talk about suicide. Most respondents reported a favorable response to the experience.

Pfeffer and colleagues (1997) developed a program called Children's Attitudes, Responses, and Emotions Toward Suicide (CARES), a specialized bereavement program for children, adolescents, and their families. Ten weekly 1.5-hour sessions were conducted by mental health professionals simultaneously for the suicidally bereaved children and their parents or caretakers. Prior to beginning the intervention, the children and parents were clinically evaluated regarding their present symptoms, current social functioning, concerns about the suicide, prior development, and psychosocial and family history. As a prerequisite to the intervention, the children were not required to know that suicide was the cause of death. The children were given weekly homework assignments relevant to the group themes and often required the support and participation of their parent. As an adjunct to the group, the children also worked with a coloring book that included a formatted letter to their deceased family member, pictures for the children to color that depicted different emotions, pages that explained about death and saying goodbye, and descriptions of coping skills for stressful events.

The children's group goals included helping the children understand death and suicide, exploring their fantasies and fears, decreasing the stigma and isolation by being with other children with a similar loss, and developing coping skills and strategies. Parent group sessions focused on similar issues, but also emphasized psychoeducation about assisting the children with their process of bereavement and any potential psychopathology. Since the group intervention included only individuals bereaved by suicidal deaths, the participants were able to empathize and share with each other around the themes of shame, guilt, trauma, anger, helplessness, and despair generated by the suicides. Most of the group members felt that they benefited from the experience.

Pfeffer et al. (2002) studied the efficacy of a manual-based version of this bereavement group intervention for 52 families (75 children), who were alternately assigned to receive or not receive the intervention. Anxiety and depressive symptoms were significantly more improved among children who received the intervention than in those who did not.

## Intervention guidelines for children and adolescents whose family members committed suicide

There are no empirically tested and proven guidelines for informing children of the suicide of a family member. A clinically relevant guideline is to be truthful and clear in discussing the cause of death with children. Truthfulness and clarity of the information bolster children's trust and security in their adult caretakers and make it possible for them to understand and process the important knowledge being presented to them. Furthermore, gaining an understanding of the universality, irreversibility, and permanency of death are essential to beginning the process of recovering from bereavement (Black, 1996). Children will need to be able to ask questions and try to master the concepts for themselves.

Faced with the trauma of suicide, however, parents' ability to communicate with their children often falls short of this ideal. Cain (1972) found that communications between children and a surviving parent were often highly distorted. For example, 25% of the children studied had witnessed some aspect of the suicide, yet within hours the surviving parent had explained and insisted that the death was a result of an illness or accident. For example, "a boy who watched his father kill himself with a shotgun was told later that night by his mother that his father died of a heart attack . . . . It was not unusual to find upon exploration that children whose parents insisted the children could not possibly know the death was a suicide knew some of the smallest, most intimate details of the suicidal act" (Cain, 1972, p. 102). Often the ostensible reason given for omission or distortion of information is to spare the children, but this can further lead to confusion and conflicts.

A second guideline is that participation in the family's funeral and burial rituals is an important bereavement intervention, even for children as young as four years old (Wessel, 1978). In preparing children to attend a funeral, they need to know what will happen, who will be there, and that people will be sad. It often helps to have less grief-stricken friends or relatives take the responsibility to be with the children and to attend to their children's distress. It is important to be aware that funerals of suicide victims have unique issues to be addressed. Funeral directors have observed that, compared to other funerals, mourners attending the funerals of suicide victims behave differently in a variety of ways: " . . . [T]here is greater social discomfort, more curiosity, and significantly less confidence about how to act toward the bereaved family" (Calhoun et al., 1976, p. 218). If after hearing a description of what will occur, children express a desire not to go, they should not be pressed to attend. Nonetheless, continued communication about the death is important to help them adequately initiate the process of mourning.

A third guideline is that attention be focused on the immediate experience of children who have had a suicidal death in the family. These immediate experiences may involve the children's feelings, behaviors, and their social context. As the process of bereavement evolves, bereaved children have changes in neurovegetative state, especially sleep and appetite, fears of abandonment, fears of the death of those they love and of themselves, as well as guilt and anger at person who died and at other family members. Children benefit from the support and attention to their experience. When the parent that committed suicide had been violent, abusive, harsh, frightening, or chronically ill, the child and other family members may also experience, alongside of grief, feelings of guilty relief; survivors may not initially be aware of, or may hesitate to express, these powerful, ambivalent feelings, and dealing with them requires attention to issues of tact and timing.

It is also important to be aware of and assess the concrete stressors that the suicide may entail for the child and surviving family members. Increased family disruption and stress, with loss of economic stability, relocation, and decreased emotional and practical availability of the surviving parent (Pfeffer et al., 1997) are common immediate sequelae for bereaved families following the suicide of a parent. These concrete issues greatly influence the life of the children, and become significant stressors for them.

A fourth clinical guideline is that children who have experienced a suicidal death should be monitored during the course of bereavement for possible manifestations of significant psychiatric symptoms or social impairment. From a clinical perspective, a thorough evaluation for depressive, posttraumatic and anxiety symptoms, suicidal ideation and acts, and developmental disruptions or regressions needs to be conducted. Because the nature of the death was suicide, often these families have significant premorbid pathology and patterns of psychosocial adjustment that place the children at risk for psychological difficulties. This may mean that the assessment of the family's prior functioning and possible psychopathology may be critical in determining the impact of the subsequent tragic deaths.

Part of the initial assessment is to ascertain the children's involvement in the immediate death process from both the parents and children. What the children remember is often very different from what the adults remember, and afterwards children are often left with concerns and ideas that are confusing. For example, one child who was not asked to attend the funeral services believed this was because his father had instructed his mother to leave him home as a punishment for his misbehavior prior to the suicidal death. Often communication is distorted and confusing for the family. Clarifying the methods of conveying information between family members is important.

Children are prone to feeling guilty, abandoned, angry, resentful and at times relieved by the suicidal death. These feelings need to be explored and validated. Unfortunately, children are often exposed to cruel and insensitive comments and taunts by their peers or adults in the community. When children are aware of feeling pained or shamed, they may not share their experiences with their parents for fear of hurting their feelings as well. Validating the child's distress and desire to protect the family can be valuable to the child's sense of reality. Therapists "should be particularly attuned to conscious and unconscious feelings of guilt due to anger or to perceived failures to save the deceased person" (Ness and Pfeffer, 1990, p. 284). Specifically, Cain (1995) reported that some children who lost a parent to suicide developed identificatory symptoms derived from the child's own fantasies and developmentally constrained understanding of the parent's death.

Melges and DeMaso (1980) identified nine obstacles to normal grieving likely to perpetuate grief in an unresolved state: "persistent yearning for recovery of the lost object, over identification with the deceased, the wish to cry or rage at the loss coupled with an inability to do so, misdirected anger and ambivalence toward the deceased, interlocking grief reactions, unspoken but powerful contracts with the deceased, unrevealed secrets and unfinished business, lack of a support group and alternative options, and secondary gain or reinforcement to remain grief stricken" (Melges and DeMaso, 1980, pp. 53–54). Furthermore, as Cain (1972, p. 14) observed "given the potent factors of denial, concealment, and evasion in the face of suicide, as well as the shame and guilt-engendered avoidance of communication, and the mutual withdrawal of and from friends, neighbors and relatives the gradual working through of mourning is severely hampered if not made impossible." Support and exploration can prevent further suffering and isolation.

### School intervention

The child is surrounded by a community network that is both affected by and responds to a suicidal death. School professionals are vital facilitators of information and models for community response. The American Association of Suicidology (AAS) (1997) has developed suicide postvention guidelines for school administrators following the suicide of a student or faculty member. The goals of the postvention program are to facilitate the students', faculty's and staff's understanding and begin the grieving process in a positive fashion, to prevent subsequent "copy-cat" suicides and attempts, and to recognize and refer at-risk individuals for psychological assistance. By having a plan of how to intervene and support those individuals impacted by such tragedies, whether intimately or more remotely, community members can begin healing and processing the loss rather than remaining numbed and isolated.

## Conclusion

A significant number of children today have experienced a suicidal death of a relative. Numerous factors such as premorbid psychiatric history, family history of psychiatric illness, and stability of caretakers influence the psychological outcome of such a loss for a child. The reactions and responses to a suicidal death are complex and include an increased risk of depression and PTSD. Clinicians need to be vigilant to recognize these treatable conditions. The most effective intervention techniques, however, remain areas requiring further research and evaluation. In broad outline, the relevant interventions include: alertness for and education about potential adverse emotional sequelae, fostering developmentally appropriate communication concerning the death and its implications for the child and family, and supporting the functioning and emotional availability of surviving family members.

## Acknowledgements

The authors wish to acknowledge the support from Nanette Laitman and the William and Mildred Lasdon Foundation, a fund established in The New York Community Trust by DeWitt-Wallace, The Klingenstein Third Generation Foundation, and The Brickell Foundation.

## REFERENCES

American Association of Suicidology (AAS) (1997). *Suicide Postvention Guidelines*. Washington DC: AAS.

American Psychiatric Association (APA) (1994). *Diagnostic and Statistical Manual of Mental Disorders*, 4th edn. Washington, DC: American Psychiatric Association.

Black, D. (1996). Childhood bereavement. *British Medical Journal*, **312**, 1496.

Brent, D. A., Perper, J., Moritz, G., Allman, C., Schweers, J., Roth, C., Balach, L., and Canobbio, R. (1993a). Bereavement or depression? The impact of the loss of a friend to suicide. *Journal of the American Academy of Child and Adolescent Psychiatry*, **32**(6), 1189–1197.

Brent, D. A., Perper, J. A., Moritz, G., Allman, C., Liotus, L., Schweers, J., Roth, C., Balach, L., and Canobbio, R. (1993b). Psychiatric sequelae to the loss of an adolescent peer to suicide. *Journal of the American Academy of Child and Adolescent Psychiatry*, **32**, 509–517.

Brent, D. A., Perper, J. A., Moritz, G., Liotus, L., Schweers, J., Roth, C., Balach, L., and Allman, C. (1993c). Psychiatric impact of the loss of an adolescent sibling to suicide. *Journal of Affective Disorders*, **28**, 249–256.

Brent, D. A., Perper, J., Moritz, G., Liotus, L., Schweers, J., and Canobbio, R. (1994). Major depression or uncomplicated bereavement? A follow-up of youth exposed to suicide. *Journal of the American Academy of Child and Adolescent Psychiatry*, **33**(2), 231–239.

Brent, D. A., Perper, J. A., Moritz, G., Liotus, L., Richardson, D., Canobbio, R., Schweers, J., and Roth, C. (1995). Posttraumatic stress disorder in peers of adolescent suicide victims: predisposing factors and phenomenology. *Journal of the American Academy of Child and Adolescent Psychiatry*, **34**(2), 209–215.

Brent, D. A., Moritz, G., Bridge, J., Perper, J., and Canobbio, R. (1996a). The impact of adolescent suicide on siblings and parents: a longitudinal follow-up. *Suicide and Life-Threatening Behavior*, **26**(3), 253–259.

Brent, D. A., Moritz, G. et al. (1996b). Long-term impact of exposure to suicide: a three year controlled follow-up. *Journal of the American Academy of Child and Adolescent Psychiatry*, **35**(5), 646–653.

Cain, A. C. (ed.) (1972). *Survivors of Suicide*. Springfield, IL: Charles Thomas.

Cain, A. C. (1995). Identificatory symptoms in bereaved children: a diagnostic note. *Developmental and Behavioral Pediatrics*, **16**(4), 282–284.

Cain, A. C., and Fast, I. (1966). Children's disturbed reactions to parental suicide. *American Journal of Orthopsychiatry*, **36**, 873–880.

Calhoun, L. G., Selby, J. W., and King, H. E. (1976). *Dealing with Crisis: a Guide to Critical Life Problems*, Englewood Cliffs, NJ: Prentice-Hall.

Caplan, M. G., and Douglas, V. I. (1969). Incidence of parental loss in children with depressed mood. *Journal of Psychology and Psychiatry*, **10**, 225–244.

Centers for Disease Control (CDC) (2002). Unpublished mortality data from the National Center for Health Statistics (NCHS) Mortality Data Tapes, CDC website www.cdc.gov/ ncipc/factsheets/suifacts.htm [updated September 9, 2002].

Cerel, J. Fristad, M., Weller, E. B., and Weller, R. A. (1999). Suicide-bereaved children and adolescents: a controlled longitudinal examination. *Journal of the American Academy of Child and Adolescent Psychiatry*, **38**, 672–679.

Cerel, J. Fristad, M., Weller, E. B., and Weller, R. A. (2000). Suicide-bereaved children and adolescents: II. Parental and family functioning. *Journal of the American Academy of Child and Adolescent Psychiatry*, **39**(4), 437–444.

Clark, D. C., and Goebel, A. E. (1996). Siblings of youth suicide victims. In Pfeffer, C. R. (ed.) *Severe Stress and Mental Disturbance in Children*. Washington DC: APA Press.

Cleiren, M. P., and Grad, O. (1994). Mode of death and kinship in bereavement: focusing on "who" rather than "how". *Crisis*, **15**(1), 22–36.

Cleiren, M. P., and Grad, O. (1996). Psychosocial impact of bereavement after suicide and fatal traffic accident: a comparative two-country study. *Acta Psychiatria Scandinavica*, **94**(1), 37–44.

Constantino, R. E., and Bricker, P. L. (1995). Nursing postvention for spousal survivors of suicide. *Issues in Mental Health Nursing*, **17**, 131–152.

Gould, M. S., Fisher, P., Parides, M., Flory, M., and Shaffer, D. (1996). Psychosocial risk factors of child and adolescent completed suicide. *Archives of General Psychiatry*, **53**, 1155–1162.

Grossman, J. A., and Clark, D. C. (1995). Child bereavement after paternal suicide. *Journal of the American Academy of Child and Adolescent Psychiatry*, **8**(2), 5–17.

Jordan, J. R. (2001). Is suicide bereavement different? A reassessment of the literature. *Suicide and Life-Threatening Behavior*, **31**(1), 91–102.

Kaffman, M., and Elizur, E. (1983). Bereavement responses of kibbutz and non-kibbutz children following the death of the father. *Journal of Child Psychology and Psychiatry*, **24**, 435–442.

Kaffman, M., and Elizur, E. (1996). Bereavement as a significant stressor in children. In Pfeffer, C. J. (ed.) *Severe Stress and Mental Disturbance in Children*. Washington DC: APA Press.

Kaplan, H. I., Sadock, B. J., and Grebb, J. A. (1994). *Kaplan and Sadock's Synopsis of Psychiatry* (7th edn.) Baltimore, MD: Williams & Wilkins.

Kranzler, E. M., Shaffer, D., Wasserman, G., and Davies, M. (1990). Early childhood bereavement. *Journal of the American Academy of Child and Adolescent Psychiatry*, **29**(4), 513–520.

Lewis, M. (ed.) (1996). *Child and Adolescent Psychiatry: A Comprehensive Textbook* (2nd edn.). Baltimore, MD: Williams & Wilkins.

Melges, F. T., and DeMaso, D. R. (1980). Grief-resolution therapy: reliving, revising, and revisiting. *American Journal of Psychotherapy*, **34**(1), 51–61.

Ness, D., and Pfeffer, C. (1990). Sequelae of bereavement resulting from suicide. *American Journal of Psychiatry*, **147**(3), 279–285.

Osterweis, M., Solomon, F., and Green, M. (eds.) (1984). *Bereavement: Reactions, Consequences, and Care*. Washington, DC: National Academy Press.

Parkes, C. M. (1980). Bereavement counseling: does it work? *British Medical Journal*, **281**, 3–6.

Pfeffer, C. R., Martins, P., Mann, J., Sunkenberg, M., Ice, A., Damore, J. P. Jr., Gallo, C., Karpenos, I., and Jiang, H. (1997). Child survivors of suicide: psychosocial characteristics. *Journal of the American Academy of Child and Adolescent Psychiatry*, **36**(1), 65–74.

Pfeffer, C. R., Karus, D., Siegel, K., and Jiang, H. (2000). Child survivors of parental death from cancer or suicide: depressive and behavioral outcomes. *Psycho-Oncology*, **9**(1), 1–10.

Pfeffer, C. R., Jiang, H., Kakuma, T., Hwang, J., and Metsch, M. (2002). Group intervention for children bereaved by the suicide of a relative. *Journal of the American Academy of Child and Adolescent Psychiatry*, **41**, 505–513.

Polak, P. R., Egan, D., Vandenbergh, R., and Williams, W. V. (1975). Prevention in mental health. *American Journal of Psychiatry*, **132**, 146–149.

Raphael, B. (1982). The young child and the death of a parent. In Parkes, C. M., Stevenson-Hinde, J. (eds.) *The Place of Attachment in Human Behavior*. London: Tavistock.

Rogers, J., Sheldon, A., Barwick, C., Letofsky, K., and Lancee, W. (1982). Help for families of suicide: Survivors Support Program. *Canadian Journal of Psychiatry*, **27**, 444–449.

Schneiderman, G., Winders, P., Tallett, S., and Feldman, W. (1994). Do child and/or parent bereavement programs work? *Canadian Journal of Psychiatry*, **39**, 215–218.

Shepherd, D. M., and Barraclough, B. M. (1974). The aftermath of suicide. *British Medical Journal*, **2**, 600–603.

Shepherd, D. M., and Barraclough, B. M. (1976). The aftermath of parental suicide for children. *British Journal of Psychiatry*, **129**, 267–276.

Tennant, C. (1988). Parental loss in childhood. Its effect in adult life. *Archives of General Psychiatry*, **45**(11), 1045–1050.

Van Eerdewegh, M. M., Bieri, M. D., Parilla, R. H., and Clayton, P. J. (1982). The bereaved child. *British Journal of Psychiatry*, **140**, 23–29.

Weller, R. A., Weller, E. B., Fristad, M. A., and Bowes, J. M. (1991). Depression in recently bereaved prepubertal children. *American Journal of Psychiatry*, **148**, 1536–1540.

Wessel, M. A. (1978). The grieving child. *Clinical Pediatrics*, **17**(7), 559–568.

# Index

Numbers in italics indicate *tables* and *figures*.